D0850076

READING ENGELHARDT

READING ENGELHARDT

ESSAYS ON THE THOUGHT OF H. TRISTRAM ENGELHARDT, JR.

Edited with an Introduction by

BRENDAN P. MINOGUE

Youngstown State University,
Youngstown, OH, U.S.A.

GABRIEL PALMER-FERNÁNDEZ

Youngstown State University,
Youngstown, OH, U.S.A.

JAMES E. REAGAN

Department of Veterans Affairs,
White River Junction, VT, U.S.A.

KLUWER ACADEMIC PUBLISHERS
DORDRECHT / BOSTON / LONDON

A C.I.P. Catalogue record for this book is available from the Library of Congress

ISBN 0-7923-4572-X

Published by Kluwer Academic Publishers,
P.O. Box 17, 3300 AA Dordrecht, The Netherlands.

Sold and distributed in the U.S.A. and Canada
by Kluwer Academic Publishers,
101 Philip Drive, Norwell, MA 02061, U.S.A.

In all other countries, sold and distributed
by Kluwer Academic Publishers Group,
P.O. Box 322, 3300 AH Dordrecht, The Netherlands.

Printed on acid-free paper

Printed in the Netherlands

To Judith Minogue
B.P.M.

To Thomas Shipka, Ph.D. and Rebecca Dale
G.P.-F.

To W. R. Kennedy, Ph.D., Susan Schorsten, M.S.N., H.M., Margaret
Drummond, M.S.N., William G. Palmer, M.D., Benjamin Hayek, M.D.
and Barbara Royko.
J.E.R.

CONTENTS

ACKNOWLEDGMENTS

The editors here gratefully acknowledge the contribution of several individuals and institutions to the conference in which the papers contained in this volume were first presented, and to the preparation of the volume. Thomas Shipka, Professor and Chairperson, Department of Philosophy & Religious Studies, James Scanlon, Provost, and Melvin North, Office of University Outreach, all of Youngstown State University, provided the encouragement and many of the resources without which that conference and this volume would not have been possible. Many thanks are due to Hendrik-Jan van Leusen of Kluwer Academic Publishers for his interest in this project, to the Sisters of the Humility of Mary, sponsors of St. Elizabeth Health Center of Youngstown, Ohio, for their financial and secretarial support, to Cathy Clagett, research assistant to Gabriel Palmer-Fernández, who gave much of her time and talents to the preparation of this volume, and to Youngstown State University for a University Research Council Grant to Gabriel Palmer-Fernández.

Foreword: A Professional and Personal Portrait of H. Tristram Engelhardt, Jr.

Laurence B. McCullough

This book is about reading the work of H. Tristram Engelhardt, Jr., Ph.D., M.D. The chapters that follow present critical assessments of Engelhardt's work in bioethics and the philosophy of medicine. In this foreword to the volume I provide a professional and personal portrait of Tris Engelhardt. I have the privilege to count Tris one of my teachers, one of my best friends, and the finest colleague with whom I have served in academic life. Academic tradition discouraged me as a colleague from contributing a critical essay to this volume. After all, I would be unduly biased. I have been having–and cheerfully losing–arguments with Tris Engelhardt for a long time now. So, let the reader be duly warned. I am indeed biased, in all of the right ways. Be assured, though, that everything that follows in the next few pages is true. As to the critical essays, I believe that Engelhardt in the final chapter of this book has something to say about whether they are true.

Tris Engelhardt has earned the status of being one of the leading international figures in bioethics and philosophy of medicine. The first edition of *The Foundations of Bioethics* was translated into Japanese and Italian. The second edition, which appeared only in 1996, has already been translated into Chinese and Spanish, with other translations in preparation. I recall that the Spanish translation of the second edition arrived here in our offices at the Center for Medical Ethics and Health Policy before the English-language second edition. No other book in the field, to my knowledge, has been translated into as many languages or has become as important in as many countries as *Foundations*.

In addition to *Foundations*, Tris has written an enormous amount, including two other books,[1] all of it important and itself in many cases the foundations for the *Foundations*. Tris has also undertaken major editorial projects, all of them in collaboration with others, particularly Stuart F. Spicker, his colleague and friend of many years. Tris co-edits three book series, of which the oldest (22 years as of this writing) and largest (52 volumes in print as of this writing) is the *Philosophy and Medicine* series issued by Kluwer Academic Publishers. He also edits the *Journal of Medicine and Philosophy*. He recently helped to launch the journal, *Christian Bioethics*, for the purpose of "Non-Ecumenical Studies in Medical Morality." As editor in these and other capacities he has done more to build the fields of bioethics and philosophy of medicine and to advance the academic careers of others than anyone else.

B. P. Minogue et al. (eds.), Reading Engelhardt, xi–xix.

Tris has held faculty appointments at Tulane School of Medicine (while a medical student), the University of Texas Medical Branch (1972-1977), and Georgetown University, where he held the Rosemary Kennedy Professorship of the Philosophy of Medicine from 1977-1982 in the Kennedy Institute of Ethics. Then he came to his senses and returned to Texas, where he has been at the Baylor College of Medicine since 1983, as Professor in the Departments of Medicine, Community Medicine, and Obstetrics and Gynecology, as well as the Center for Medical Ethics and Health Policy. He also serves as Professor of Philosophy at Rice University. During the 1988-89 academic year he had the high honor to be made a Fellow in the prestigious Wissenschaftskolleg zu Berlin, during which time he began to turn his attention to the preparation of the second edition of *Foundations*.

Under "Civic and Other Awards" on his curriculum vitae, Tris would, I am sure, want the reader to know that he includes: Honorary Citizen of Galveston, Texas, 1977; Honorary Harbormaster of Galveston, June 3, 1977; and Honorary Deputy Sheriff of Galveston County, since 1988. What powers of arrest the latter grants him I fear to learn.

I first met Tris Engelhardt–I hail him regularly by his first name, Hugo, always looking forward to his hearty "Laurence!" in reply–in the spring of 1974, at the dissertation defense of his good friend, Thomas J. Bole, III. Tom had invited me to his defense, such being public events in the Department of Philosophy at The University of Texas at Austin, where I was then beginning the work on my own dissertation, on Leibniz. Tris served on Tom's dissertation committee and in spirited exchanges during the defense Tom held his own with Tris, not an easy thing to do, it struck me then. Afterwards, to celebrate Tom's becoming Doctor Bole, a number of us repaired to English's restaurant on the upper Drag, near The University, where conversation flowed freely and beautifully, full of wit and humor, reflecting an evident, deep friendship between Tris and Tom. In the glory of a Texas evening in spring and the after-glow of a first-class intellectual salon I went back to my dissertation work. Tom moved ahead to the blissful freedom of those marked by the privation of that burden. Tris went back to the University of Texas Medical Branch at Galveston, where he was teaching what I then thought were rather exotic subjects, medical ethics and philosophy of medicine, in the equally exotically named Institute for the Medical Humanities. Tris, I learned that afternoon and evening, had both a Ph.D. in Philosophy and his M.D., then a rare double degree in the United States. My memory of Tris from this first encounter is of a philosopher and physician, the order is important, I think; a philosopher and scholar of enormous intellectual capacity; one of the smartest, most well-read individuals whom I had ever met; master of German, Spanish, and Latin (speaking, not just reading; if asked on March 17th he will sing, after a fashion, the "Wearin' o' the Green" in Latin; I have heard this myself; it is a truth); intense, really intense; generous, without limit, I came later to learn; deeply loyal to friends; a real gentleman; and, from hat to boots, a Texan.

All of these, and more, are really important for appreciating Tris, but let me start with the last, because Tris is indelibly a Texan. Tris' ancestors came to Texas before it had ceased to be a state of Mexico and became a Republic in 1836. They settled first in Harrisburg, then near Brenham, and later in Comal County. Readers of his books will notice Tris' expressions of gratitude to these ancestors. Visitors in his home will meet many of these folks in a wall full of photographs, some very old, about which Tris will hold forth in a learned, respectful, and obviously affectionate way, if asked. Ask, if you ever get the chance; you'll be glad you did.

Tris' course syllabi carry such essential information as dates of reading assignments, tests, and term paper submission, as well as the Battle at Coleta Creek, the massacre at La Bahia, Independence Day (no, not the one in July), and the Battle of San Jacinto.[2] It is not widely known that Tris was not actually born in Texas, rather in New Orleans. In defense of Tris, he was not responsible for this event, because non-persons cannot be accountable for events in the world. Tris carries a Texas Passport, which he will present upon entry from Texas into the United States and which has been stamped by passport and immigration control authorities of more than a few nations. Unlike the passport issued by the government of the United States–against which we Texans continue, rightly, to chafe–a Texas Passport never expires. Even though he is very well traveled indeed, Tris should not be read as a cosmopolitan citizen of the world, but as a Texan.

One of Tris' teachers in Austin, his *Doktorvater*, Irwin C. Lieb, has written that none of us is wholly present; we are also partly past and future.[3] Now, I know Tris thinks that philosophers shouldn't, because, after Kant, they cannot, do metaphysics, but this didn't stop Chet Lieb and it won't stop me. I often think that Chet must have had Tris in mind when he made his metaphysical arguments about time, because to a very great extent, Tris is partly past and not just in being Texan. His gentlemanly ways, his courtliness, his ease with his own intellectual abilities and a level of scholarship only a handful of human beings ever accomplish, and–above all–his deep philosophical commitments in Kant and Hegel all make him, to my mind at least, an *ante-bellum* Texas gentleman. The *"bellum"* in question, I have learned from Tris, I was mistakenly taught as a school child to call the American Civil War. I now call it also (Tris' influence remains incomplete in this respect) the War Between the States or the War of Northern Aggression, linguistic matters about which Tris is very serious. If you read Engelhardt simply as a late-twentieth century intellectual, doing bioethics and philosophy of medicine, in the current fashion, without a past, you will make a big mistake.

Tris reveres his teachers. He knows and freely acknowledges that and how deeply they have shaped him personally, intellectually, and professionally. When you read Engelhardt, you read the work of a philosopher-physician deeply respectful of and willingly indebted to his teachers. Let me tell you about some of them.

In the 1960s Tris enrolled at The University of Texas at Austin, first as an undergraduate in Zoology and then as graduate student in Philosophy. In the latter capacity he studied under Chet Lieb, John Silber, Marjorie Grene, John Findlay, Charles Hartshorne, and Richard Zaner. Chet Lieb mentored Tris' dissertation and I know that Chet's death in 1992 shrank Tris' world, as it did for all of us who were made better philosophers in Chet's seminar room and conversations at the Schultz Garten, one of the great academic institutions in Texas.[4] John Silber taught Tris Kant and brought to Austin Tris' other teachers. He studied philosophy of science with Marjorie Grene, and Findlay, Hartshorne, and Zaner completed the dissertation committee that Chet Lieb directed.

Tris completed his Ph.D. in just over three years, making him a legendary figure among graduate students who came to Austin in the later 1960s and early 1970s. To my knowledge no Philosophy graduate student at The University before or since has matched this extraordinary accomplishment. In Austin, Tris first studied with Klaus Hartmann, the great Hegel scholar, with whom Tris would go on to do a Fulbright Graduate Fellowship in Bonn University after completing his degree in Philosophy. Hartmann's influence on Tris has been immense, as Tris himself freely acknowledges.[5]

Before starting his graduate study of Philosophy, Tris entered Tulane Medical School, his father's alma mater. Two teachers were especially important to him there. John Duffy taught Tris the history of medicine. James Knight taught Tris psychiatry. As Dean of Students at Tulane, Jim approved

Tris' request for a leave that interrupted his clinical clerkships, so that he could undertake his graduate studies in Austin. The field, not just Tris, owes Jim Knight a hearty "thank you" for his decision to approve Tris' request, which was unusual, to say the least, in the conservative world of medical education at the time.

When he returned to Tulane to complete his medical degree, Tris undertook with Richard Zaner the translation of Alfred Schutz's and Thomas Luckmann's *The Structures of the Life-World*.[6] Tris did this work while on his clinical rotations, including obstetrics and gynecology. In between delivering babies, most of whom were delivered by medical students at New Orleans' Charity Hospital, he worked on this translation. Tris once told me that, as a medical student, he had delivered scores of babies alone. I can see him sitting with a patient in the labor area or maybe in the hall, attending to her, monitoring her progress in labor and the fetus' status, and translating from German, which is his first language, as well as that of his children.

As this translation indicates, Tris believes in texts and scholarship about texts in a way that is decidedly not post-modern. This is also plain to anyone who has read his work. For example, the two editions of *The Foundations of Bioethics*, whatever else one might think of them, are monuments of scholarship in the histories of philosophy, medicine, theology, and ideas generally, not to mention excellent primers on Texana. These books are packed with references and footnotes.

Tris learned footnotes from Klaus Hartmann. In explaining how, Tris goes on record as noting a deficiency in Texans. This is startling, unnerving even; I can find no other such reference in his work:

> I can still recall vividly Hartmann's reaction after reading the final version of my dissertation. He found me irredeemably a neo-neo-Kantian rather than a Hegelian. My dissertation he considered impoverished of footnotes, at least from the standpoint of his understanding of good scholarship.[7]

To which passage the following footnote, of course, is appended:

> Professor Hartmann suggested that my dissertation was good as the work of a Texan or an American, but anemic when it came to footnotes by any standard he would take to be appropriate. As a good student, I set about remedying this defect. My first book (which I completed during a fellowship studying under Hartmann in Bonn) sported one footnote commanding two-thirds of the bottom of three pages.[8]

In *Foundations* Tris surely improves on this promising start of following the instructions of his beloved Klaus Hartmann. When you read Engelhardt, you are reading the work of an accomplished scholar with few peers in the field.

Family counts a great deal to Tris. He is deeply in love with his wife of 31 years, Susan, who works with him on many of his scholarly projects. They speak German at home and raised their three daughters in German, with Texan and American English coming as second and third languages. I can recall dinners at his home in Galveston when I was his research assistant–I realized years later when I read his tribute to Hartmann that he was treating me as he had been treated, forging another link in the great chain of teachers into our past–where, with my paltry ability to speak, much less comprehend spoken German, I was not quite sure what was going on around me or how to get more to eat. Tris worked with his daughters each evening, often returning to his own work after their homework was done and they had gone on to the sensible chore of getting a good night's sleep. I could tell when this had happened; my phone would ring and he would tell me that he just needed five minutes and just one more thing. There was, sometimes, an uncharacteristic imprecision to such requests.

Like Chet Lieb and Klaus Hartmann, Tris is thoroughly devoted to his students, especially those who come to work for him as his research assistants. All of us quickly discovered that for the duration the Thirteenth Amendment did not reach into our lives and its protections were replaced by unstinting work, the highest intellectual expectations, the thrill of striving for and being part of excellence, and the deep bonds of friendship. This was more than a fair trade, I can, with confidence, say for all of us. Tris has in this way brought more people into the field than anyone else, I believe. We are fiercely proud to have been his students.

When you work for Tris you help him read what needs to be read for his work and then you read what he writes. You write with him, too. He has helped all of us launch our academic careers, and so he made us his colleagues as well. You argue with him tooth and nail and in the process of doing so you receive an unmatched philosophical education. As his student, Tris wants you not to think as he thinks but as you think for yourself when you strive for the intellectual standards that he sets for you. Tris, I am convinced, would think himself a failure if he were to produce intellectual clones. As you argue with him about what he has given you to read–and, in its umpteenth draft, to read again, usually at some impossibly late hour–Tris listens and he rewrites what he has written. I started in 1974 to read what became the first edition of *Foundations* and other students later read what became the second edition. So when you read Engelhardt you read someone who is a master teacher. He wants you to argue with him. So do so; you will be a better thinker for the effort.

Tris is a physician and a very good one. He reads medicine, well and widely. I have taken my own and family members' health problems to him and he has helped me understand them and come to terms with them. He has a deep grasp of human illness, disease, suffering, and dying. He is a superb teacher of medical students and residents, in lecture halls and clinical services alike. He is also a serious student and published scholar of the history of medicine. His elective course on the subject here at Baylor annually attracts a large student enrollment and many faculty auditors. He has thought long, hard, and well about medicine–as a social institution, about its history, about the epistemological claims that it can make, about its value-laden character, as a way of life. That he has two doctorates shapes his work fundamentally, so read Engelhardt also as the physician committed to the well-being of patients.

Tris lives a deeply religious and spiritual life, as he makes plain in the second edition of *Foundations*. He is a creature of God who thrives in an ancient Christian faith community and its defining, sustaining spirituality of transcendence. He marks the days by the great rhythms of the calendar of the Orthodox saints and can tell you something important about almost all of them. When you read Engelhardt on religion and spirituality and the importance of the content-full morality that they make actual in human lives, when you read him expressing concern for the spiritual emptiness of some ways of human endeavor, take him very seriously.

The papers here were first presented at a conference hosted by the editors at Youngstown State University. I watched Tris closely as the two days of discourse and celebration unfolded. He was altogether in his element. He listened to the papers intently and responded to each of them in the closing session of the conference. He is allowed a last word in this book, too. Almost all of his students were there. Kevin Wm. Wildes, S.J., came from Georgetown and John Moskop from East Carolina University, and both contribute papers to this volume. One evening four of us put together a panel in tribute to our teacher, mentor, colleague, and friend. Mary Ann Cutter came east from Colorado Springs and spoke beautifully of how her students responded to reading Engelhardt. George Khushf came north from Columbia, South

Carolina and described the rewards of being Tris' most recent student, displaying with no small pride and delight his framed instrument of manumission. Stephen Wear came west from Buffalo in the person and full regalia of his forebear, General John Streeter of the First New Hampshire Volunteers, and–defiantly unregenerate Yankee that he is–instructed Tris on the mistaken ways of General Hood and his Texans at a faraway place and longago time called the Battle of Gettysburg and other important matters. One of Tris' present students, who has come from the People's Republic of China to study with Tris, Dr. Ruiping Fan, traveled from Houston. We gathered later that evening for a photograph, the first time that so many of us had been together with Tris. Tris' other students, George Agich, Tom Bole, Eric Juengst, and Mark J. Cherry were not able to be there but were, I like to think, there in spirit. They were a glorious two days. Read this book as a reflection of a very special time in academic life.

Watching all of this, especially the panel, one of the conference organizers remarked to me, as the conference drew to its close, that it was unusual in academic life these days for students to show such respect and regard for their mentor, all the more so, because he knew, Tris had, with the exceptions of Mark and Ruiping, not directed our dissertations. Tris had taught us after that work had been done, making our evident high regard for Tris very special in our colleague's judgment. More, our colleague said, we obviously had great affection for Tris, an even more unusual relationship to one's mentor these days in academia, our colleague noted. He got it all just right. When you read Engelhardt, you read the work of a philosopher-physician who is respected, revered, and loved by his students, who look forward, as we hope the reader will, to the next argument with Tris.

NOTES

1. H. Tristram Engelhardt, Jr., *Mind-Body: A Categorial Relation* (The Hague, The Netherlands: Martinus Nijhoff, 1973) and *Bioethics and Secular Humanism: The Search for a Common Morality* (Philadelphia: Trinity Press International, 1991).

2. If you don't recognize the latter four references, you have, in the language of *Foundations*, chosen the wrong content-full morality, e.g., being a Yankee. To avert the disaster that, as a consequence, certainly impends, remove yourself to Texas with all speed and undertake our re-education program–but not too many of you.

3. I. C. Lieb, *Past, Present, and Future: A Philosophical Essay About Time* (Urbana and Chicago: University of Illinois Press, 1991).

4. For those unfortunate to find themselves moral strangers, Schultz Garten and its Sacngerrun-dehalle are located on San Jacinto (see note no.1), just south of The University. Schultz's, as its denizens know it, claims the title of the oldest, continuously operating tavern in Texas, haven to students, professors, and legislators–the latter to be regarded, Tris has correctly taught me, as public menaces and threats to free people everywhere.

5. H. Tristram Engelhardt, Jr., "Klaus Hartmann and G. W. F. Hegel: A Personal Postscript," in H. Tristram Engelhardt, Jr. and T. Pincard, eds., *Hegel Reconsidered* (Dordrecht, The Netherlands: Kluwer Academic Publishers, 1994), 225-29.

6. Alfred Schutz and Thomas Luckmann, *The Structures of the Life-World*, trans. and intro. Richard M. Zaner and H. Tristram Engelhardt, Jr. (Evanston, Illinois: Northwestern University Press, 1973).

7. Engelhardt, "Klaus Hartmann and G. W. F. Hegel: A Personal Postscript," 225-29.

8. Engelhardt, "Klaus Hartmann and G. W. F. Hegel: A Personal Postscript," 229 n.1.

BRENDAN P. MINOGUE, GABRIEL PALMER-FERNÁNDEZ, AND JAMES E. REAGAN

Reading Engelhardt has been an extensive enterprise. The book completes a project that includes the conference, "Ethics, Medicine and Health Care: An Appraisal of the Thought of H. Tristram Engelhardt, Jr.," held at Youngstown State University on the weekend of September 30, 1995. It is comprised of essays first presented at that conference.[1]

The conference was organized by The Dr. James Dale Ethics Center of Youngstown State University to recognize the publication of the Second Edition of *The Foundations of Bioethics*, and to express the editors' affection for its author. *Foundations* has become part of the modern bioethical cannon. It is frequently cited and discussed in many works in various fields, and it is difficult to imagine how a bioethics course can proceed without reference to Engelhardt. Furthermore, *Foundations* is an international text translated into Italian, Chinese, Japanese and Spanish. Finally, the Second Edition of *Foundations* includes new material, and therefore warrants close reading and commentary throughout the bioethics community.

Our affection for Engelhardt began in 1981 when he made the first of fifteen annual visits to Youngstown, Ohio. At first his primary host was the Department of Family Medicine of Youngstown's St. Elizabeth Health Center. He was enormously well-received by local healthcare providers and educators, especially at The Northeastern Ohio Universities' College of Medicine and at Youngstown State University, where he was conscripted to hard labor in the Department of Philosophy & Religious Studies and The Dr. James Dale Ethics Center. Faculty members from these institutions subjected Engelhardt to challenging dialogue and, in the process, many of us were fortunate to become his friends.

Engelhardt surprises academics because he speaks not only intelligently but also humorously. His good cheer invites students and readers to participate in an important conversation, and consequently the serious work of bioethics becomes a joyful event. He has a gift for playful seriousness that signals to all that they may join safely in a discussion where each person's interests are heard, no one's ability is demeaned, and everyone's dignity is preserved.

For nearly a decade, often in sleep-deprived conversation in our homes, in sober offices or in other spirit-filled settings, Tris responded to our continuous criticisms of his views. He listened to our ideas and encouraged us to pursue

1

B. P. Minogue et al. (eds.), Reading Engelhardt, 1–14.
© 1997 *Kluwer Academic Publishers. Printed in the Netherlands.*

them. We also shared stories of our lives, and none became the worse for that. In short, we came to know the person Tris Engelhardt as one who deeply loves philosophical conversations, and in 1994 we decided to express our accumulating affection and respect by sponsoring the conference and editing this book.

The conference showed that our experience with Engelhardt is not unique. Over seventy participants from around the country and abroad explored and criticized Engelhardt's thought. Those who did not know him were surprised at the spontaneous play that infused the program. Many who attended the conference told us that they had anticipated the philosophizing but not the fun. A few asked why we, the editors, who are not students of Engelhardt, had organized this conference. We replied then as we explain now: Tris Engelhardt is a friend to us, and his work is central to any adequate understanding of the field of bioethics.

OVERVIEW OF *FOUNDATIONS*

As a moral and political philosopher, H. Tristram Engelhardt, Jr. is deeply influenced by Kant and Hegel, as well as by the skepticism that operates within our secular society. In *Foundations* Engelhardt explores several philosophical justifications of contemporary secular bioethics. He argues that secular ethics aims to identify criteria for peaceably regulating the behavior of persons living in our type of society, a society that does not presuppose the truth of any specific content-full view of the good and the right (a religious, hedonistic, or perfectionistic view of morality, for example). So conceived, *Foundations* undermines two important accounts of ethics. The first account views ethics as a search for a distinct moral authority such as a holy book or a prophet. The second treats ethics as grounded in rational moral intuitions, dispositions, and theories. Both views suffer in the hands of secular skepticism. Persons living within a secular society simply cannot agree on either authority or intuition, and, given Engelhardt's proscription of the use of force, both approaches are impossible within such a society.

Engelhardt then engages his reader in a dialectical account of what secular bioethics should accomplish. The Kantian Engelhardt thinks that secular bioethics should establish a transcendental account of how free persons can derive rational (i.e., universalizable and impartial) justifications for specific moral rules involving individual liberty and the common good. But the skeptical Engelhardt argues that secular bioethics can establish few of the moral rules that might bind men and women in a common effort. For Engelhardt, we live amidst the ruins of two centuries of failed transcendental proofs of these moral rules and values.

The condition of a modern, secular and pluralistic society is characterized by the strong view that most coercion is unjustifiable, including the kind which seems to be necessary to win agreement about who are the correct moral authorities and which are the correct moral intuitions. Engelhardt's skeptical attack on contemporary secular ethics exposes the difficulties in justifying a universally binding and coherent morality. More generally, he holds that content-full views of the good fail because they "attempt to justify a particular moral vision (which itself) presupposes exactly what it seeks to establish so that moral theoretical arguments are at best expository, not justificatory."[2] Some of these views include a distinct moral authority, such as God; others assume agreement on the definition of the good. But because persons are so deeply divided in their views about the good, concrete universal definitions of the good are impossible to identify.

Engelhardt, however, does not deny the possibility of a secular bioethics. On the contrary, we can deduce a thin or, as he puts it, content-less secular bioethics. The concept of agreement, Engelhardt argues, can provide rules necessary for peaceable living. Engelhardt makes this concept explicit by identifying two principles, the principle of permission and the principle of beneficence. The principle of permission requires respect for the necessary and constitutive role of the will in achieving agreement generally and in achieving particular agreements. Violations of this principle involve acting on others without their consent. The principle of beneficence permits persons to attend to the interests of others. Violations of this principle involve disrespect for these interests. Disrespect, however, is not the same as ignoring the interests of others. It occurs only if one has agreed to attend to the interests of others. For Engelhardt, ignoring others' interests must be permitted for persons who choose neither to enter into nor benefit from beneficent-based agreements. There is, therefore, a clear conceptual priority to the principle of permission over beneficence that gives Engelhardt's bioethics its *quasi*-libertarian flavor.

The importance of permission can be illustrated with Engelhardt's doctrine of personhood. All known persons are human beings, but not all human beings are persons, because some humans lack the rationality necessary to enter into agreements. For Engelhardt, human beings lacking rationality are outside the clear boundaries of persons. Fetuses, infants, young children, severely retarded individuals and irreversibly comatose and vegetative patients are outside of these boundaries and, therefore, are not persons in the strict sense. How we should treat nonpersons is itself a matter of agreement and, therefore, bioethical questions regarding abortion, definition of death and a host of other issues need to be approached within the context of the priority of permission.

Although Engelhardt approaches libertarianism, his version of libertarianism is neither pure nor absolute. For example, he subscribes to a Lockean view of the universal ownership of property that allows for two-tiered health care systems. Nor does he celebrate a gratuitous libertarianism. To the contrary, he repeatedly argues that persons need not and should not always seek to be free from all responsibilities for others.

Criticisms of Engelhardt's work often focus on the status of permission. For some, Engelhardt's bioethics presupposes the priority of the ethical value of individual freedom and of its political correlate, individual liberty. In response, Engelhardt claims that "within secular philosophical reasoning, ultimate questions cannot be answered. Even the project of secular philosophical reason cannot itself be valued or endorsed, at least in general secular terms."[3] For Engelhardt, the principles of permission and beneficence are necessary not for all forms of life, but only for secular rights and secular obligations. In this sense they are *principia*: they indicate the source and origins of particular areas of the secular moral life.

OVERVIEW OF THE ESSAYS

In "Everything Includes Itself in Power: Power and Coherence in Engelhardt's *Foundations of Bioethics*," James Nelson argues that Engelhardt's principles are too lax in what they permit persons to do and too stringent in what they prohibit persons from regulating. He challenges both the necessity and sufficiency of "agreement" as a basis for intelligible and adequate regulation. Given that persons reach opposing agreements, how are agreements that themselves cause conflicts ranked? How are persons bound by agreements to which they do not consent but to which they find themselves subjected nonetheless? What counts as consent? How can persons be necessarily represented as actually giving consent to specific agreements? Does inequality among persons require an equivocal account of consent?

Given these misgivings, Nelson questions whether Engelhardt's claim that "agreement" (the principle of permission) is in fact any different from other traditional bases used to defend the exercise of power. For Nelson, permission is as arbitrary as other forms of power which Engelhardt has criticized for being arbitrary. He points out that Engelhardt simply asserts that for persons who avow peace as the defining characteristic of morality, departure from the principle of permission is morally blameworthy. Nelson, however, finds this assertion "a purely stipulative use of 'moral'... devoid of any resources for explaining what it is about the ability of persons to permit and agree that ought to command our respect."

Stanley Hauerwas offers a theological appraisal of Engelhardt's work. He acknowledges similarities between Engelhardt's project and his own work in Christian theological ethics, but in this essay he wants to identify important differences. Hauerwas finds Engelhardt more ethically attentive to order than morality, to exchange than trust, to politics than economics, and he draws his distance from Engelhardt by making these differences explicit.

Hauerwas concurs with Engelhardt's assessment that the distinctive moral convictions of Christian believers cannot be rationally deduced from general secular philosophical concepts. He also finds Engelhardt's attempt to characterize Christian communities within secular terms problematic. For example, Christian communities cannot be understood as arising from choice. For Hauerwas God chooses the Christians; they don't choose Him. Engelhardt sees these communities as emerging from the voluntary choice of their members, while Hauerwas finds himself a Christian in much the same way he finds himself a Texan. Furthermore, for Hauerwas Engelhardt's comparative account of Christian and secular ethics undermines the Christian task of living an alternative life by positing secular grammar as itself a morally sufficient source of authority. For Christians, moral authority does not come from secular culture, and the assumption that morality can be secular does violence to those Christian communities that pursue or resort to secular ideals.

Hauerwas questions not only Engelhardt's account of moral authority, but also his account of moral rationality. MacIntyre and Foucault, he notes, give non-Enlightenment accounts of rationality, and Engelhardt does not address these accounts. Hauerwas also rejects Engelhardt's notion of the state as a morally neutral and tolerant bureaucratic agency deliberately designed to allow peaceful pursuit of private goods by free agents. Real states have always had more substantive values. Finally, Hauerwas disagrees with Engelhardt's urging that today's physicians and other health care providers should aspire to be peaceable but otherwise morally empty Hegelian bureaucrats. That vision, says Hauerwas, can sustain neither providers nor patients in the difficulties and tragedies they face.

Haavi Morreim, in "Medicine's Monopoly: From Trust-Busting to Trust," employs some familiar Engelhardtian principles to explore several aspects of contemporary medical economics. She argues that for many years the medical profession has "exercised a virtual monopoly" on medical goods and services, a monopoly that has produced rising inflation and inappropriate restrictions on the autonomy of patients and practitioners. The tools used to secure this monopoly include control over licensure, prescription, education and the legal definitions of standards of care. This monopoly has reduced human liberty by restricting patients' access to alternative treatments, increasing the costs of conventional treatments, and neutralizing the power of the market to establish costs.

This monopoly has also decreased the autonomy of physicians to treat patients according to their best clinical judgment. For example, physicians cannot prescribe narcotics for hopelessly addicted patients. Nor can they prescribe Prozac for the purpose of life enhancement. Morreim appeals to Engelhardt's principle of permission to justify her view that medicine will benefit from increased freedom of individual patients and physicians to create "mutually agreed upon" plans of care. She also appeals to Engelhardt's interpretation of disease as a value-laden social construction. Treatments, she argues, must be at least as value-laden as the diseases they are designed to reduce. Morreim closes by asserting that the value of mutual trust is essential in achieving good care and that our society can enhance trust by restoring authority in medicine to physicians and patients.

In "Engelhardt's Communitarian Ethics: The Hidden Assumptions," Kevin Wildes, S.J. contends that Engelhardt is a "libertarian by default." According to Wildes, Engelhardt's libertarian principles are all that remain after the demonstrated failures of several substantive and community-based theories of ethics. These theories fail to achieve the level of universal assent and sanction required to comprehend the secular societies of the twentieth and twenty-first centuries. Neither Jonsen and Toulmin's casuistry nor Beauchamp and Childress' principles achieve universal approbation because they presuppose a common or shared concurrence of moral values that does not exist in a pluralistic, secular state.

Wildes argues that Engelhardt's critique of communitarian ethics presupposes a particular juridical view of "community" which is not reflected in the existence of real communities. Communities, for Engelhardt, are constituted by metaphysical beliefs, but, according to Wildes, it would follow from this that Franciscan Friars and Dominican Preachers would have to belong to different communities since they differ over important metaphysical doctrines. But they do not belong to different communities. Both orders belong to the Roman Catholic community, just as Roman and Orthodox Catholic believers are both Christian. Wildes notes that many diverse particular communities with important differences are nonetheless found to be far more unified than Engelhardt's juridical perspective permits. Wildes then suggests that suspicion of ecumenism and moral fideism ground Engelhardt's metaphysical interpretation of community.

In "*Monopoly* With Sick Moral Strangers," Wade Robison criticizes Engelhardt's libertarian interpretation of morally praiseworthy and blameworthy allocations of health care resources. For Engelhardt, the principle of permission is a necessary condition for the possibility of peaceably providing and receiving health care. This principle, Engelhardt contends, transcends all possible particular moral values. For example, values involving rights, goods, freedoms and order are secondary to permission. Engelhardt claims that his permission principle does not presuppose or arbitrarily privilege any such value. Since liberty is the highest order value, Engelhardt requires that libertarian free market models of exchange take precedence over other models for the distribution of health care.

Robison challenges Engelhardt's claim that liberty is prior or more basic than other values. He thinks Engelhardt's principle of permission, like all contingent principles, is conditionally true or conditionally false: permission is important but not absolutely so; peace is important but not unconditionally so. For Robison, neither liberty nor any other single moral value is the secular correlate of a God. Rather, particular moral values (e.g., intuitions, rules, goods, dispositions, attitudes) gain or lose priority relative to specific activities in which persons engage. Robison uses the game of *Monopoly* to illustrate the idea that all values including liberty have a contingent quality. He shows that this particularly libertarian game takes liberty as a vitally important value, but not as the exclusive or unconditional value. *Monopoly* can be imagined as a game with different conditions depending on the status of the players. For example, we may choose to let young players have twice as much money as experienced players. We may not allow young players foolishly to spend their money on worthless properties. In short, the situation at the beginning of the game may require different conditions or rules. Otherwise it would be less fun. If freedom is capable of being restricted for purposes of fun within this arch-libertarian game, then freedom may be restricted in the game of life when there are good reasons that require us to do so. For Robison, sickness is a reason for limiting liberty in life just as youth is a reason for limiting freedom in monopoly.

In "Beyond Forbearance As The Moral Foundation For A Health Care System: Analysis of Engelhardt's Principles of Bioethics," Rory B. Weiner argues, first, that Engelhardt's principle of permission must be complemented by a principle of cooperative beneficence in order for persons peaceably to negotiate agreements, and second, that the principle of cooperative beneficence combines with the principle of permission to establish a universal positive right of access to health care.

According to Weiner, Engelhardt's deduction of the principle of permission as a necessary and sufficient grounding for secular morality is mistaken because inequality among persons is genuine and deep. Inequalities in education, wealth, health, security and access to information jeopardize the freedom of some persons to enter agreements. Forbearance or non-interference with others' choices, by itself, is not a sufficient moral principle for secular society. We must add something to the non-interference rule. Cooperative beneficence, through which all members (i.e., moral strangers) of a secular society accept the duty to collaborate in helping the least well-off, is also necessary. Furthermore, since cooperative beneficence "is as basic as the principle of permission, we may use coercive power to assure its compliance."

Weiner seeks to undermine Engelhardt's transcendental confidence. He argues that free but deeply disadvantaged moral strangers will not primarily value their freedom, but rather may find that freedom futile for improving their relative position in society. Weiner also notes that Engelhardt's analytical silence about how inequality undermines freedom belies Engelhardt's claim that his principle of permission is ethically non-normative, neutral or value-free.

Mary Ann Gardell Cutter, in "Engelhardt's Analysis of Disease: Implications For A Feminist Clinical Epistemology," turns to Engelhardt's "constructivist" analysis of medicine and disease to develop a feminist clinical epistemology. A successful feminist clinical epistemology, she argues, would clarify the gender biases of particular medical accounts of health, disease and illness. These clarifications would reduce injustices and harms currently visited upon women and also improve their prospects for better health care in the future. According to Cutter, Engelhardt holds that scientists, physicians, citizens and patients construct rather than discover facts and the meanings of medicine, health, disease and illness. Furthermore, they construct them using subjective (i.e., selective, and historically conditioned and contingent) criteria, methods and ideals of description, evaluation, explanation and social significance. In any particular construction, these components overlap. Hence, such constructions necessarily require specific agreements among the relevant parties regarding what counts as factual, rational, moral and meaningful.

Cutter recognizes Engelhardt's contribution to clinical epistemology, especially his efforts to deconstruct medicine by showing the genesis and transformations of the concept of disease in the history of Western European society. She follows suit with an outline of her own deconstruction of contemporary Western medicine and exposes a gender bias that both harms women and prevents progress in treating patients. Cutter's outline is shaped by Engelhardtian themes which emphasize differences among individual patients and value-laden assumptions that often harm women. She notes that gender has been excluded as a significant criterion in treating patients and in designing and implementing research protocols. Therefore, the possibility that women and men suffer diseases differently has been neglected, obscured or denied. For Cutter, medical observations and findings are often gender dependent, that is, they presuppose theories of evidence, explanation, significance, appropriateness and control that exclude consideration of women's experience.

In "*The Magic Mountain*: A Prelude To Engelhardt's Phenomenology Of Illness," Richard M. Owsley looks to Engelhardt's phenomenological depiction of illness to interpret Thomas Mann's novel, *The Magic Mountain*. A phenomenology of illness, Owsley says, attends to the structures and textures of the afflicted person's conscious appropriation of the disease. According to Owsley, Engelhardt asks the right questions. How does the patient experience herself as sick? What changes of dispositions and attitudes, and alterations of relationships occur when the individual becomes ill? How do sick persons encounter and adapt to their situation? Mann, as interpreted by Owsley, explores just these questions in *The Magic Mountain*. The principal character, Hans Castorp, becomes ill with tuberculosis while visiting a sanatorium. In interaction with other patients and caregivers, Castorp observes and experiences many aspects of patients' appropriation of the sick role: withdrawal from work, family, home, employment, and functioning; increasing investment in medical care, human sympathy and pessimism. Chronically sick people continuously exhibit disparate feelings: frivolity and depression, hope and resignation, pride and degradation, normality or aberrancy. For Owsley, Mann's characters personify and convey changing sentiments shaped by the fluctuations in their disease. Owsley interprets Castorp as reconstituting himself from "healthy" to "ill," and notes that this change includes the replacement of innocence by sophistication. He concludes that Mann's characters experience their illness as something "other," thus causing disorientation, estrangement, dislocation and isolation. Disease also alters their experiences of time, space, and quality of life.

John C. Moskop, in "Persons, Property Or Both? Engelhardt On The Moral Status Of Children," examines Engelhardt's two opposing views of the moral status of young children. The more basic and clear Engelhardtian thesis is that in a secular society young children are not persons and do not possess the moral rights of persons. Parents of young children possess the same freedom and responsibility toward them that pregnant women possess toward their fetuses. The second and more complex Engelhardtian thesis is that in secular society young children may be recognized as "future persons" or "social persons" or "property" and therefore possess moral rights. Moskop acknowledges that Engelhardt's two views seem irreconcilable. He recommends the second view. Moskop admits that representing children as social persons and/or property seems odd, alarming and offensive. However, he argues that this representation does not mean that the power of parents is unrestricted, since property owners are often profoundly restricted in what they can do to their property. Saying that parents own their children means that parents have some rights of dominion over their children.

In "Tris Engelhardt And The Queen Of Hearts: Sentence First, Verdict Afterwards," Margaret Monahan Hogan examines and rejects Engelhardt's view that fetuses are not persons and lack the basic moral right to life. She counters his neo-Kantian concepts of potentiality, personhood, human relations, rights and responsibilities with a neo-Aristotelian account that depicts fetuses as persons who possess the right to life. Hogan proposes that practical reason suggests that autonomy is more limited than Engelhardt allows, and that personal relations are more internally regulated than Engelhardt describes. She argues that autonomy is considerably more limited than Engelhardt seems to realize. In addition, "potentiality" is a much more complex state of being than Engelhardt acknowledges. Regarding fetuses and persons, Hogan interprets Engelhardt's potentiality-actuality distinction as "an all or nothing affair" which fails to understand the nature of human fetuses. She proposes an alternative account of fetal development, one that depends on the Aristotelian notions of efficient, formal and final causality. This account implies that because fetuses are potential persons they are already natural, actual, purposeful, and progressive beings who are persons.

Cynthia Brincat, in "The Foundations of *The Foundations of Bioethics*: Engelhardt's Kantian Underpinnings," questions Engelhardt's understanding of Kant's civil and ethical commonwealth. Despite the presence of apparent similarities between Engelhardt's and Kant's visions of the state, she argues that there is a crucial difference between the two views. Kant and Engelhardt both recognize the profound semantic, logical and conceptual gaps which emerge from differences among people engaged in moral discourse within a pluralistic society. As a consequence, both Kant and Engelhardt endorse a separation between general and content-specific moral tiers. This distinction allows for the creation of a framework of mutual respect, which in turn allows for the peaceful resolution of moral differences through respectful negotiation. Peaceful resolution is possible only if we admit a two-tiered moral system in which differences in definitions of the good are managed by an appeal to mutual respect.

Despite these similarities, Brincat asserts that Engelhardt has failed to recognize that Kant's articulation of the two separate tiers of moral discourse includes a profound teleological notion. According to Brincat, Kant's ethical commonwealth allows progression towards moral integration. This teleological element shows the impossibility of treating the distinction between the public and private moral tiers as absolute. Hence both Engelhardt's depiction of Kant and Engelhardt's own moral discourse are static and incomplete.

Thus Brincat argues that Engelhardt is mistaken when he says that Kant "smuggles moral content" into the civil commonwealth. Kant's civil commonwealth includes a teleological notion allowing for progressive integration of the different tiers within social life. For Brincat, Engelhardt's critique of Kant misses the fact that Kant saw something that Engelhardt cannot see, namely, that for any civil community devoid of moral integration, peaceful negotiations would at best consist only of cessations of conflict. A true and lasting peace, by contrast, requires a "consummate moral community" made manifest through the ethical commonwealth.

In "Engelhardt, Historicism And The Minimalist Paradox," Brendan P. Minogue argues that differences between the first and second edition of *The*

Foundations suggest that Hegel's influence on Engelhardt is overtaking Kant's. At the heart of Engelhardt's bioethical program, he argues, is a paradox, which he calls the minimalist paradox. It asserts that, for Engelhardt, the secular state is both ignorant and not ignorant of such things as active euthanasia, infanticide and commercial surrogacy. According to Minogue, Engelhardt resolves this paradox by assuming the Kantian idea that once we are ignorant of something we are necessarily obligated to permit it. But historical states do not follow this rule because they do not think that there is an actual necessary connection between ignorance and permission. Hegel is deeply aware of this problem, especially in his critique of Kant's formalism. According to Hegel, there is no formal way to determine what we should do when we cannot prove to everyone's satisfaction that something like active euthanasia is wrong. For Minogue, the difficulty with any purely formal minimalism is that there is no way to determine what is included or excluded from the minimalist program. Is a national health care program included or excluded? Minogue argues that Engelhardt himself is aware of this difficulty. In the first edition he seems to reject national health care but in the second edition he favors a two-tiered health care system which requires individuals to pay taxes for a minimally decent health care system. This change is at odds with Engelhardt's reputed libertarianism and implies that the state is indeed free to create a health care system despite the presence of vast moral ignorance.

In "The Unjustifiability Of Substantive Liberalisms And The Inevitability Of Engelhardtian Procedural Liberalism," Ruiping Fan argues that Engelhardt's program of "thin" or non-substantive political liberalism which assumes no particular intuitions, sensibilities or concepts of the good life is a necessary and sufficient guiding philosophy for contemporary secular states and societies. Fan reviews three schools of "thick" or substantive political liberalism: deism capitalism, utilitarianism and social contractarianism. He finds each of them unsatisfactory. He sees Adam Smith as a deist capitalist who appeals to a distant but benign God to buttress the view that the selfish pursuit of wealth by individuals generates optimum social welfare. Fan responds that appeal to God wields no justifiable authority in a religiously pluralistic society. John Stuart Mill's utilitarianism does not rely on God, but it does authorize interference with the free market to secure public welfare. Fan replies that public welfare is a value always indeterminate and therefore essentially contestable, and as such never a source of justifiable limitation of the permission principle. John Rawls avoids appeals both to God and to a substantive account of public welfare, but posits an "overlapping consensus" among secular citizens about certain particular moral values, a consensus that some Rawlsians call "wide reflective equilibrium." Fan counters that such consensus and equilibrium simply do not extend to all secular societies, and he poses examples of Singaporean political structures, values and trade-offs to demonstrate the point. Given the deep substantive moral divisions that characterize the lives of moral strangers in secular societies, Engelhardtian procedural liberalism alone is capable of morally underwriting peaceable politics.

Faith L. Lagay, in " Secular? Yes; Humanism? No: A Close Look At Engelhardt's Secular Humanist Bioethic," argues that Engelhardt bids to admit his bioethics to the humanist tradition, and that we ought to reject the plea. Lagay comes to grips with Engelhardt not over *Foundations*, but over *Bioethics and Secular Humanism: The Search for a Common Morality*. She summarizes both Engelhardt's leveling critique of traditional sources of moral authority and his formal procedural bioethics, and observes that absent welfare considerations, this bioethics "serves as a political expedient for keeping the peace rather than serving as a common morality." Lagay closely tracks Engelhardt's exegesis of ten historical types of Western humanism and gives particular attention to the humanism in which he situates his bioethics. She then argues that Engelhardt's bioethics is not a humanism because it discredits and degrades humanistic moral reasoning, and undercuts the presumption of positive beneficence, the deployment of value judgment, cultivation of morality through education and the arts, the appreciation of the importance of "context," and the values of rhetoric and emotion.

Finally, Engelhardt, in "The Foundations of Bioethics and Secular Humanism: Why Is There No Canonical Moral Content?" responds to many of the criticisms leveled against him in the above essays by articulating and then stressing the refusal of their authors to acknowledge what precious little is left of morality in light of the failure of the modern philosophical project and the sociological fact of diverse and incommensurable moral visions. When we meet as moral strangers we are bound neither by God nor a content-full view of the good and the right. Although we want more, as moral strangers we are bound only by a modest or sparse morality of permission, the authority of which is drawn from our agreements. Engelhardt warns that if we assume more than this modest morality we may well repeat this century's bloody history.

NOTES

1. We gratefully acknowledge the assistance of our colleagues, Drs. Thomas Shipka and Bruce Waller, in the planning of the conference and their helpful suggestions on an earlier draft of this Introduction.

2. H. Tristram Engelhardt, Jr., *The Foundations of Bioethics*, 2nd ed. (Oxford and New York: Oxford University Press, 1996), 7.

3. Engelhardt, *Foundations*, 58.

1

EVERYTHING INCLUDES ITSELF IN POWER: POWER AND COHERENCE
IN ENGELHARDT'S *FOUNDATIONS OF BIOETHICS*
=====

JAMES LINDEMANN NELSON

> *Then everything includes itself in power*
> *Power into will, will into appetite;*
> *And appetite, an universal wolf,*
> *So doubly seconded with will and power,*
> *Must make perforce an universal prey,*
> *And last eat up himself.*

Troilus and Cressida, Act One, Scene Three

A way of understanding an important theme in the history of ethics, at least since the Enlightenment, is to see it as an attempt to chain Shakespeare's universal wolf. Somehow, power must be kept from dissolving without residue into will and appetite. Otherwise, we run the risk of various kinds of war, which few regard as an efficient way of achieving their ends, and fewer still desire for its own sake. Further, we lose what strikes me as a deep human hope: that there are ways of living that are *legitimate*. By this I mean that the circumstances and projects that form our lives are not merely expressions of a purely contingent play of historical forces with which we will have to either put up if we must or pull down if we can. Rather, we hope that our lives can be made to reflect, even if darkly, something that is true about the way things ought to be, quite independently of whatever you or I or anyone else might think or wish. The way things ought to be, according to this hope, will at least constrain and perhaps even guide our power, turning it to ends other than whatever we or others just might happen to desire, steering it toward what in fact we should yearn for. Should this hope fail, we face not only Hobbes' prospect of the war of each against all, but an even profounder threat: the loss of a deeply important feature of our notion of ourselves as agents. For if there is only power, and only will and appetite to guide it, if there is nothing to be said for any goal or end or form of life that would distinguish it as more worth pursuing than any other, then what is to prevent us from slipping into a kind of inertness, in which all pursuits are comparatively indifferent, and any pursuit

15

B. P. Minogue et al. (eds.), Reading Engelhardt, 15–29.
© 1997 *Kluwer Academic Publishers. Printed in the Netherlands.*

seems ultimately vain? The will, as David Wiggins has noted, craves objective reasons in determining what is worth pursuit: "often it could not go forward unless it thought it had them."[1]

For H. Tristram Engelhardt, the world and our strivings in it are redeemed from ultimate vanity by God, who speaks with relative clarity to Orthodox Catholics, more obscurely to other Christians, more obscurely still to non-christian believers, and altogether unintelligibly to many of us. Because, as Engelhardt acknowledges, God has not chosen to make the truth plain to all, the goals sought and constraints observed by Orthodox Catholics will seem, to one extent or another, undermotivated, confused, misunderstood, regrettable, perverse, or even evil, and any exercise of power toward these goals will seem, insofar as it affects a nonbeliever such as me, and in the absence of the grace of conversion, more or less alien and arbitrary. Orthodox Catholics will, of course, have similar views about how I live my life, and the same problem will, *mutatis mutandis*, confront all of us.

So, at least as regards our social lives in a pluralist state, we all hear the howl of Shakespeare's wolf. Engelhardt's work stands in a long tradition of efforts to forge out of reason a chain for power. "A goal of ethics," he tells us, "is to determine when force can be justified."[2] But it is a tradition that, at least as he and many others see it, is just about out of gas. The idea that we could somehow find out how to domesticate the wolf, direct our power, appetite, and will toward ends that were (demonstrably) really good in ways that were (evidently) really right, relying for those demonstrations and that evidence on the exercise of faculties common to all persons, is not only unlikely in fact, but, according to Engelhardt, impossible in principle. Human reason has no canonical vision of how we all should live tucked away in its hat. Reason might help us better understand the implications of some constellation of normative commitments we accept on other grounds, set them in better, more perspicuous, more coherent order. But it cannot provide us with a guaranteed-to-be-correct transcendental blueprint of the good life. Nor, apparently, can it even justify the selection of plausible contenders for that role.

Any such blueprints as we have are the result of our participation in traditions much more specific than the point of view of reason as such, that come installed with more-or-less rich conceptions of what is worth living for. Within such traditions–with our "moral friends"–reason may be useful in its underlaborer role, helping resolve unclarity or disagreement about what the vision of the good requires. But between one tradition and the next there is grave and irresolvable disagreement concerning the good. What reason can do on its own, however, is to justify rigorously a few minimal, but at the same time quite far-reaching, constraints on both our actions and our motivations. In rough summary, Engelhardt takes reason as competent to reveal, with apodictic certainty, the following: we must not act in ways that involve other people without their permission (the *permission principle*), and we must be motivated to act in ways that seek the good of others, although what such motivation will concretely involve is impossible to specify outside the context of certain conceptions of the good which are not themselves determinable by reason (the *principle of beneficence*).[3]

The world that ensues as ordered by these principles alone is nightmarish. It is not merely a world in which a Canadian-style system of health care is seen as so coercive as to be immoral[4]–that's a comparatively trivial result. It is a world in which toddlers, rather than veal calves, could be fattened for the table in factory farms, and in which our desire to witness violence need not be sublimated via football, but could be more robustly gratified by the spectacle of gladiators hacking each other to death. All that would be needed, apart from a good deal of money, is the permission of the morally considerable parties to these practices, bolstered by assurances that the motivations involved were not flat-out malevolent.[5] As toddlers are not, in the world ordered by the permission principle, morally considerable, and as all kinds of nonmalevolent motivations for blood sports can be offered, these activities would have to be tolerated.

The horror stems not merely from the laxity of the permission principle, but also from its stringency, coupled with the emptiness of the beneficence principle. It would always be blameworthy, Engelhardt says, to kill one innocent, unconsenting person, even if failure to do so caused the deaths of billions; indeed, it would seem implied by his position that it would never be permissible merely to *shove* an unconsenting, innocent person slightly to the left were that somehow the necessary condition required to avert mass destruction. The assessment that the supposed catastrophe were worse than inconveniencing an unconsenting, innocent person would necessarily draw upon certain rationally undemonstrable and in the present case, unshared ideas of how certain outcomes should be valued, and hence, could not confer secular moral authority.[6]

One lesson that emerges from this overview is that Engelhardt, while sincerely lamenting the poverty of its implications, is still a true fan of the methodology of modern philosophy. Not for him, for example, the tempered ambition of many contemporary mainstream moral theorists, who incline to the view that achieving coherence among our principles, our best conceptions of the world overall, and our considered moral judgments lends reasonableness, and perhaps even warrant to those judgments.[7] He will have a foundationalist system of ethics, no matter how shockingly out of step it is with deeply held and widely shared moral convictions.

The basic motivation for this deeply disturbing view is that there is simply no ranking of goods for which reasons can be given of a kind that would show anyone who rejected them to be irrational. If we attempted to shut down the baby slaughterhouses, or even nudge a recalcitrant gentleman to his left to spare the rest of creation, without such reasons at our disposal, we would be guilty of what is virtually the only thing we can know (in a publicly defensible way) to be a moral enormity: treating persons–or, more precisely, innocent persons–in ways in which they have not in some significant way consented.

In proper foundationalist fashion, Engelhardt spends much of his book displaying the implications of his view for problems in bioethics. But, learned, thoughtful, and imaginative though it be, this is not the feature of his work that will engage my interest here. I will consider Engelhardt's attempt to demonstrate that the permission principle is binding on all rational agents insofar as they would be moral.

ENGELHARDT'S TRANSCENDENTAL DEDUCTION

In the crucial second chapter of the *Foundations*, Engelhardt categorizes the possible ways in which one might provide general secular reasons for moral conclusions, and finds them all wanting. No such reasons will ever be able to show how we ought to live our lives in any detail; we cannot know on such grounds what we ought to strive for, what we should attempt to avoid, what is noble, what base, or what we are to make of our dependence on others, and theirs on us. The answers to such questions reside in specific moral traditions, whose adherents may well share the kind of commitments to a notion of the good that can both guide a life and make thinking about morality profitable. Some of the answers to be found in such communities are true (Orthodox Catholicism), some false (those of every other community insofar as they disagree with Orthodox Catholicism) and some simply incoherent (cosmopolitan yuppies, who survive off an ill-fitting, badly understood and unsupported melange of Judeo-Christian moral precepts which cannot be justified outside the metaphysical commitments of those religious views). But all are rationally indemonstrable.

It might seem bold to claim that it can be known that no effort to rationally assess, refute, reform or justify the moral understandings of the traditions or quasi-traditions in which we find ourselves could ever be successful. But Engelhardt's argument is forceful. In essence, he claims that whatever system of normative justification you favor–intuitionistic, casuistical, consequentialist, rational choice, game theoretic, natural law, or what have you–will always presuppose the very thing it is trying to justify: a particular moral understanding, in terms of which intuitions, cases, consequences, and so forth assume their moral salience. For instance, regarding intuitionism, Engelhardt generates examples which bring home both the conflict in intuitions among moral agents, and the fact that the intuitions of a given agent may underdetermine the choices she faces. How can we resolve these conflicts without relying on some notion of the good for which intuitionism cannot itself account? In considering consequentialist approaches, Engelhardt points out that theoretical options within that family of views will always bespeak some commitment to values for which the theories cannot account. Should we be hedonic or agathistic utilitarians? Average or total? What discount rate should we use in considering the impact of actions on the future? The theory seems incapable of resolving these issues without drawing on the resources of some sense of value not itself vindicated by the theory.

Engelhardt presses the same point against other standard approaches relentlessly. This is not to say that he leaves not a stone upon a stone: intuitionists, for instance, might reply that the existence of disagreement and underdetermination among agents does not by itself show that there are no intuitions generally recognized as having moral authority; implications for unclear cases might be teased out analogically, not in a way that guarantees apodictic certainty, but which yields strong presumptions for or against other courses of action and understanding. Utilitarians, for example, might choose to maximize preferences rather than pleasure, happiness, or interests, precisely in order to side-step making general normative commitments, locating these outside the theory, in individuals. But it surely isn't clear that any of these moves would be successful against Engelhardt's critique. Preferences as such may simply leave me cold; I may have epistemological views which make the prospect of relying on an intuition ridiculous. Yet however it stands with general proofs of the categorical impossibility of ever demonstrating the correctness of a

particular system of moral justification, it surely must be granted that disagreement about these matters in the present state of knowledge need not
escape the bounds of what is reasonable.

However, despite the fact that no "content-full" moral notion is generally
available, we are not, as Engelhardt sees it, reduced altogether to moral
nihilism in our dealings with those who do not share our particular view. There
remains the permission principle (his principle of beneficence is too vacuous
to do much work in this context). Even in the face of reason's failure to defend
any content-full notion of morality, we can still morally guide interchanges
among strangers in terms of what they have agreed to, and hence, at least thus
far, chain the wolf.

Engelhardt takes on a pretty stiff epistemic burden in defending this view;
there needs to be proof against the skeptical strategy he advances against the
standard accounts. One might say, for example, that he has an analogous
problem with "future discount rates" to that with which he has taxed con-
sequentialists; do my agreements bind me as stringently twenty years after they
are made as they do now? He seems to incline to the view that they do, but
there are contrary intuitions–Parfit's, for example–and the whole matter seems
to rest on very complex issues in the theory of identity over time.[8]

Other questions suggest themselves. Am I to regard all agreements, no
matter what turns out to be the consequences of keeping them, as equally
sacrosanct? Or do agreements come in different flavors, from the profound to
the trivial? Certainly, some of my authoritative agreements are tacit–Engelhardt
says as much in his analysis of the justification of adolescent children remaining under the authority of their parents.[9] Mightn't it be said that my agreement
not to engage in buying or selling luxury health care in Ontario, or to put up an
English sign over my business in Quebec, is tacitly given by my continued
residence in such places? The police power of neither government will hinder
me from leaving, after all. Why, on the other hand, should I pay any attention
to the distribution of property I encounter as I emerge into awareness of the
social conventions of my society? It affects my life in major ways, I did not
explicitly agree to it, and even if current distributions could be understood in
terms of free agreements (a dubious idea) there seems little reason to regard a
Lockean view of property as itself true beyond the possibility of a reasonable
doubt. Why should not property holdings be regarded as usufructs, for
example?[10]

Again, I think general answers to these questions emerge out of Engelhardt's text, but it is surely inviting to imagine that many of them involve a certain understanding of the value of keeping commitments that is presupposed in his version of the view, not justified by it. Or, as in the case of his views of personal identity and the analysis of property, they rest on other, eminently contestable philosophical views.

I propose, however, to refrain from examining metaphysical issues concerning how best to understand just what these persons are who make longterm agreements, or what is the limit of their decision-making authority, and try to take seriously Engelhardt's claim that the permission view does not stem from any notion that "permission"–or "persons," for that matter–have any particular moral value (as any such assignment to these notions of moral value would be contestable and indemonstrable).

Engelhardt claims that, in the free agreements of "moral strangers" we see disclosed "a transcendental condition of the possibility of a general domain of human life and of the life of persons generally...[namely, the domain composed of] speaking of blame and praise with moral strangers, and...establishing a particular set of moral commitments with an authority other than through force."[11] Although Engelhardt refers to this domain as "unavoidable,"[12] the nature of the imperative involved in taking a moral point of view seems distinctly hypothetical. He allows that the moral authority of free agreements requires a decision to collaborate. So the position actually seems to be the following: if we wish to interact with others on terms other than those of force, then we need to see our agreements with them as possessing moral authority.

I take the invocation of "moral authority" to mean something of this sort: even if it turned out subsequent to my making such an agreement that it did not serve my interests, and even if it were the case that I could fail to adhere to the agreement in a way that would make me better off (for example, circumstances in which I could depart from the agreement undetectably) I should still adhere to the agreement.

Now, why ever should I do that?

My question is not a version of the "Why should I be moral?" chestnut. What I am asking is this: what in the desiccated moral world with which Engelhardt leaves us, makes according with agreements moral, reneging, immoral?

What is there in what Engelhardt has said which would provide me with anything that I could rationally count as a moral reason–a secular, public kind of moral reason–for sticking to an agreement? One answer that springs quickly to mind is that doing so will be more likely to preserve a peaceable community than not doing so. Engelhardt, however, is very explicit that this is not *his* reason–"This view of ethics and bioethics is not grounded in a concern for peaceableness," he writes.[13] While it may be true that accordance with commitments will tend to preserve peaceable communities, one could only see that as a reason for action against a backdrop that put a positive value on such communities, and, as Engelhardt sees it, there's no secular ground for thinking that any such view is more reasonable than views that despise peaceable communities, that see divergence in moral understandings as the perfect pretext for the exercise of the heroic virtues that only conflict can nurture. Some folks may well prefer to kill the infidel, even if that means pulling the temple down on top of them, too.[14]

Another possible candidate for a reason here is that securing a reliable way of arranging terms of cooperation with others apart from force should be very attractive to any agent. I have excellent reason to believe that, whatever it is that I value, in the long run I will be more likely to obtain it if peaceable, reliable coordinated action with others is a standard feature of life. Accordingly, I act irrationally if I do that which undermines peaceable coordination. But this reason still leaves me thinking strategically rather than morally: if I am very powerful, or extremely subtle, or know I will die soon anyway, then it may well be very much an open question whether it is in my long term best interests to keep my word. The key here is my making a prudential judgment about the impact of my departure from the standing terms, and, as I am confident Engelhardt would say, what constitutes prudence here is unintelligible apart from my adherence to a rationally underdetermined sense of what is good.

The straw still floating at this point seems to be the idea that it is necessary that I regard my agreements as authoritative and keep to them (or, at least, see myself as bound by them, and recognize that I am a worthy target of censure and other blame if I renege) if I am appropriately to describe my relationships to others as moral. In other words, standing by my agreements simply is what it is to act morally (as this notion is understandable in secular contexts). This seems to me closest to what Engelhardt means in this chapter. But it also is unlikely to keep the wolf from the door, for it seems a purely stipulative use of "moral." Apart from strategic considerations, it is curious indeed why anyone advantageously positioned would see herself as having any reason to care about whether her conduct is so describable.

In sum, then, my criticism of Engelhardt is this: in relegating morality (in the secular realm) to a matter of coordinating various kinds of permission-giving and agreement-keeping among those able to give permission and make agreements, devoid of any resources for explaining what it is about the ability of persons to permit and agree that ought to command our respect (since any such account would draw on some content-full, and therefore unjustifiable, conception of the value of persons and their deeds), it seems impossible to understand how permissions and agreements, as such, count as moral reasons for action.

As this point is so central to understanding and assessing what Engelhardt is up to in the *Foundations*, and as the critical reply I here make to his position seems so natural, I want to spend some further time trying to understand how the viewpoint expressed in the permission principle could reasonably have moral authority. I'll consider two possibilities. One concerns Engelhardt's attempt to analogize his notion of the conditions for the possibility of moral discourse with conditions for the possibility of empirical enquiry. The other has to do with the possibility that those moral strangers who meet together to resolve what Engelhardt does, after all, call moral problems, all bring just the kind of understanding of what morality is at base so as to fit with unique snugness into his framework.

THE ANALOGY WITH SCIENCE

In his third chapter, Engelhardt writes, "The concrete fabric of morality must then be based on a will to a moral viewpoint....The secular moral point of view...will be that intellectual standpoint from which one understands that conflicts regarding the propriety or impropriety of a particular action can be resolved intersubjectively by mutual agreement, and which viewpoint one then embraces in order to enable an intersubjectively grounded practice of blaming and praising, of mutual respect, and of moral authority. The moral fabric sustaining the various forms of the moral life is then a general practice that is as unavoidable as is the interest in resolving moral disputes. In terms of that morality, mutual respect becomes understood as using others only with their permission."[15]

One way of understanding this passage is to see it as signaling Engelhardt's resignation of yet another of the traditional hopes of moral philosophy: providing good reasons why we should take up a moral point of view at all. The suggestion seems to be that morality depends on the will, not the intellect, on a will to a moral viewpoint that is motivated, so I suppose, by nothing other than the attractiveness of morality itself.

But invoking the autonomy of morality is not the problem. The problem is that what will is supposed to light upon in seeking a moral point of view–the binding force of agreement–is not even an intelligible candidate for that role without some further reason for thinking that agreements with persons ought, for nonstrategic reasons, be kept.

Engelhardt's talk of enabling blaming or praising and mutual respect and moral authority seems otiose. He may indeed be describing a language game in which such phrases as "you are to blame" can be appropriately used only in relation to a person's behavior with respect to other person's agreements, and in which notions of authority and respect are also defined in these terms. But there is no reason given for thinking that we should invest these phrases with anything like the salience that we do in our ordinary contexts of moral discourse. When I blame someone for breaking a promise, this makes sense because promise breaking, in the absence of very serious reasons of certain restricted kinds, expresses contempt, or at least insufficient respect, toward beings I regard as worthy of respect in virtue of their value and vulnerabilities. For Engelhardt, blaming someone for breaking an agreement seems to involve marking one's failure to respect another being who is worthy of respect solely in virtue of their being able to make agreements. While my account surely needs to be filled in, Engelhardt's seems to have nowhere to go.

Engelhardt claims that his principle of respect for permission is somehow analogous to accepting the principle of induction to ground empirical knowledge claims. I understand this claim along the following lines. Suppose someone were to say, "The sun will rise in the East tomorrow," and cite for evidence the fact that it always has done before. Imagine a skeptic replying, "Look, that it has done so before is absolutely no evidence that it will in the future. What you really need here is some metaphysical claim to the regularity of nature. But apart from special revelation from God, we know that there is no reason to believe that any such argument will ever succeed; Hume showed that. So this claim about the sun is completely unsupported." From what I can make out, Engelhardt thinks the appropriate response to the skeptic's reply should run this way: assuming the regularity of nature is simply part of what it is to make an empirical generalization, a condition of the possibility of this region of discourse, or something of that sort.

So the analogy here is supposed to be, just as making an empirical generalization presupposes induction, making a secular moral assessment presupposes
the permission principle. But the analogy limps. Whatever might be said about
the ultimate bonafides of induction, clearly a minimally coherent life presupposes some degree of regularity; we simply are not at liberty, in any
practical sense, to act as though we did not believe that the past was a guide to
the present. And, as a matter of fact, we do believe it: I see no reason to think
that acceptance of the idea that the future will resemble the past in ways we can
identify and project is not a part of common sense metaphysics. But one could
easily imagine, and even live, a life in which one's relationships with moral
strangers was not moral in any ordinary sense, nor even in the sense of granting
nonstrategic authority to agreements. One might be perfectly strategic about
the whole matter, acting in accord with one's agreements insofar as one had
self-interested reasons for doing so, and not otherwise; international relations
gives us a good view of this writ large.

We could, then, make agreements, and respect each others' extendings and
withholdings of permissions in the manner of an enlightened egoist. We might
even agree to arrange things in the world to make respecting permissions and
agreements more likely to be in one's own interest. I'd be very happy not to
call the resulting system a moral one, but it is far from being impossible. If one
gives up the necessary conditions for the very coherence of the physical world,
one has given up on sanity. If one has given up on Engelhardt's candidate for
a necessary condition for the very coherence of the (public) moral world–the
principle of permission–you've got plenty left. In addition, of course, there
seems no reason to accept that such a "moral world," erected on such a slender
and unlovely basis, has anything attractive enough about it that we should
worry about its coherence, unless it is its promise of avoiding conflict. But
that, of course, may not always matter to us. And it may not always be at issue.

THE RELATIONSHIP BETWEEN SECULAR AND CONTENT-FULL MORALITIES

Perhaps what I have regarded as unjustifiable stealing from the forbidden
territory of content-full moral views is not at all illicit on Engelhardt's view.
Perhaps what he really thinks is that our motivation to be moral stems from our
diverse repositories of moral content, and that, in coming to disagreements with
strangers with a community-based motivation to avoid conflict and do what
there are good reasons to do, or something of that sort, we come to realize on
reflection that the only features of our moral commitments that survive the

corrosive skepticism of postmodernity are those which can be expressed in the principle of permission. On this reading, I will keep my agreements with Engelhardt for roughly Kantian reasons, and he will keep his with me because God so commands, but when we meet as strangers, we leave behind both Kant and God and merely keep a sense of the moral seriousness of agreements with others.

But little seems to be gained by this move. Recall that we want secular morality to be able to lend some principled, defensible coordination to human life. For example, the state is empowered to enforce contracts, and its coercions here are supposed to be justified by reason. But on the interpretation we are now considering, the moral warrant for the coercive enforcement of agreements is not simply the permission principle as it may be understood in a secular light; it is a permission principle which is motivated by what might be called an overlapping consensus among the partisans of many content-full moralities. But ultimately, no secular reason can be given for accepting any of the content-full moralities which motivate secular allegiance to the permission principle; hence, there ultimately is no secular reason which permits coercion of those who dissent. It is, after all, false to think that everyone is going to regard agreements and permissions as morally authoritative, albeit on distinct and incommensurate grounds; some may not regard them as morally significant at all. Many others will regard them as having some kind of moral authority, but not in ways that cohere with Engelhardt's understanding of their form and force. On its own terms, then, the secular moral world as envisaged by Engelhardt acts wrongly if it acts coercively toward those who do not accept the permission principle, and it cannot be assumed that all will, or even that they should.

Try as I may, then, I cannot see how to invest the permission principle with the magic Engelhardt sees for it. Apart from some no doubt local and contestable belief that people and what they do are morally important, it is hard to grasp why their agreements matter.

APRÈS MOI, LE DELUGE?

If the permission principle, understood as a delivery of transcendental reason, lacks any kind of moral authority worth caring about, then it is vain to attempt to understand it in that fashion anymore. All it reflects, then, is a specific understanding of what is of value in human lives; hence, the permission principle slips back into the pack with all the other attempts to make sense of ourselves as moral agents. It seems to me important to acknowledge that it does so; apart from the philosophical imperative of trying to get straight about such things for their own sakes, the permission principle–at least hooked up with certain views of property acquisition with which it is often associated and which Engelhardt seems quite willing to espouse–will generally tend to justify distributions of power in private hands in their present, highly inegalitarian fashion. If this is morally justifiable, then it will have to be shown to be so in contrast with other competing, content-full notions of justice, and not handed the palm because of some claim to a unique form of rational grounding. Reason is not guiding power here; indeed, it looks much more as though we have yet another instance of power gobbling reason up.

But this returns us to Engelhardt's skepticism. Without his transcendental archimedean point, have we any way of engaging in moral discourse with those who do not share our traditions? And, to my mind, an even more disturbing question follows hard on: absent good reasons, have we any way of understanding why we ourselves should espouse our own traditions, particularly if we lack faith that their truth is guaranteed by God?

Engelhardt's concern is that all the ways that people make sense of and direct their lives involve commitment to values and to rankings of values that are widely various among individuals, communities, cultures, traditions, and so forth. All attempts to rationally justify any of these systems simply assume what is to be proved, and hence are useless, except perhaps as devices to explicate a given vision. As universal conversion to any specific tradition is not a realistic hope, and as there can be no argument proving that people should accept the aspirations and constraints of any tradition, there can be no moral authority outside the communities informed by given traditions, either. The play of power is all that we can rely upon in public space.

This strikes me as a fear that is motivated by the same hope that the Enlightenment bred: in the absence of transcendental grounds of some sort for constraints on our behavior, anything goes. A view from nowhere, or blindness. If God is dead, all is permitted. It seems to me that we needn't live on such dramatic heights. Rather, we can approach the task of making sense of, refining, and even justifying the moral understandings by which we live immanently, rather than transcendentally. We must start from where we are, elucidating what we value, relating our various commitments, striving for greater coherence among our moral, philosophical, and empirical beliefs, regarding disagreements with others, insofar as we can, as chances to increase the power and scope of our own understandings. This is, of course, an impressionistic sketch of a wide reflective equilibrium approach to moral justification.

Would this sort of a procedure, even in ideal terms, ever leave us any better off in terms of the rationality of our moral beliefs? Would it ever put us in a position where we could close the baby-abattoirs, call a halt to the gladiatorial games, or even tax citizens in service of a schedule of goods with which they may not fully agree–universal health care, for example–and not simply be ravening the slaughterhouse owners, the eager gladiators, or the dissenting citizens, Shakespeare's universal wolf striking yet again?

The project of postmodernity is to make sense of reason in the face of our confinement to the circle of this world; this is a project that faces us in science, as much as it does in ethics. If we are to understand our judgments, be they moral, empirical, or conceptual, as nonarbitrary–and it is essential to our continuing to make sense of ourselves as rational agents that we do so–we will have to understand "nonarbitrariness" immanently. This, I think, may be most difficult for thinkers such as Professor Engelhardt, who have allegiance to a very robust notion of the transcendental, and who see the postmodern condition, I suspect, as a function of the Fall. The rest of us who think that it matters deeply how we live our lives, on our own, and with others, who resist being devoured by appetite and power, may take some heart from a trenchant observation with which Derek Parfit concludes his *Reasons and Persons*: nonreligious moral philosophy is a very young study. The complaint that it has failed to provide us with decisive and evidently warranted ways of living and understanding, with an unbreakable chain for the wolf, may be as premature as an analogous complaint would have been had it been lodged against the science of the 18th Century.

NOTES

1. David Wiggins, "Truth, Invention, and the Meaning of Life," *Proceedings of the British Academy* (1976), reprinted in his *Needs, Values, Truth* (Oxford: Basil Blackwell and the Aristotelian Society, 1987), where the quote appears on p. 341. For discussion, see James Lindemann Nelson, "Desire's Desire for Moral Realism: A Phenomenological Objection to Non-Cognitivism," *Dialogue* 28 (1989): 449-460.

2. H. Tristram Engelhardt, Jr., *The Foundations of Bioethics*, 2nd ed. (Oxford and New York: Oxford University Press, 1996), 67.

3. See the discussion in *Foundations*, Chapter Two, especially p. 67ff, and Chapter Three. It may be worth noting that Engelhardt is committed to the view that acting does not include refraining. Otherwise, it would seem impossible not to act in ways that sometimes involve others without their permission.

4. As Engelhardt suggests on p. 385.

5. One could, for instance, justify consensual gladiatorial contests with reference to the "delectation" of the spectacle, and the "refined recall of the kill" with other fans of the game. See Engelhardt on hunting, *Foundations*, 141.

6. See p. 130 of *Foundations*. Engelhardt does say that it would be permissible to use deadly force against someone who was an innocent threat to my life. Is the key difference here that in the first case, I–the agent who alone could interfere with the threat–am not personally at risk of life and limb?

7. The image described is, of course, that of Rawls. For a manageable statement, see his "The Independence of Moral Theory," *Proceedings and Addresses of the American Philosophical Association* 48 (1974-75). See also Norman Daniels, "Wide Reflective Equilibrium and Theory Acceptance in Ethics," *Journal of Philosophy* 76, no. 5 (1979), and Michael R. DePaul's *Balance and Refinement* (New York and London: Routledge, 1993).

8. Derek Parfit, *Reasons and Persons* (Oxford: Oxford University Press, 1984).

9. Engelhardt, *Foundations*, 156.

10. See, for a relevant discussion, Clark Wolf, "Contemporary Property Rights, Lockean Provisos, and the Interests of Future Generations," *Ethics* 105, no. 4 (1995): 791-818.

11. Engelhardt, *Foundations*, 70.

12. Engelhardt, *Foundations*, 69.

13. Engelhardt, *Foundations*, 70.

14. Of course, such folks are choosing not to be moral in Engelhardt's terms (that is, in what he takes to be the only terms open to a secular morality), and thus opening themselves up for what he regards as the appropriate censure of rational beings from other parts of the universe, and the violent response of others. While one might well wish to avoid either response, that surely is different from seeing either as deserved. In other words, I might refrain from violating the permission principle if I feared the wrath of those I violated or the scorn of observing aliens. What seems unintelligible is refraining from living out my warrior ethic simply and solely because it violated the principle.

15. Engelhardt, *Foundations*, 104.

2

NOT ALL PEACE IS PEACE: WHY CHRISTIANS CANNOT MAKE PEACE WITH ENGELHARDT'S PEACE

STANLEY HAUERWAS

WHO WROTE THE SECOND EDITION OF *THE FOUNDATIONS OF BIOETHICS*?

I begin with a confession. Like most confessions it is difficult to make. More-over, it involves others, and in particular Tris Engelhardt, whom I am honored to call a friend. I am hesitant to cause him embarrassment, but I simply can no longer live with the deception. Tris Engelhardt is not the author of the Second Edition of *The Foundations of Bioethics*. I am the author of the Second Edition. I confess I think it was a clever idea for me to write the Second Edition and on the whole I am pleased with the execution, but I now see that the truth should prevail. I am, of course, indebted to Tris for his cooperation and I hope I have not damaged his well deserved reputation.

You may well ask, "How did you ever come up with such an outrageous idea?" Actually it is all Robert Paul Wolff's fault. He wrote a devastating review of Allan Bloom's, *The Closing of the American Mind* in which he suggested Bloom's book was actually written by Saul Bellow.[1] According to Wolff, Bellow wrote "an entire coruscatingly funny novel in the form of a pettish, bookish, grumpy, reactionary complaint against the last two decades. The 'author' of this tirade, one of Bellow's most fully realized literary crea-tions, is a mid-fiftyish professor at the University of Chicago, to whom Bellow gives the evocative name, 'Bloom.' Bellow appears in the book only as the author of an eight-page 'Foreword,' in which he introduces us to his principal and only character. *The Closing of the American Mind* is published under the name 'Allan Bloom,' and, as part of the fun, is even copyrighted in 'Bloom's' name." Wolff proceeds to show that Bellow has written this novel to make fun of the Straussians and, in particular, Strauss' strange theory of concealment.

When I read the first edition of Engelhardt's *Foundations*, I not only thought his account of what a secular bioethics entails was right but I also was impressed that others found his position persuasive. Yet when I say what Engelhardt says I am dismissed as an unreflective Christian theologian. For example, when I say there is no reason on secular grounds to prohibit suicide or even to call it suicide, I am accused of being "against the world." When I have suggested that attempts to ground secular ethics in "reason" have not been

B. P. Minogue et al. (eds.), Reading Engelhardt, 31–44.

successful I am accused of fideism. When I argue that liberal political arrangements cannot provide an account of legitimacy I am described as a "sectarian." In short when I say what Engelhardt says I am classified as an indiscriminate basher of liberalism and the Enlightenment.

So I got this great idea. Why should I not write a new edition of the *Foundations*, confessing my Christian faith, but trying to show constructively what a secular world ought to say or can say about ethics and in particular bioethics. I would not have to create a character as Wolff alleges Bellow had to do because we all know that Engelhardt is all too real. I hope I did not misuse Engelhardt's charitable spirit by assuming he would approve of my use of his name, but I saw no other way I could ever expect to get a hearing. Without such a strategy I would always be accused of wanting to make matters worse than they are in order to make Christians and the church look better than they are. So assuming Engelhardt's persona, I rewrote the *Foundations*.

Accordingly I argued that all attempts to justify a content-full secular ethic could not help but fail because any such content cannot help but beg the question of the standard by which the content is selected (41).[2] I confess I took particular pleasure in showing how Kant smuggled moral content into his attempt to ground ethics in reason alone, but it was even more fun exposing Kant's absurd views about masturbation (105-108). I could even claim that "we live in a century in which more people have been slaughtered in the cause of secular visions of justice, human dignity, ideological rectitude, historical progress, and purity than have ever been killed in religious wars" (15) and have some hope of being heard.

It was an absolute joy to write the chapters dealing with issues like abortion, death, informed consent, refusal of treatment, the distribution of health care assuming the permissive character of secular bioethics. I was able to show on purely secular grounds there was little reason to prohibit what many continue to assume are reprehensible actions and results. Then I could end each chapter with a paragraph like this:

The difficulty is that in the ruins of a collapsing Judeo-Christian moral vision it is difficult for individuals to assemble coherent moral intuitions regarding how one should approach life and death decisions. Once moral sentiments are disarticulated from the content-full moral and metaphysical framework in which they had once been embedded, they no longer can provide reliable guidance. On the one hand, in general secular terms it will appear as if there is nothing morally improper in assisting suicide or supporting voluntary euthanasia. On the other hand, since this life will appear to be all there is, it can take on an absolute significance. Previous moral concerns regarding murder and in favor of the respect of human life may be transferred to a particular content-full moral assertion regarding the importance of saving lives at all costs. However, even in secular terms, individuals may have values that outweigh their concerns to preserve their own lives. In the absence of a coherent, content-moral vision, there will be at best confusion within which the only general secular guidance will be that derivable from the consent of those involved (344).

I was not trying to make people "Christian" or even to make them appreciate Christian practices by suggesting the anomalies produced by the consistent working out of a secular ethic. Rather I wanted to remind those Christians who continue to be so enthusiastic about secular arrangements that we may be losing our soul. To suggest a secular ethic can give you no reason for having children is not to judge those who represent such an ethic, but rather to remind Christians why it is so important for us to maintain our communities in which such practices are not lost (277). Indeed I hoped in the light of "Engelhardt's" Second Edition that my suggestion that Christians must begin to think about what a Christian practice of medicine might look like would not be so easily ignored.[3] I could say more about the various strategies I employed in writing the Second Edition, but I am sure enough has been said to convince you that in fact I am the author.

WHY YOU CANNOT "CHOOSE" TO BE A CHRISTIAN

Now that I have completely convinced you that I am the author of the Second Edition of the *Foundations*, I now must say that I have been putting you on. I did not write the Second Edition. Engelhardt must be given credit for that feat and accept the praise and criticism he so richly deserves. I realize that you may be a bit put out at me for so skillfully convincing you that I wrote the Second Edition, but I did so only because I thought serious philosophical and theological issues were and are at stake. By suggesting I could have written the Second Edition, I hope to have shown why some (and perhaps most of all, Engelhardt!) may think Engelhardt's and my views similar. That is not the case, but why it is not is difficult to get clear. Having convinced you I could have written the Second Edition, I must now indicate why I could not have done so.

I begin with what I take to be the deepest difference between us, namely our understanding of Christianity. Our difference is not simply that Engelhardt is

Orthodox while I represent the more ancient tradition of Methodism. Rather our difference is quite simply I think being Christian is more like being Texan than he does. Let me explain by quoting from the Preface to the Second Edition a paragraph I think is destined to become one of the most famous in contemporary philosophical literature.

> If one wants more than secular reason can disclose and one should want more, then one should join a religion and be careful to choose the right one. Canonical moral content will not be found outside of a particular moral narrative, a view from somewhere. Here the reader deserves to know that I indeed experience and acknowledge the immense cleft between what secular philosophical reasoning can provide and what I know in the fullness of my own narrative to be true. I indeed affirm the canonical, concrete moral narrative, but really it cannot be given by reason, only by grace. I am, after all, a born-again Texan Orthodox Catholic, a convert by choice and conviction, through grace and repentance for sins innumerable (including a first edition upon which much improvement was needed). My moral perspective does not lack content. I am of the firm conviction that, save for God's mercy, those who willfully engage in much that a peaceable, fully secular state will permit (e.g., euthanasia and direct abortion on demand) stand in danger of hell's eternal fires. As a Texan, I puzzle whether these are kindled with mesquite, live oak, or trash cedar, but this is a question to be answered on the Last Day by the Almighty. Though I acknowledge that there is no secular moral authority that can be justified in general secular terms to forbid the sale of heroin, the availability of direct abortion, the marketing of for-profit euthanatization services, or the provision of commercial surrogacy, I firmly hold none of these to be good. These are great moral evils. But their evil cannot be grasped in purely secular terms. To be pro-choice in general secular terms is to understand God's tragic relationship to Eden. To be free is to be free to choose very wrongly (XI).

I hesitate to assert the superiority of theology to philosophy, but I must begin by noting that there are some things theologians know that philosophers cannot know. Any theologian would know that God stokes the fires of hell with trash cedar. God would never use the beauty of a live oak tree or the determination of the mesquite to fire hell. Moreover, there is the further question of the place of fire in hell since I prefer to believe that Dante is right to think ice, not fire, insures the absolute loneliness that makes hell a loneliness that, I might add, looks very much like Engelhardt's society of strangers. But these are not matters he should be expected to know.

The problem is quite simply in his language. Listen again, "one should join a religion and be careful to choose the right one." The issue involves the presumptions, peculiar to a liberal culture, that shape the language of "choice." Of course from a secular point of view one may describe someone becoming a Christian or a Unificationist as a matter of choice, but that is not how those becoming Christian are taught to understand what is or has happened to them. To be baptized in Christ's death and resurrection is to be made part of a people, part of God's life, rendering the language of choice facile.

Notice that Engelhardt did not use the language of "choice" to characterize what it means for him to be a Texan. He knows such language is surely a distortion of the great and good reality that comes from finding one's life constituted by such a land and people. Along with me, Engelhardt never knew a time when he did not know how to "talk right." Of course being born amid the riches of being Texan does not mean that one can take such a gift for granted. We must learn the skills necessary to make what we are ours, but such skills are only intelligible because we know being Texan comes first as gift not choice.

I am aware I may be making far too much of Engelhardt's language of choice. He does say that "only by grace" is he a "born-again Texan Orthodox Catholic." Yet the issue does not turn finally on the choice of words, though what words we use is all important, but rather on the narratives and the material conditions that such narratives presume. My worry about Engelhardt's Second Edition is that the narrative that shapes the position of the Second Edition is insufficiently determined by his Christian convictions. It is so because his account of Christianity remains far too "voluntary." As a result Christians are robbed of the resources we need to resist the subtle temptations of Engelhardt's "peaceable society," a society I believe designed to render the Christian worship of God puerile.

Engelhardt, good Christian that he is, certainly does not desire that result. He explicitly claims that the "libertarian character of a defensible general secular morality is not antagonistic to the moralities of concrete moral communities whose peaceable commitments may be far from libertarian (e.g., the communism of monasteries). The arguments in *The Foundations of Bioethics* are not opposed to such sentiments within particular, peaceable, moral communities. Strictly, with respect to such sentiments, the arguments are neutral" (X). In the next section I will explore whether Engelhardt's "peaceable society," built as it is on the ruins of the Enlightenment project, is really so benign, but first I need to develop what I find problematic about his understanding of Christianity and its relation to the kind of society he depicts.

When I was asked to blurb the First Edition of the *Foundations*, I said "as a Christian theologian, I welcome Engelhardt's profound account of what a secular ethic in medicine should entail. It will show Christians why good pagans have seen the church as a threat to the peace of polytheistic and secular societies, while those who take a 'secular point of view' will find its full implications explored in the book."[4] Actually that is not what I first sent to the publisher. My first blurb had said, "If you want to know why the pagans rightly thought they should kill the Christians, read this book." The publishers thought that was a little too direct.

I think, however, the point is still valid and the changes in the Second Edition have not made me change my mind. Pagans understood (as Engelhardt well understands) that the great problem with Christians is we have no use for tolerance. We are not going to validate a public polytheism even if it buys us a peace which is just another way of saying we are not being physically killed at the moment. The God we worship as Christians wants it all. "Render unto God the things that are God's and unto Caesar the things that are Caesar's" is not what Caesar wants to hear. Caesar also wants it all, particularly, when Caesar has become "democratic."

For example, Engelhardt says that the position put forth in the *Foundations* requires the "privatization" of all particularistic convictions (VIII). Accordingly the moral life must be lived in two dimensions: (1) that of a secular ethic that strives to be content-less and thus is able to span numerous moral communities and (2) the particular moral community within which one can achieve a content-full understanding of the good life (78). Lutherans have long had a theology to underwrite such a division, but neither Engelhardt nor I am persuaded by the Lutheran distinction between orders of creation and redemption, between law and gospel. Given the results of this century, moreover, most Christians find such a distinction questionable since we now know the horror which it proved powerless to resist.

The issue is not the misuse of such a distinction, but rather the distortion of Christian convictions implicit in it. When Christians allow their faith to be privatized, we discover we can no longer maintain the disciplines necessary to sustain the church as a disciplined polity capable of calling into question "the public." Of course Engelhardt can respond that is not his problem since such a result is not entailed by his religious convictions. I think, however, that he cannot avoid the issue so easily as can be seen from the language of "choice" I highlighted above. The great challenge before Christians in Engelhardt's world, and I believe it is in fact the world in which we exist, is how our lives as Christians can be as involuntarily constituted as being Texan. To be Christian means we must be embedded in practices so materially constitutive of our communities that we are not tempted to describe our lives in the language offered by the world, that is, the language of choice. Only then will Christians be able to challenge an all too tolerant world that celebrates many gods as alternatives to the One alone who alone is worthy of worship.

Note that my concern is not to try to reconstitute Christendom or advocate Christian "rule" in late Enlightenment societies like the one called America. Rather the issue is service to our non-Christian brother and sister. If, for example, we believe abortion is sin that injures not only child and mother but our very ability to be parents then we must find ways to help one another, Christian and non-Christian alike, not to be subject to the terror of that alternative. What alternatives to abortion might look like will differ from context to context, but Christians surely cannot promise those committed to a peaceable society that our alternative will appear "peaceable" because such views are allegedly only our private opinion.

For example, we owe it to our non-Christian sister and brother to try to help them live lives that are as life giving as that which God has made possible for us to live. Excluding violent alternatives from the common life of a society is not a bad thing. I certainly wish for the Pentagon not to exist. I work for it not to exist. Of course that work must always be a witness that we hope others will find compelling, but I certainly do not assume that such witness might not take publically defensible forms that make, for example, military funding more difficult. From my perspective you cannot put enough bureaucratic controls on military spending to insure "we the people" are not ripped off.

Of course Engelhardt may respond that the kind of peaceable society he thinks necessary is one that will allow just the kind of witness I want Christians to make. I doubt that, but to show why I will need to look more closely at Engelhardt's peace. Before I do so, however, I want at least to mention one issue that I suspect lies at the bottom of some of my deepest disease with Engelhardt. Engelhardt assumes that witness is what you need when your position cannot be "rationally" defended, but I assume that witness is one of the most determinative forms of rationality.

At several points Engelhardt observes that Roman Catholicism made the mistake of trying to provide rational grounds for being Catholic. He suggests that prior to the Reformation the Christian West envisaged a single authoritative point of view available not only through grace, but also rational argument (68). According to Engelhardt as a result Western Christianity, and in particular Catholicism, undermined its own roots by trying to establish by reason what only faith can show (94).[5] I am not unsympathetic with Engelhardt's argument at this point. I have argued in a somewhat similar fashion that attempts to base Christian morality on some kinds of natural law theory can lead to violence.[6]

Yet I think Engelhardt owes us a fuller account of reason than he has supplied if we are to understand his position as well as knowing what might be wrong with it. To suggest that it is a mistake to base faith on reason depends on what you mean by reason. Certainly Aquinas did not think knowing God as Trinity was of the same status as knowing God exists, but neither did he think that belief in the Trinity lacked rational warrant. Aquinas assumed that theology was faith seeking understanding, but faith did not name the necessity of an irrational starting point. Rather, faith is that which is established by the most trustworthy witnesses.

In *Bioethics and Secular Humanism* Engelhardt suggests a "rational perspective is that which can be defended on the basis of general principles. If one rejects a rational perspective for the resolution of controversies, one can still appeal to force, prayer, inducements, and seduction. But one will not be able to explain why any of these alternative approaches is correct without giving reasons on its behalf."[7] Christians believe we can give "reasons on behalf" of that which we believe that should not only be persuasive, but understood as true. To be sure such "reason giving" is a complex activity requiring the transformation of our lives through location in the Christian tradition, but as MacIntyre has helped us see any account of rationality cannot be otherwise.[8] I am aware that Engelhardt may well disagree with MacIntyre at this point, but at least I think it is clear that he owes us a more developed account of rationality.

THE VIOLENCE OF ENGELHARDT'S PEACE

I am a pacifist, so it is hard for me to be against peace. Yet not all peace is peace and, in particular, it is not the peace of Christ. I am not at all convinced that the peaceable society Engelhardt desires exists, can exist, or if it did exist, would be peaceable. What I fear Engelhardt gives us is not peace, but order. He observes that "until a general conversion to the Faith or to a particular ideology, or to a generally imposed orthodoxy, one will need to search for common grounds to bind rational peaceable individuals and to direct health care decisions"[9] (35). One of the goals of ethics is to find a way to avoid the use of force for resolving moral controversies, or when that is not possible, to determine when and how to limit the use of force (67).

Engelhardt wisely, I think, no longer calls the fundamental principle necessary for such a project the "principle of autonomy," but rather the "principle of permission" (XI). This change rightly indicates that the "peaceable society" Engelhardt desires can only "be derived from the concurrence of individuals. Because the only morally authorized social structures under such circumstances are those established with the permission of the individuals involved, the majority that binds moral strangers has by default an unavoidable libertarian character. However, this is not out of any value attributed to freedom or individual choice. The plausible scope of societal moral authority is limited because of plausible limits of the consent to be governed by others" (X).

I admire what I can only describe as the monkish intellectual austerity that governs Engelhardt's development of the contours of his peaceable society. I have my doubts whether he can in fact show that the principle of permission is the "core" of the morality of mutual respect (117) because such an account seems too close to Kant for someone who has disavowed the Kantian deduction. That is not, however, my worry about Engelhardt's understanding of the peaceable society. Rather my concern is Engelhardt's presumption that his peace is in fact institutionalized through democracy. I challenge Engelhardt's claim that the principle of permission provides only an "empty process" for generating moral authority for sustaining a minimum ethic of praise and blame (109).

Engelhardt claims that liberal democracies are "morally neutral by default. They cannot acquire the authorization to establish a particular moral vision, religion, or ideology. After all, given the failure of reason to discover the rational, canonical, content-full moral vision, establishing a morality or ideology as a government's concrete morality or moral vision has no more secular moral plausibility or authority than would the establishment of a particular religion. Limited democracies are therefore morally committed to not being committed to a particular vision of the good; they are committed rather to being the social structure through which, and with the protection of which, individuals and communities can pursue their own and divergent visions of the good" (120). All I ask of Engelhardt is to name just one such "social structure" that actually exemplifies his "neutral public square." When it comes to government nature abhors a vacuum and if the secular square is alleged to be empty you can be sure that is an ideology for a quite particular set of interests.

Engelhardt may mean for his peaceable society to be a thought experiment, a utopian creation to enrich our imaginations. I would certainly not want to disparage the importance of utopian schemes, but I do not think that is what Engelhardt is about. He seems to believe that the liberal democracies of the West approximate his libertarian ideal. If they do, however, they are anything but benign. More importantly, even as a thought experiment Engelhardt's "peace" remains far too coercive.

Engelhardt has read Foucault, but has chosen to ignore Foucault's understanding of power. The supervisory strategies necessary to sustain Engelhardt's peace are simply coercion called freedom. For example, people whom we call tribal cannot help but find the necessity of being an individual in order to be part of Engelhardt's peaceable arrangements but a form of violence. Tolerance, which Engelhardt identifies as the primary cardinal virtue of the morality of mutual respect, cannot help but kill (419). People are, of course, quite literally killed in the name of tolerance, but it is equally the case that tolerance kills the soul.

It is to Engelhardt's credit that he understands that his peaceable society must produce character types whose virtue is their moral vacuity.[10] Yuppies become the prophetic vanguard of the "coming worldwide secularity in public policy," because they see themselves as bound to no parochial, history-bound tradition, belonging as they do to no one or no place. That Engelhardt, at least the Engelhardt that supports his peaceable society, should find such people desirable should not be surprising. They are, after all, exactly the kind of people he needs to supply the bureaucracies that control the lives of those who continue to persist in more determinative ways of life.

I cannot help but think Engelhardt's world, like other liberal accounts of social cooperation, can only be imagined because he continues to presume continuing Christian habits and institutions. For example I simply do not see how he can account for why some people will think they ought to care about other people simply because they fall ill. Why should those that constitute Engelhardt's peaceable society, who moreover embody the virtues of that society, think it important to set aside some people to do nothing with their lives other than to be present to and care for the sick? He says that his social world can only supply "a general abstract understanding of what it means to be a physician or nurse" (294). Any more determinative conception must come from within a particular community of physicians and nurses. Yet why would the latter understand themselves to be in the same practice as the former. Indeed given his own analysis of the variability of what "ill," "health," and "disease" can mean, there is no reason to assume they would even be acting in the same world of illness or health.[11]

Engelhardt suggests that physicians are "often cast into a role analogous to those of bureaucrats in a large-scale nation. They must come to terms with the moral commitments and views of individuals from various moral communities while preserving the moral fabric of a peaceable, secular, pluralistic society. It is for this reason that Hegel identified civil servants as the universal class (in contrast to this, Marx assigned the role of the workers.) Civil servants are committed to the general realization of freedom in the nation according to Hegel... Letter carriers must deliver mail to all on their routes and not discriminate against some on the grounds of their political commitments... To ensure this takes place, one may need bureaucratic rules that clearly establish in general what will be done, for whom, and under what circumstances. Physicians and other health care professionals are often in the position of civil servants, in that they must make clear to patients what will be done for them, to them, and under what circumstances" (298-299). Accordingly patients and physicians who meet one another as strangers will need to know what safeguards are present to protect the patient as well as what services the physician is committed to providing.

Engelhardt's yuppies may well become such civil servants, but I see no reasons why Christians would imitate them in doing so. Even more important I do not think Christians as patients could or should trust their lives to such civil servants. Indeed what seems missing from Engelhardt's account of the kind of medicine possible in his peaceable society is how to account for trust. His whole project seems to be an attempt to substitute exchange for trust while still trusting that some people will continue the habits of trust. I see no reason to believe that trust, and in particular the kind of trust that has made medicine as we have known it medicine, will continue in a world of exchanges.

The language of exchange, moreover, introduces the most profound violence I think presupposed in Engelhardt's peaceable society. Engelhardt is way ahead of the game insofar as he knows that ethics, and in particular bioethics, cannot be separated from politics, or perhaps more accurately put, is a politics. But missing from his account of the peaceable society, missing from his account of democracy, is economics. Such an omission, moreover, is not innocent if you believe, as I do, that nothing is more violent than the capitalist market.[12] But it is exactly such a market that Engelhardt seems to presuppose as central to his peaceable society. I am, of course, aware that such a market dominates all our lives. What is important for those of us who are Christians, however, is not to call good the fact that we currently feel we have no alternative to that market.

O.K., IF YOU ARE SO SMART, WHAT ALTERNATIVE DO YOU HAVE?

I realize that the kind of criticism I have made of Engelhardt's account of the peaceable society cannot help but appear unfair. It seems unfair because with the best will in the world Engelhardt is striving to help us find an alternative to what he fears is the coming violence. If you do not like his alternative it seems you must be expected to at least provide an alternative of your own. Yet I do not have an alternative to offer to Engelhardt's peace. At least I do not have an alternative to offer at the theoretical level of Engelhardt's proposal.

Our task, as Christians, is not to offer such theoretical alternatives, but rather to be an alternative. Christians provided such an alternative when they thought it was a good thing to provide houses of hospitality for people who would have otherwise died alone. Christians provided such alternatives when they did not kill their children who were born deformed. Christians provided such alternatives when as patients they exemplified the virtue of patience by not asking physicians to do more than they could or should. Without such fundamental practices, practices that those who are not Christian can imitate, theoretical constructions of Engelhardt like peaceable societies can too easily give Christians the presumption we know more than we do and even worse we can do more than we can.

I fear we Christians must be content to live out our lives in the world as we find it. It is a world, I fear, that descriptively resembles Engelhardt's peaceable society. Our task as Christians is not to make such a world more terrible than it has a tendency to be, but to survive in such a world. Which is finally why, as much as I would have found it an attractive possibility, I could not write the Second Edition of *The Foundations of Bioethics*.

NOTES

1. Wolff's review appeared in the *New Republic*.

2. H. Tristram Engelhardt, Jr., *The Foundations of Bioethics*, 2nd ed. (Oxford and New York: Oxford University Press, 1996). All references will appear in the text.

3. That is, of course, one of the purposes of my *Suffering Presence* (Notre Dame: University of Notre Dame Press, 1986).

4. Engelhardt rightly observes that the failure of the modern moral philosophical project "returns us to the polytheism and skepticism of ancient times with a remembrance of the philosophical monotheism and Faith that fashioned the West" (11). Secular people too often assume that once Christianity is rendered irrelevant, the world will be free of the gods. The truth is exactly the reverse as we see in our own time the defeat of Christianity becomes the time for the rebirth of the gods. The problem with the secular is it is so hard to keep it secular.

5. Engelhardt footnotes Michael Buckley's *At the Origins of Modern Atheism* in support of this point. I am not sure Buckley's argument is the same as Engelhardt's. It was not Aquinas who produced the rationalism that in turn gave us modern atheism, but later Scholastic developments. Everything depends on what you take reason to be.

6. Stanley Hauerwas, *The Peaceable Kingdom* (Notre Dame: University of Notre Dame Press, 1988), 50-71.

7. H. Tristram Engelhardt, Jr., *Bioethics and Secular Humanism: The Search for a Common Morality* (Philadelphia: Trinity Press International, 1991), 16.

8. MacIntyre has developed this account most fully in his *Whose Justice? Which Rationality?* (Notre Dame: University of Notre Dame Press, 1988) and *Three Rival Versions of Moral Enquiry: Encyclopedia, Genealogy, and Tradition* (Notre Dame: University of Notre Dame Press, 1990). Crucial to understanding MacIntyre's position is his claim in *Whose Justice? Which Rationality?* that the "concept of tradition-constituted and tradition-constitutive rational enquiry cannot be elucidated apart from its exemplifications" (p. 10). Too often criticisms of MacIntyre try to separate his account of rationality from the story he tells, but the whole force of his position is to deny such a distinction can be made. "Tradition" does not name a new epistemological option to that of the encyclopedist and the genealogist, but rather is an attempt to show why you cannot begin with epistemology for an account of rationality. In other words MacIntyre is developing philosophically the theological claim of what faith seeking understanding looks like.

9. Who is this "one" that takes up this project? Is it a Christian? One of the troubling aspects of Engelhardt's position is its historical abstractness.

10. Engelhardt, *Bioethics and Secular Humanism*, 35-40.

11. Engelhardt observes that "a traditional Roman Catholic community is likely to have under-standings of health, disease, disorder, deviance, and disability quite different from those of a community of secularized cosmopolitans. Their different constructions of medical reality can then be embedded in alternative health care systems, which carry with them quite different understandings of what should count as a disease to be treated and of what treatment expenses should be sustained by the community" (227). What Engelhardt needs to justify is why given his account he thinks he can still speak of "medical reality" and "health care systems" as if they are simply "there."

12. See, for example, Alasdair MacIntyre's, *Marxism and Christianity*, Second Edition (London: Duckworth, 1995) and in particular the new Introduction. MacIntyre observes that in premodern societies markets were auxiliary to production, but in "the markets of modern capitalism prices are often imposed by factors external to a particular market: those, for example, whose livelihood has been made subject to international market forces by their becoming exclusively producers for some product for which there was, but is not longer, international demand, will find themselves compelled to accept imposed low prices or even the bankruptcy of their economy. Market relationships in contemporary capitalism are for the most part relations imposed both on labor and on small producers, rather than in any sense freely chosen" (XII).

3

MEDICINE'S MONOPOLY: FROM TRUST-BUSTING TO TRUST

E. HAAVI MORREIM

In his revised *Foundations of Bioethics*, Engelhardt has provided a rich and far-reaching account, not just of the moral foundations of bioethics, but of their implications in a wide array of areas. From issues of birth, life, and death, to defining the concept of disease, to patients' prerogatives in choosing and refusing their health care, to the shape and future of the nation's health care system, Engelhardt offers a coherent picture of the ways in which particular controversies should be addressed. Even the most comprehensive account, however, cannot discuss every issue. This chapter takes up a significant challenge in the changing economics of health care, one whose resolution has already begun but whose future directions need careful consideration. The chapter is not a critique, but rather an extrapolation of the ways in which Engelhardt would probably regard this issue.

The discussion begins with a major but relatively unnoticed transformation that is taking place in American health care. It is spurred largely by economic changes, but has implications ranging far further. For many years, the medical profession has exercised a virtual monopoly over the training, tools, and even concepts of illness and healing, primarily through laws of licensure and prescription, and a nearly unilateral economic control over volumes, kinds, and prices of services. Although it has helped to promote great progress in medical science and health care, such a monopoly has also had its disadvantages. It has diminished citizens' access to alternative healing approaches and, reciprocally, it has also increasingly served to box physicians into awkward conflicts of personal and professional integrity as they find themselves caught between patients' demands for the tools they control and societal values that restrict the use of those tools. And it has fostered a level of economic extravagance that can not be sustained indefinitely.

However, the situation is now changing. As those who pay the costs of care reconsider what they will buy and how much they will pay, the medical profession's influence over consumers' options for treatment of their maladies is weakening rapidly. Physicians are becoming just one–even if still first–of many who now have power over how illness is defined, diagnosed, and treated. These changes open up a new pluralism that may enhance freedom and health care for everyone. It is a shift of which Engelhardt can approve. At the same

B. P. Minogue et al. (eds.), Reading Engelhardt, 45–75.

time, this economically prompted "trust-busting" is raising profound questions of trust throughout health care.

MEDICAL AND ECONOMIC MONOPOLY

Under United States law, physicians have exercised an almost unilateral power to define what disease is, to ascribe it to individuals, to determine what therapeutic interventions will be provided for whom, and even to determine how much money will be spent in the process. Of relatively recent vintage, this control has arisen from science, law, and economics.[1] Though medicine does not claim to be the only approach to healing illness, it does claim to be the one founded on empirical science while other approaches, such as acupuncture or Christian Science, are generally based on metaphysical or religious frameworks. Therefore, to the extent that people want scientifically warranted methods to diagnose and treat their ailments, medicine will naturally enjoy priority. Since this demand has been substantial in twentieth century Western society, medicine has earned a significant measure of its dominance by high-quality performance, bringing steadily expanding scientific understanding and technologies, and finely honed skills to the cure and care of human maladies.[2]

Dominance has been enhanced by legal and economic arrangements, as highlighted in the following list.

Licensure and control of education, accreditation, entry, and discipline. Physicians' legal authority is largely seated in laws of licensure that give the medical profession the exclusive right to define, diagnose, and treat disease and, beyond this, to determine who may enter the profession, how they will become qualified, and under what conditions they may be forced to leave.[3] Indiana's medical practice act is fairly typical as it broadly defines the practice of medicine:

(1) Holding oneself out to the public as being engaged in the diagnosis, treatment, correction or prevention of any disease, ailment, defect, injury, infirmity, deformity, pain or other condition of human beings, or the suggestion, recommendation or prescription of administration of any form of treatment, without limitation, or the performing of any kind of surgical operation upon a human being, including tattooing, or the penetration of the skin or body orifice by any means, for the intended palliation, relief, cure or prevention of any physical, mental or functional ailment or defect of any person; (2) The maintenance of an office or place of business for the reception, examination or treatment of persons suffering from disease, ailment, defect, injury, infirmity, deformity, pain or other conditions of body or mind.[4]

Only those licensed to practice medicine are permitted to engage in these activities, and only those who complete accredited courses of medical education and certification can be awarded licenses. The medical profession controls both this accreditation process and also the various state medical practice boards that grant and revoke licenses.

Power of prescription. In the past few decades medicine has developed powerful tools that are likewise under exclusive control of physicians. With the exception of relatively low-risk over-the-counter remedies, only a physician's prescription can grant citizens access to medical drugs and devices. Similarly, the entry of new agents into the realm of accepted prescription remedies is significantly influenced by physicians on the federal Food and Drug Administration boards that give or withhold approval for testing and marketing of new drugs and devices.

Control of allied professions. Though physicians do not literally provide all science-based means of diagnosis and healing, most ancillary providers' functions are defined in terms of their relationship to physicians, and many remain under direct medical control and supervision. Thus, "[m]ost state licensure laws proceed by creating an exclusive province for physicians and then carving out narrow enclaves within that province for various other licensed occupations."[5]

Practice acts governing nurses and physicians' assistants exemplify. The Missouri nursing practice act permits nurses to engage in the "assessment, nursing diagnosis, nursing care, and counsel of persons who are ill, injured or experiencing alterations in normal health processes,"[6] and permits nurses to administer treatments prescribed by physicians, to educate patients about health matters, and the like.[7] It is interesting to note that, in a number of instances, once a state practice act has stated that physicians alone are permitted to diagnose disease, nurses are then permitted to engage in "nursing diagnosis"–without defining the difference.

Physicians' assistants are more dependent, permitted to practice only under the direct supervision of a physician,[8] while other kinds of providers, such as physical therapists, may be accorded considerably more independence.[9] Laws vary from state to state. Nonallopathic providers such as chiropractors are governed by their own statutes, and historically the medical profession's efforts to suppress them have sometimes been forceful.[10]

Power over payment. In most cases a physician's order is necessary for patients to receive third-party coverage for medical expenses, since most insurers and managed care organizations insist that they will cover only "medically necessary" services, not over-the-counter or folk remedies. For many years those orders also were almost always sufficient to assure payment. Insurers did engage in limited retrospective review, mainly to ensure that claims fit within their general rules for reimbursement–payments for home health care, for instance–would not be made if the policy did not cover them. But rarely did insurers deny payment for physician-ordered products or services.

Physicians and other major providers such as hospitals were also able to determine how much, not just when and for what, they were paid. Thanks in large measure to retrospective, fee-for-service payment based on "usual, customary and reasonable" charges, these providers enjoyed a cost-plus pass-through system in which they determined how much they would be paid for whatever care they chose to provide.[11] This payment system was significantly reinforced in the mid-1960s with the adoption of Medicare and Medicaid. On some observers' view, it is no accident that the costs of health care rose dramatically thereafter.[12]

Additionally, physicians largely set the tone for rapid addition of new technologies. Several factors contributed: physicians' professional commitment to bring their patients the latest and best tools of treatment; their personal concerns about tort litigation, inclining them to practice defensive medicine; payers' willingness to cover all medically necessary care, as determined by physicians.[13] As a result, "medical need" came to be defined as virtually anything that is technically feasible and might possibly benefit the patient without causing undue harm, regardless of cost.[14] New technologies were quickly adopted and paid for as standard care, thereby encouraging manufacturers to develop still greater technological feats of diagnosis and treatment.

Control over the structure of health care delivery. Until recently, organized medicine was powerful enough even to restrict the systems by which health care is delivered. The growth of prepaid health plans was significantly impeded, for instance, by the profession's ethical proscription on salaried practice. That prohibition was principally supported by the argument that physicians who are employees of lay organizations will have dual allegiances, generating potential conflicts between obligations to patients and those to their employers, thereby commercializing the profession in unhealthy ways.[15] The profession's exclusion of these plans began to erode with a 1943 antitrust suit in which the American Medical Association (AMA) was held to have engaged in unlawful boycott and restraint of trade by forbidding member physicians from becoming employees of, or even from professionally associating with, physicians in a Washington, D.C. prepaid plan.[16] Not until the 1970s, however, did federal legislation open the door to widespread growth of health maintenance organizations (HMOs) and other alternative delivery systems.

A major obstacle to that change was a restriction on delivery systems, one that persists in many states: laws banning the corporate practice of medicine. As the rationale goes, only physicians with the requisite knowledge can actually practice medicine–not hospitals, insurers, HMOs, or any other entity under lay control. Lay ownership of physician services allegedly would cause poorer quality of care, a commercial exploitation of medical practice, and a split of the physician's loyalty between patients and employers.[17] These laws are now undergoing significant change, to be discussed below. Still, those that remain impede the formation of alternative delivery systems such as hospital-owned integrated delivery networks.

Authority over the legal standard of care. Physicians also define medical standards for legal purposes. In tort litigation, the duty of care a physician owes a patient is determined mainly according to customary practice–what reasonable physicians generally do under the same or similar circumstances, with some room for exceptions such as reputable minorities. In this way physicians, unlike virtually any other profession, tell the courts what the law should expect of them.[18]

Physicians also have primary authority over other legal matters. They are legally empowered to declare death, and their testimony is often decisive in other contexts, such as courts' determinations about whether someone should be civilly committed as a danger to himself or others, whether someone is competent to govern his own affairs, and so forth.

In sum, the twentieth century medical profession has enjoyed a remarkable degree of autonomy not just over its own services, but over the broad span of legal and financial arrangements that govern health care. The arguments supporting such control are familiar. Medicine involves such esoteric knowledge and skills that ordinary lay people are not equipped to determine their own needs, provide their own care, or appraise the quality of practitioners or their services. Patients may also be too ill to shop around, and so they need to be assured that they will receive at least a basic quality of service from any member of the profession.[19] Reciprocally, medicine and other professions have suggested that if they are not permitted special exemptions from competition, their dedication to service could become tarnished.[20] Because the necessary conditions for a free market can not be met in this very special area,[21] they propose that we leave the regulation to those who know what they are doing.[22]

These arguments should not be dismissed. Patients are indeed vulnerable in matters of health and health care, not only because illness can impair one's usual level of competence, but also because there is an unavoidable disparity of knowledge and power between those who are ill and those who provide these complex forms of care. There is much opportunity for harm by those who do not know what they are doing. Furthermore, the medical and allied professions, unlike some other purveyors of healing, have avowed an ethic of service that places patients' interests paramount, even above their own welfare. And in matters as complex as scientific medicine, there is room to doubt seriously whether anyone lacking the relevant training can appraise the quality of providers and services. These important arguments on behalf of shielding health care from traditional market structures will warrant further discussion below. Nevertheless, medicine's monopoly has also spawned some important problems.

PROBLEMS WITH MEDICINE'S MONOPOLY

Medicine's monopoly has come under increasing scrutiny. Critics argue, for instance, that the actual procedures and tests governing entry to the profession have remarkably little documented correlation with clinical proficiency; at the other end, disciplinary procedures for removing incompetent, unethical, or impaired physicians are alleged to be inadequate, sometimes geared more to protecting colleagues and suppressing competitors than to ensuring quality within the profession.[23] Beyond this, the medical profession's considerable power to limit the number of available physicians is said to have caused scarcities and maldistribution of service, as seen in the relative scarcity of physicians in rural and inner-city areas. In some cases these scarcities drive consumers toward injurious self-help and charlatans. Physicians' power to limit the kinds of services that allied and alternative providers can offer has arguably raised the costs of care, for instance by requiring patients to pay a physician in order to gain access to a nurse practitioner or physical therapist or psychologist.[24] And it may likewise have impeded the development and usage of less costly, perhaps even more effective, kinds of services, providers, and health care systems.[25]

While these criticisms are important,[26] the problems go deeper. Medicine's monopoly has significantly limited the concepts of illness and healing available to understand the maladies of humankind. Perhaps even more important, it has intruded on the values and freedom of patients and physicians alike.

Concepts. Medicine takes great and legitimate pride in its scientific foundation, the tools and skills of which have brought longer and better living to millions of people. And yet the scientific approach has limits. First, it inherently excludes concepts that are not subject to measurement and quantification. Metaphysical or spiritual concepts, as where disease is seen as the product of separation from God, cannot be encompassed.

Second, medical science excludes or minimizes dimensions of illness that are difficult to quantify, even when recognized to be important. Many features of quality of life are notoriously difficult to quantify, for example, and when they cannot be conveniently measured or connected with a fairly clearcut constellation of signs and symptoms, they are more likely to be ignored.[27]

More generally, scientific medicine systematically minimizes the role of human emotion and interpersonal relationships as a part of healing. And not by accident. It is well known that the placebo effect–a phenomenon reflecting the biological power of human relationships, emotions, and expectations–can alter the results of research undertaken to test a particular drug, device, or procedure. Accordingly, some of the best scientific research favors the randomized, double-blind, controlled trial, which is explicitly designed to exclude the placebo effect from interfering with the accuracy of results. In other words, medical research expressly excludes this powerful effect from its research in order to ensure that research looks just at the drug, device, or procedure, and not at the "noise" created by researchers' or patients' hopes and expectations. At the same time, however, there is rather little study of the placebo effect itself: what it is, how it works, and how best to elicit the healing powers of the human mind. The result is ironic: though excluded from research trials because it is so powerful, the placebo effect is not ordinarily used as an explicit or systematic tool of healing, because it is so difficult to study scientifically.[28] And so physicians tend to ignore, downplay, or relegate it to "the art of medicine"–since, after all, "we have no data on that." Placebo thereby assumes a dubious role in ordinary medical practice, mainly construed as the ethical dilemma of whether to deceive patients with a "nothing"-pill in order to quell their demands for inappropriate medications or to deflect them from treatments that might do harm.[29]

Third, scientific study in medicine has historically been confined to a rather limited array of topics, leaving much of medical practice unsupported by the careful research that is ostensibly the hallmark of medicine. Again, not by accident. Science is expensive. Although the federal government funds some research, much of it has been undertaken by manufacturers of drugs and devices hoping that their new products will be successful in the marketplace. So long as health care reimbursement was generous, there was little reason to spend precious science funds on ways to save money or enhance efficiency.[30] And so long as most scientific research therefore focused on the costliest and newest products, medicine as a scientific discipline naturally came to emphasize expensive new drugs and devices. If there is no research to show that an older generic drug is just as effective as the new drug, and if the latest drugs and devices will be readily reimbursed by payers, then physicians have naturally felt compelled to use it. Medicine became the science of the expensive. As a further result of this dearth of research into ordinary remedies for ordinary problems, physicians' routine clinical practices show wide variations that cannot be supported by objective factors such as differences in the patients or their illnesses, leaving many medical routines more a product of fashion and ideology than of empirical research.[31]

Freedom and values: restrictions on patients. Medicine's authority over diagnosis and treatment has created powerful restrictions on the freedom of patients and even, as discussed in the next section, of physicians.

Patients' diminished freedom is seen most immediately in the restrictions on availability of alternative kinds of treatment. Despite the recognized inability of science to capture every important dimension of human illness and healing, and despite the lack of funding to support research into all the areas suitable for scientific inquiry, medicine's monopoly has tended to suppress alternative healing. For example, acupuncture, which is based on a Chinese metaphysic, was largely spurned until scientific trials began to show its effectiveness in a variety of contexts.[32] In the 1960s the AMA aggressively tried to eradicate chiropractic, even while acknowledging that it was "effective, indeed more effective than the medical profession, in treating certain kinds of problems, such as back injuries."[33] As recently as 1990, the North Carolina Supreme Court upheld a decision by the state's medical licensing board to revoke the license of a physician who had included homeopathy in his practice–even though everyone involved acknowledged that there was no evidence that this practice had ever harmed a patient.[34]

The suppression of alternatives to mainstream medicine does not, of course, render them entirely unavailable. In fact, citizens use them to a considerably larger degree than many observers had realized.[35] And of course, spiritual concepts are not outlawed. Competent adults can refuse even life-saving medical interventions for any reason they wish, including religious beliefs. A number of states expressly permit parents to use spiritual forms of healing for their children, declaring that such an approach will not be construed as child abuse or neglect.

But permission to seek religious rather than science-based healing is significantly circumscribed. Parents have permission to use spiritual healing only as far as the courts allow. If a physician believes that child needs a life-saving blood transfusion, most judges readily override the refusal of his Jehovah's Witness parents. Christian Science parents have been criminally prosecuted for failure to use medical science to aid an ill child;[36] parents who refuse chemotherapy for their child's cancer on religious grounds have been forced to accept it;[37] and pregnant women whose near-term fetuses are in distress have been forced to undergo caesarian delivery, even against their religious objections.[38]

Medicine's monopoly has also contributed to the high cost of care that renders treatment less available to anyone lacking adequate insurance. This arises through several channels.

Physicians' legal authority in setting the medical standard of care, combined with the law's expectation that this standard be uniform for all patients, regardless of their (in)ability to pay, drives up health care costs substantially. Propelled by science and defensive medicine to adopt the newest treatments and then compelled by law to do so for everyone equally, physicians have found themselves providing an ever more technological and costly level of care. This uniformity hides the often marginal character of the improvement provided by some newer modalities, and the widely variable value of such interventions in specific circumstances. A high-cost clot lysis agent for heart attack patients, for example, may (or may not) save a few more patients, but at vastly higher cost.[39] An older, generic hypertensive agent may be just as effective as newer agents for many patients, so that the costliest new agents might be safely reserved for more selective patients–yet often only the costlier agents are used.[40] So long as the law expects uniformity, and the majority of patients have the insurance to afford a generous level of care, cost-conscious adjustments in care are difficult to make, and patients everywhere must pay the price.

Another cost-driver arises from physicians' power of prescription. Because they almost unilaterally determine which patients will receive how much of which drugs and devices, manufacturers mainly market directly to physicians. Gifts, gadgets, and slick promotions, sometimes lavishly expensive, have been used to win physicians' time and attention and, in some cases, their gratitude.[41] Though most physicians conscientiously resist such pressures, and deny that these promotions truly influence their prescribing habits, evidence suggests that the subtle influence may be greater than physicians realize.[42]

A further cost-driver comes from restrictions on scope of practice. As one commentator notes, "[p]rofessional licensure laws have long made the provision of most personal health services the exclusive province of physicians. Obviously, such regulation limits consumers' options by forcing them to use highly trained, expensive personnel when other types might serve quite well."[43] In other cases, nonphysicians are permitted to perform services, but only under the "supervision" of a physician, and often billed at the physician's rates rather than at the ancillary provider's scale. Similarly, many services in this country that are provided by specialists, and charged at commensurately higher rates, could safely be provided by generalist physicians.[44]

In sum, the dominance of orthodox medicine has made alternate care more difficult to find and nearly all care at least somewhat more difficult to afford. Even more troubling is the presumption, underlying many of these restrictions, that the dominance is necessary because citizens are not really capable of making their own decisions. This presumption is found on a general level regarding the populace as a whole, and appears in a more restrictive version when particular individuals are diagnosed as ill.

On that more general level, the presumption has appeared in antitrust cases in which members of various professions have sought to preserve control by restricting the free availability of information and options. Several of these cases feature attempts to avoid even having to compete with other members of the same profession, let alone competing with alternative professions. Typically in such cases, the profession argues both that clients are too ignorant and vulnerable to make their own decisions in the market, and reciprocally that if their profession is not granted special exemptions from competition, they may themselves become unprofessional.

For instance, in *Virginia Pharmacy Bd. v. Va. Consumer Council,*[45] pharmacists defended their policy of proscribing all advertising of drug prices:

services such as compounding, handling, dispensing "are time consuming and expensive; if competitors who economize by eliminating them are permitted to advertise their resulting lower prices, the more painstaking and conscientious pharmacist will be forced either to follow suit or to go out of business";

"advertising will lead people to shop for their prescription drugs among the various pharmacists who offer the lowest prices, and the loss of stable pharmacist-customer relationships will make individual attention–and certainly the practice of monitoring–impossible";

the professional image of the pharmacist as a skilled and specialized craftsman will be damaged making it more difficult to attract talent to the profession and reinforce the better habits of those who are in it; "[p]rice advertising...will reduce the pharmacist's status to that of a mere retailer";

pharmacists who advertise "will be taken up on by too many unwitting customers. They will choose the low-cost, low-quality service and drive the 'professional' pharmacist out of business. They will respond only to costly and excessive advertising, and end up paying the price. They will go from one pharmacist to another, following the discount, and destroy the pharmacist-customer relationship. They will lose respect for the profession because it advertises. All this is not in their best interests, and all this can be avoided if they are not permitted to know who is charging what."[46]

The Supreme Court rejected these arguments. "There is, of course, an alternative to this highly paternalistic approach. That alternative is to assume that this information is not in itself harmful, that people will perceive their own best interests if only they are well enough informed, and that the best means to that end is to open the channels of communication rather than to close them."[47]

In *Bates v. State Bar of Arizona,*[48] attorneys who advertised their prices at a legal clinic were disciplined by the state bar for violating a ban on self-promotion through advertising. The state bar was concerned about advertising's adverse effects on professionalism. "The key to professionalism, it is argued, is the sense of pride that involvement in the discipline generates. It is claimed that price advertising will bring about commercialization, which will undermine the attorney's sense of dignity and self-worth. The hustle of the marketplace will adversely affect the profession's service orientation, and irreparably damage the delicate balance between the lawyer's need to earn and his obligation selflessly to serve. Advertising is also said to erode the client's trust in his attorney: Once the client perceives that the lawyer is motivated by profit, his confidence that the attorney is acting out of a commitment to the client's welfare is jeopardized. And advertising is said to tarnish the dignified public image of the profession."[49] However, the Supreme Court struck down the ban, noting that if the public is unsophisticated, then more information, not less, is the remedy. And the Court poked at the profession's ethical arguments: "It is at least somewhat incongruous for the opponents of advertising to extol the virtues and altruism of the legal profession at one point, and, at another, to assert that its members will seize the opportunity to mislead and distort."[50]

Medicine's monopoly over diagnosing disease poses significant hazards to the freedom of the people to whom illness is ascribed. To begin with, the lavish economic support of medicine has tended rather markedly to expand the concept of disease according to what is treatable, thereby redefining many otherwise-routine human conditions as illnesses. Many young people who previously were regarded as juvenile delinquents have been reclassified as emotionally disturbed, once ample funding became available to hospitalize them.[51] And childbirth, menopause, obesity, jet lag, even baldness become "medical conditions" once surgical and pharmacological interventions are available.[52]

This medicalization of human conditions in turn threatens a curtailment of human freedom. When an annoying adolescent is declared to be ill, for instance, he can be hospitalized against his will, and not necessarily to his benefit.[53] The serious abuses of psychiatry in the Soviet Union have been well documented.[54] Reciprocally, the increasing classification of human conditions and conduct as illness erodes human responsibility. As noted by Dan Callahan,

> matters get out of hand when all physical, mental and communal disorders are put under the heading of "sickness," and all sufferers (all of us, in the end) placed in the blameless "sick role." Not only are the concepts of "sickness" and "illness" drained of all content, it also becomes impossible to ascribe any freedom or responsibility to those caught up in the throes of illness. The whole world is sick, and no one is responsible any longer for anything. That is determinism gone mad.[55]

Freedom and values: restrictions on physicians. Medicine's domination of the concepts, diagnosis, and treatment of disease also poses troubling and somewhat ironic threats to the freedom and integrity of physicians themselves, both as persons and as professionals. On the one hand, although society has given control over the tools of healing to orthodox medicine, it is only with significant strings. The ostensible purpose of physicians' control over these wonderful but dangerous drugs, devices, and procedures is to ensure that they benefit patients without causing undue harm. But society sometimes takes the lead in defining harm. Although physicians are free to prescribe most drugs as they see fit, for instance, they must follow detailed rules regarding controlled substances such as narcotics, amphetamines, depressants, and stimulants. Society has decided that people should not spend their lives as drug users, even if they are free to pursue a wide variety of other risky or unhealthy lifestyles. And society has appointed physicians to be the first-line police for this value, on pain of losing their licenses if they do not.[56] As a result, even patients who clearly need and deserve such medications, including those suffering pain postoperatively or in the terminal stages of cancer, may be denied adequate pain relief by physicians who fear that they may lose their licenses by overzealous medical boards guarding narcotic use.

Because of this societal oversight, physicians are in a terribly difficult position when patients or their families request a treatment that has been spurned by society or the profession. Many women, for instance, still would like to have breast augmentation surgery, even with silicone implants. Yet society will not currently let them make this risk-benefit decision for themselves.[57] Similarly, some physicians perceive a societal obligation to deny treatment to patients whose lifestyles cause or contribute to their medical problems. Some surgeons would deny coronary artery by-pass surgery to smokers,[58] for instance, or liver transplants to alcoholics,[59] or repeat heart valve replacements to chronic intravenous drug abusers.[60]

Other societal values can likewise circumscribe patients' choices. Consider psychoactive drugs such as Prozac, which apparently can render many people more confident and happy, with virtually no side-effects in most cases. On the one hand, physicians are expected to prescribe drugs only for "proper" and "medically necessary" purposes. And those purposes may not embrace personal enhancement through drugs, an activity regarded by some observers as a kind of cheating that bypasses the salutary character-building effects of pain and anxiety. Accordingly, many physicians decline to prescribe Prozac for patients who have no standardly diagnosed psychopathology: if it is not a treatment for an illness, it must not be used. On the other hand, much of medicine is devoted to improving quality of life, even at a purely cosmetic level, and it is not clear why a physician should let such "pharmacological

Calvinism" stand in the way of someone's desire to enjoy better living through chemistry.[61]

The value/power struggle comes to a peak in the so-called futility cases. Here, the physician's control over medical technology is the very thing that renders him susceptible to a powerful reciprocal force exercised by patients and families. In such situations, a physician may feel that endless prolongation of a purely vegetative existence is not "medically indicated," indeed incompatible with the very integrity of the medical profession, and accordingly may refuse to order such interventions as cardiopulmonary resuscitation or ventilator-assisted respiration in an intensive care unit. However, the family who disagrees and wants to insist on endless aggressive life-support may actually use the physician's monopoly over this technology as a weapon against him. Since the physician is the only one who can prescribe such treatments, so that the family cannot secure them from anyone other than a physician, the family can attribute the patient's "premature" death directly to the physician's refusal. The physician is uniquely blamed when the patient dies today, rather than tomorrow, for lack of heroic care. The prospect of civil or even criminal litigation in such scenarios often prompts physicians to defer to such families, even against their own better judgment and personal values. Thus the unique power that permits physicians to implement their values can become the very thing that preempts it.[62]

In sum, although medicine's monopoly endows physicians with a remarkable degree of control over the concepts, tools, laws, and economics of health and healing, they sometimes find this same power turned against them, creating difficult personal and professional dilemmas.

ENGELHARDT'S APPRAISAL OF MEDICAL MONOPOLY

Engelhardt would agree that medicine's monopoly is problematic, for reasons very basic to his philosophy. Observing the intensely value-laden nature of medicine, Engelhardt argues that there is no single, demonstrably correct, canonical way of discovering these values. As he shows in Chapter Five of *Foundations*, for example, even such ostensibly clear matters as defining and classifying disease entities, and diagnosing them in particular individuals, is normatively loaded. One cannot appeal to some sort of "design" or "ideal environment," because people can differ in their description of the way things are "meant" to be. Neither can one invoke statistical normality, because what is typical is not necessarily good, nor is the atypical necessarily bad. "There is no canonical content-full secular vision of medical reality, of illness and disease, of health and proper health care."[63] Indeed, because our disease language can shape as well as reflect reality, descriptions and ascriptions of illness must undergo the same sort of discussion and negotiation required to resolve other value differences throughout our lives as people in a pluralist society.

If defining disease is value-laden and therefore irreducibly controversial, choosing treatments is even more so. Even if it is true that medicine as a profession espouses certain substantive values–an ongoing controversy in itself–it is even clearer that not all patients subscribe to their physicians' values. Accordingly, Engelhardt argues forcefully on behalf of the moral necessity of obtaining patients' permission before undertaking treatment. Though he does not address the issue directly, he also would quite surely decry physicians' monopoly control over prescription drugs and devices, which permits them to let their personal or professional values stand in the way of patients' ability to seek the treatments they want. Very likely, therefore, so long as society reserves these for physicians' control, Engelhardt would en- dorse a robust black market in prescription drugs and other therapeutics, and similarly an open market for citizens to purchase services such as laboratory tests without the necessity of first obtaining a physician's permission.

In the same vein, Engelhardt will also oppose the substantial control that physicians have exercised over the levels and directions of resource allocation. The scope of practice laws that can require a person to patronize physicians instead of nurse practitioners or iridologists should be forgone, perhaps in favor of a system in which each purveyor of health care provides clear and detailed information about its healing modalities. Similarly, in a more Engelhardtian world, neither courts nor physicians would mandate that every citizen receive the same quality and quantity of care, regardless of ability to pay. Engelhardt is emphatic on this point:

> The imposition of a single-tier, all-encompassing health care system is morally unjustifiable. It is a coercive act of totalitarian zeal, which fails to recognize the diversity of moral visions that frame interests in health care, the secular moral limits of state authority, and the authority of individuals over themselves and their own property. It is an act of secular immorality. A basic human secular moral right to health care does not exist–not even to a 'decent minimum of health care'. Such rights must be created.[64]

These observations do not imply that Engelhardt would permit patients to force physicians to behave in ways that violate the latter's own values and consciences. Physicians as moral agents are entitled to give or withhold their permission, just as patients are. Thus, a surgeon must not be forced to perform an operation that he considers too risky, just as a right-to-life obstetrician should not be forced to provide abortions. Neither should an internist be pressured to lie to an insurer so the patient can receive resources to which his health plan does not entitle him. And neither should surrogates be able to coerce physicians to provide endless heroic care to patients in a persistent vegetative state.

Quite possibly, on Engelhardt's view, the surest way to mitigate the coercion that physicians can exert on patients, and reciprocally the coercion that patients sometimes exercise over their physicians, is to remove or at least substantially reduce the monopoly control that physicians have traditionally exerted over diagnosing and treating disease, and over the nation's resources. Physicians might present themselves more as one kind of healer among others, even if perhaps still first among equals. Instead of purporting to define what constitutes disease, they could simply describe "clinical problems,"[65] identifying the kinds of conditions they can help, the ways in which they do it, and at what cost.

Engelhardt, or any of the rest of us, may or may not agree with a complete dissolution of medicine's monopoly. But interestingly, recent economic changes are rapidly achieving a kind of "trust-busting" that might have seemed impossible only a few years ago.

ECONOMIC CHANGES MITIGATING MONOPOLY

After decades of relentlessly escalating expenditures, those who most directly pay the costs–governments and employers–are finally beginning to gain some control over those costs. Many of them are capping or capitating the amount they pay for each beneficiary, and many are either creating or subscribing to health plans that closely control the level and intensity of services provided. At last, premium costs appear to be leveling and, in some regions of the country, actually declining. Notably, these changes are in turn spawning a marked reduction in physicians' historical power.

Current trust-busting. Medical monopoly is diminishing on several fronts. First, a host of parties now influence medical practices. Insurers, developing their own criteria of medical necessity, have become much more aggressive in denying payment for treatments and procedures. Managed care organizations (MCOs) likewise implement tight guidelines, or incentivize physicians to develop their own. Large businesses that self-insure instead of purchasing existing health plans are similarly adopting practice parameters they expect physicians to observe when caring for their employees. And malpractice insurers have still further guidelines to which their physician subscribers must adhere. These varying standards can reflect widely differing philosophies about proper medical care, and in some cases actually demand diametrically conflicting approaches to care.[66]

Most significantly for this chapter's purposes, however, these economic agents' guidelines mean that physicians now share their authority over medical standards of care. Although technically a refusal to pay for this or that intervention still leaves the physician free to order it, the lack of payment has an enormous power over what is done for a patient. Beyond this, MCOs typically limit their drug formularies to drugs the MCO considers cost-effective, restricting physicians from ordering off-formulary medications without special exemption. Concomitantly, some pharmaceutical companies are switching their most intense marketing efforts away from physicians whose prescribing power is now diminished, toward the MCOs whose formulary decisions set the parameters of prescribing. In sum, physicians no longer set medical practices unilaterally.

A second loosening of physicians' influence concerns changes in the scope of practice permitted for nonphysician providers of health care. One of the MCOs' most important ways of controlling costs is to rely on less costly workers, such as nurse practitioners (NPs), physicians' assistants (PAs), nurse midwives, and other ancillary caregivers, to provide care that they believe does not require a full medical education and extensive residency training. Accordingly, NPs and PAs provide large amounts of screening and routine care of minor illnesses; many also undertake more complex procedures, such as sigmoidoscopy, colposcopy, endometrial sampling, minor biopsies, laceration repair, joint aspiration and injections, splinting, and casting of some bone fractures.[67] A relative shortage and maldistribution of primary care physicians, particularly in rural and inner-city areas, has accelerated this shift. Additionally, many state legislatures have recently broadened their laws governing nurses and other ancillary providers, commonly granting greater independent drug-prescribing authority and sometimes even the right to bill directly for services without requiring physician authorization.[68]

In addition, nonallopathic healers are gaining recognition. As noted above, many people already use alternatives such as chiropractic, acupuncture, herbs, massage therapy, and the like.[69] In recognition that at least some of these approaches may make real contributions to human health and wellbeing, the National Institutes of Health established in 1992 the Office of Alterative Medicine to run scientific trials on these alternatives and to foster incorporation of those found to be safe and effective.[70] In the process, alternate concepts of illness and healing, and a greater array of values, gain acceptance along with the wider diversity of treatments.

A third loosening of physicians' authority emerges as states loosen their laws governing the corporate practice of medicine. Earlier exemptions were necessary to make HMOs possible, since many HMOs are corporations that hire physicians as employees rather than simply negotiating with them as independent contractors.[71] In recent years, corporate practice laws have rarely been enforced,[72] and many are now under legislative reform as hospitals and other major players in the health care industry seek to establish vertically integrated delivery systems so that they, too, can enter the highly competitive managed care market. Their integration, like HMOs', will often require hiring physicians as employees.

Fourth, patients themselves are beginning to acquire greater economic control and thereby greater medical control, at least in some settings. Instead of purchasing the usual indemnity insurance or managed care plan for their employees, a number of business corporations are now offering medical savings accounts (MSAs) combined with catastrophic insurance. In these plans, employees are provided with high-deductible insurance (typically $3000 or so) and a dedicated fund of money with which to pay those up-front deductible costs. Access to health care is preserved as employees enjoy essentially first-dollar coverage, yet because they can keep whatever money remains in the fund at the end of the year (or other designated period of time), they have substantial incentive to ensure that their care is costworthy.[73] By bringing patients into the economic consequences of their health spending decisions, such incentives also permit patients to exercise greater control over their medical decisions, and the need for outside controls such as utilization review may be commensurately diminished.[74]

Future trust-busting. There is reason to expect further diminution of physicians' authority over health matters. Employers, governments, and MCOs will continue to scrutinize medical traditions. If medical savings accounts become more widely available, patients will join the ranks of those holding the purse strings, bringing their widely varying views about what illness is, and how and when what sort of health care should be sought.[75] Further, as the health care economy becomes increasingly competitive, a greater variety of provider organizations is likely to bring a broader array of concepts about how health care ought to be conceived and delivered.

Another likely change is a shrinking of our concept of disease and with it, the appropriate range of medical treatment. As noted above, generous funding for health care, including mental health care, tended to promote a broad concept of illness. So long as treatment and payment were available, then a problem was apt to be considered a disease. But as health care funding shrinks, so will our concept of disease. MCOs are already beginning to suggest that the real cause of health care costs is not really physician behavior, so much as patients–their illnesses and injuries. And as citizens begin to appreciate that they, not some anonymous "third party," really pay for health care, we are likely to see the currently fashionable focus on victimhood and treatment replaced by greater recognition that many health problems are caused by voluntary behavior.[76] Accordingly, we should not be surprised to see some mental disorders reclassified as character flaws on the lines of orneriness, weakness of will, and the like. And we can expect to see less financial support for the illnesses and injuries that result from voluntary conduct.[77]

FROM TRUST-BUSTING TO TRUST

These changes will be a mixed blessing. On the one hand, as medicine's monopoly over defining, diagnosing, and treating illness loosens, physicians as well as patients and society as a whole can be expected to benefit. Increased diversity can foster creativity, reduce costs, and mitigate the coercion that inevitably arises when people are permitted just one official avenue of healing.

Indeed, the medical profession's grip on its accustomed control may even need further loosening. Despite evidence that allied health professionals can often serve as well as physicians in certain capacities, some members of organized medicine remain fairly adamant about retaining control. For instance, the American College of Physicians' Task Force on Physician Supply recently issued a position paper endorsing expanded roles for nurse practitioners and physician assistants, including some authority for them to prescribe drugs–but only in a system in which physicians are ultimately accountable. "Until evidence shows that advanced practice nurses can provide high-quality health care services in independent practice arrangements without accountability to physicians, the College cannot support independent practice of nurse practitioners or direct fee-for-service payments to them."[78] Thus, the College believes that the public must continue to pay physicians in order to gain access to these alternate providers. While quality of care is a legitimate concern throughout health care, the presumption that one kind of professional should be a gatekeeper permitting or withholding citizens' access to other kinds of provider needs to be reevaluated.

On the other hand, there are serious drawbacks in the current reshuffling of power and economics. Scientific medicine has provided extraordinary help in preventing, curing, and ameliorating human ailments. As professional influence and research funding become scarcer, at least some opportunities for further improvement will surely be lost. And despite the criticisms of cynics, the medical profession has sustained a high level of dedication and commitment to the welfare of their patients, including those unable to pay. Part of what has made such dedication possible has been physicians' clear access to health care resources lying well beyond their own professional services—an access to technologies and facilities that is now rapidly fading.

Further, as medicine's monopoly dissolves, the AMA's direst predictions about alternate delivery systems are at least partly coming true. The increasing corporatization really does, more often than solo fee-for-service practice, place physicians in systematic conflicts of obligation and conflicts of interest. Contractual commitments to MCOs or even to large-group physician practices, for instance, can pit physicians' loyalty to patients against their obligations to the organization. And although fee-for-service carries the obvious hazard of excessive services and costs, the conflicts of interest posed by incentives, capitation, risk pools, and other mechanisms of cost containment are much more difficult for patients to detect, and can likewise be more difficult for physicians to combat. Moreover, lay people in charge of corporate health care delivery may not always be attuned to clinical contingencies and uncertainties that can be crucial to high-quality care; their mission to promote the organization's financial success may not always embrace such nuances. And in the high-powered world of medical economics, employers and payers sometimes buy, sell, and trade blocks of patients as a virtual market commodity.[79] Continuity of care and physician-patient relationships can suffer, despite evidence that continuity of care often leads to better outcomes, lower costs, and greater satisfaction for patients and physicians alike.[80]

In sum, the more welcome benefits of trust-busting precipitate sobering challenges to trust, in two dimensions: questions about the competence of those providing care, and doubts about their motivations.

Under the old monopoly regime, competence was to be assured because physicians, whose esoteric knowledge qualified them both to care for illness and to evaluate colleagues' competence to do the same, were to ensure that only qualified providers entered and remained in the field. Admittedly, this assurance has not been entirely reliable, as evidenced by criticisms of the profession's rather poor record in disciplining errant members. Unfortunately, it is not at all clear that the current situation is demonstrably better. MCOs may use lesser-trained providers, not because they are documentably as good, but simply because they are less costly. Although there is good reason to suppose that many services traditionally performed by physicians can very capably be provided by others, a comprehensive factual basis for determining who should be doing what is still lacking.

Similarly, motivation under the old regime was ostensibly assured by the professional commitment of physicians to serve patients' interests, even above their own. Again, the realities probably have never matched the ideals. It was easy to be altruistic as long as free-flowing finances permitted physicians to provide every service of conceivable benefit, regardless of the cost. But again, current realities may pose even greater challenges to professionalism. It is more difficult than ever for physicians to hold their patients' interests paramount, as powerful market forces regularly pressure them to do otherwise.

We must consider, then, how to (re)build trust in an era of profound economic change and uncertainty. Two basic approaches provide a reasonable beginning: increasing consumers' information and enhancing their control. But even these two must be complemented by a third, namely, a renewed emphasis on professional commitment.

First, it is imperative to recognize that blind faith will no longer suffice, if ever it did. In keeping with the old proverb, "trust, but verify," patients and purchasers of care need to know more about what they are receiving in exchange for their money and for their willingness to place their bodies and health and money in the hands of this or that provider or health plan. This information should concern both competence and motivation.

Accordingly, better information must be created concerning what sorts of care work, how well, under what conditions. Fortunately, some of this information and disclosure are now emerging. Many payers, MCOs, and private foundations are undertaking systematic outcomes studies to create guidelines for care. Likewise, efforts are underway to assess the quality of care provided by health plans and by individual physicians. This information should be made as freely available as possible. New York State, for instance, reveals tallies of morbidity and mortality for both hospitals and physicians providing cardiac surgery procedures.[81] These studies and guidelines undoubtedly need considerable improvement, but major efforts are underway.

Disclosure must also cover the factors that influence motivation. Incentive systems and risk pools that reward physicians for frugality should be revealed, alongside health plans' basic strategies for keeping costs under control. As in any fiduciary relationship, these conflicts of interest must be made plain so that those who are vulnerable can take them into account in making decisions.[82]

Second, trust is enhanced through control. A lack of alternatives, just like blind faith, may sometimes have been mistaken for trust in the past, but that era is gone. The more that patients are free to tailor their care to their own needs and preferences, and the more free they are to leave a relationship that does not satisfy, the more fully will the relationships in which they remain embody a genuine trust. Accordingly, the ongoing diminution of physicians' monopoly can ultimately enhance patients' trust.

There is a variety of ways in which patients' choices and control over their care can be enhanced. As a beginning, we should remove the presumption that physicians and health care plans must provide all people with the same level of care, regardless of their ability or willingness to pay. Engelhardt is not alone in arguing that people must have far greater freedom to purchase varying packages of health benefits. Havighurst, for example, argues that the medical profession's opinions and practices should no longer be permitted to determine the contents and costs of the health plans people buy. Rather, freedom of contract should prevail. Health plans might offer various levels of care via differing guidelines, for instance.[83]

In a similar vein, people might exercise considerably greater control over the routine expenses of health care via medical savings accounts, in which people purchase catastrophic policies with high deductibles, then draw on a dedicated medical savings fund to meet the deductible expenses. In this way, people have greater reason to engage their physicians in discussions about which interventions are both medically and economically worthwhile.[84] And they would have greater financial freedom to visit alternative providers such as chiropractors and acupuncturists. The more that patients experience some level of economic accountability for their choices, the more economic control they will have, and thereby the more medical control.[85]

Greater choice for patients among various kinds of providers does not necessarily have to be blind choice. Neither must it mean a diminution in the quality and stature of the medical profession. There is no reason in principle why physicians should not continue, at least as vigorously than they do now, to monitor quality within the profession and ensure that, if someone chooses to visit a physician, that person can count on a certain level and kind of expertise. Such internal monitoring is now found particularly within medical specialty boards. These boards establish rigorous entry criteria before a physician can call himself a fellow of the American College of Physicians or of the American College of Surgeons. Many of these boards now also require periodic recertification. Arguably, the quality assurance found in such privately sponsored organizations may be better conceived and enforced than in state-sponsored licensing boards. Hence, even if states were to back away from broad, vague laws stipulating that only licensed physicians can diagnose and treat human ailments, there is no good reason why physicians could not retain or even enhance their status as providers who offer scientifically based care, with reasonable assurance of a particular level of quality.[86]

Admittedly, the above proposal is somewhat odd: that we enhance trust by alleviating the need for it–first, to help patients become better informed about their health, health care providers, and health plans, so they do not have to take claims of competent healing or altruistic motive solely on faith; and second, to present a broader array of choices, so that patients can exit more easily a relationship in which they do not feel trust. Perhaps this oddity is best understood if we recognize that an important residual of vulnerability cannot be removed from this realm. The discrepancy between providers' greater knowledge and power, and patients' emotional, intellectual, and physical impairment in the face of illness, creates a disparity of power that cannot be eradicated. The upshot of this article, however, is that this disparity is not necessarily best addressed by further increasing the power of just one sort of provider, namely the allopathic medical doctor. Rather, a greater empowerment of patients is more likely to protect them than placing virtually all the economic, legal, and healing power in one set of hands.

This discrepancy of power brings us to the third approach to preserving trust as physicians' legal and economic control fades. Professionalism and integrity, the commitment of the physician to serve the needs of the patient and voluntarily, avowedly, to give patients' interests priority, must remain a hallmark of medicine.[87] Such professionalism is vigorously defended by many physicians concerned about today's dramatic economic changes,[88] defended as our best available "antidote to the inevitability of [this] market failure in medicine."[89] At present, this traditional virtue is fragile and under challenge from many sides. And as the medical profession loses its formal power, it must and can earn back its influence by the quality and dedication of its service. Such a move would be the best way to replace monopolistic trusts with patient trust.

NOTES

The author acknowledges with gratitude the very helpful comments provided on earlier drafts by Robert M. Sade, M.D., Brendan P. Minogue, Ph.D., Gabriel Palmer-Fernández, Ph.D., and James E. Reagan, Ph.D.

1. The middle ages were known for guild control over many occupations, but the widespread use of licensing to regulate professions is largely a feature of the twentieth-century. By the mid-1800s, an antiregulatory movement in the country had opened the medical profession essentially to anyone who chose to hang a shingle. Only after the turn of the century did licensing laws emerge. See D. B. Hogan, "The Effectiveness of Licensing: History, Evidence, and Recommendations," *Law and Human Behavior* 7 (1983): 117-138, at 118-20. See also P. Starr, *The Social Transformation of American Medicine* (New York: Basic Books, 1982).

2. Howard Brody would call this power the physician's "Aesculapian power"–the mastery of facts, theories, and skills that achieves healing results. Brody distinguishes this sort of power from the "charismatic power" that a physician may win based on personal qualities, and from the "social power" that arises from the special authority that society has given physicians to determine what will count as truth and knowledge in medicine. H. Brody, *The Healer's Power* (New Haven: Yale University Press, 1992), 16-17. Brody's account of social power points toward the legal and economic power discussed just below in this essay, but does not entirely capture the force that arises when society grants physicians exclusive legal permission to define, diagnose, and treat disease, or the economic authority to determine how much others will spend on their care.

3. Hogan, "The Effectiveness," 129-30.

4. Cited in *Medical Licensing Board of Indiana v. Stetina*, 477 N. E. 2d 322 (Ind. App. 1985). In Tennessee: "Any person shall be regarded as practicing medicine who treats, professes to treat, operates on, or prescribes for any physical ailment or any physical injury to or deformity of another." T.C.A. §63-6-204. The statute explicitly does not apply to "the administration of domestic or family remedies in cases of emergency" or to dentistry, military physicians, midwives, veterinary surgeons, osteopaths, chiropractors not giving or using medicine, opticians, optometrists, chiropodists, Christian Scientists, physician assistants, registered nurses, or licensed practical nurses rendering services "under the supervision, control and responsibility of a licensed physician."

5. C. C. Havighurst, "The Changing Locus of Decision Making in the Health Care Sector," *Journal of Health Politics, Policy and Law* 11 (1986): 702.

6. Cited in *Sermchief v. Gonzales*, 660 S. W. 2d 683 (Mo 1983).

7. Comparably, the Tennessee statute defines nursing as "the performance for compensation of any act requiring substantial specialized judgment and skill based on knowledge of the natural, behavioral and nursing sciences...as the basis for application of the nursing process in wellness and illness care," and includes "nursing management of illness, injury, or infirmity including identification of patient problems." T.C.A. §63-7-103(a)(1).

8. B. R. Furrow, S. H. Johnson, T. S. Jost, R. L. Schwartz, *The Law of Health Care Organization and Finance* (St. Paul: West Publishing Co., 1991), 69 ff.

9. C. C. Havighurst, "The Changing Locus," 703.

10. See K. Leffler, "Economic and Legal Analysis of Medical Ethics: The Case of Restrictions on Interprofessional Association," *Law and Human Behavior* 7 (1983): 183-192. Chiropractors are licensed as primary care providers in all fifty states, but are limited practitioners in that they are not allowed to prescribe drugs or perform surgery; some states specify that they are not permitted to treat infectious or contagious diseases (at p. 186). See also *Wilk v. American Medical Association*, 895 F. 2d 352 (7th Cir. 1990) (cert. denied 111 S. Ct. 513 (1990)).

11. D. W. Light, "Is Competition Bad?" *New England Journal of Medicine* 309 (1983): 1316. For a more detailed discussion of this historical picture and relevant bibliographical cites, see E. H. Morreim, *Balancing Act: The New Medical Ethics of Medicine's New Economics* (Washington, D.C.: Georgetown University Press, 1995).

12. B. B. Roe, "The UCR Boondoggle: A Death Knell for Private Practice?" *New England Journal of Medicine* 305 (1981): 41-45; T. L. Delbanco, K. C. Meyers, E. A. Segal, "Paying the Physician's Fee: Blue Shield and the Reasonable Charge," *New England Journal of Medicine* 301 (1979): 1314-20.

13. Havighurst suggests: "Although the tenets of the professional paradigm of medicine are nowhere officially set down, they seem to include the following:
•Medical care should be evaluated only on the basis of safety and efficacy, without regard to cost considerations.
•Decisions concerning the appropriate utilization of medical services should be based exclusively on scientific evidence and expert opinion.
•Consumers are generally incapable of making appropriate choices about their health care.
•Patient preferences should be honored under the profession's ethical principle of informed consent but not by letting consumers choose qua consumers with costs in view.
•Consumers should look to physicians and not to other agents to protect their interests.
•Physicians, as professionals guided by scientific principles and ethical concern for patient interests, should enjoy autonomy in their professional work and be accountable only to other independent professionals.
•Professional norms alone should set the limits of physician judgment."
C. C. Havighurst, *Health Care Choices: Private Contracts as Instruments of Health Reform* (Washington, D.C.: The AEI Press, 1995), 113.

14. C. C. Havighurst, J. F. Blumstein, "Coping with Quality/Cost Trade-offs in Medical Care: The Role of PSROs," *Northwestern University Law Review* 70 (1975): 26; Havighurst, *Health Care Choices*, 117.

15. In 1932, the AMA renounced a blue-ribbon panel, sponsored by several philanthropic organizations, that concluded group practice would be desirable. "The physicians of this country must not be misled by utopian fantasies of a form of medical practice which would equalize all physicians by placing them in groups under one administration. ... It is better for the American people that most of their illnesses be treated by their own doctors rather than by industries, corporations or clinics." (editorial), "The committee on the costs of medical care," *Journal of the American Medical Association* 99 (1932): 1950, cited in K. Grumbach, "Requiem for Traditional Medical Practice in the United States," *Archives of Family Medicine* 4 (1995): 756-57.

16. *American Medical Association v. United States*, 317 U.S. 519 (1943).

17. J. M. Alexander, "Potential Legal Problems Associated with Integrated Systems," in *Integrated Health Care Delivery Systems*, ed., A. Fine, (New York: Thompson Publishing Group, Inc., 1993), 147; J. G. Wiehl, *et al.* "Legal Issues Related to Systems Integration," in *Integrated Health*, 12, ed., A. Fine; Furrow, *et al.*, *The Law of Health Care*, 189-90; Havighurst, "The Changing Locus," 703; Starr, *The Social Transformation*, 24.

18. Havighurst, "The Changing Locus," 706-7. Note how the rapid diffusion of new technology via defensive medicine, identified above, becomes a self-fulfilling prophecy: widespread adoption on the assumption that it will be expected by courts renders it a prevailing approach, therefore the standard of care.

19. Furrow, *et al. The Law of Health Care*, 41; Havighurst, *Health Care Choices*, 330; E. Rayack, "Medical Licensure: Social Costs and Social Benefits," *Law and Human Behavior* (1983): 147-156.

20. See *Virginia Pharmacy Bd. v. Va. Consumer Council*, 425 U. S. 748 (1976), *Bates v. State Bar of Arizona*, 433 U. S. 350 (1977), and *National Society of Professional Engineers v. United States*, 435 U. S. 679 (1978), discussed below.

21. W. C. Hsiao, *et al.*, "The Resource-Based Relative Value Scale," *Journal of the American Medical Association* 258 (1987): 800.

22. Starr, *The Social Transformation*, 22 ff.

23. Hogan, "The Effectiveness"; Rayak, "Medical Licensure."

24. *Blue Shield of Virginia v. McCready*, 102 S. Ct. 2540 (1982).

25. Hogan, "The Effectiveness," Rayak, "Medical Licensure"; Furrow *et al.*, *The Law of Health Care*, 41; S. E. Baker, "The Nurse Practitioner in Malpractice Actions: Standard of Care and Theory of Liability," *Health Matrix* 2 (1992): 325-55.

26. E. H. Morreim, "Am I My Brother's Warden? Responding to the Unethical or Incompetent Colleague," *Hastings Center Report* 23, no. 3 (1993): 19-27.

27. E. H. Morreim, "The Impossibility and the Necessity of Quality of Life Research," *Bioethics* 6 (1992): 218-232; I. F. Tannock, "Treating the Patient, Not Just the Cancer," *New England Journal of Medicine* 317 (1987): 1534-35; A. Coates, V. Gebski, J. F. Bishop, *et al.*, "Improving the Quality of Life During Chemotherapy for Advanced Breast Cancer," *New England Journal of Medicine* 317 (1987): 1490-95.

28. M. D. Sullivan, "Placebo Controls and Epistemic Control in Orthodox Medicine," *Journal of Medicine and Philosophy* 18 (1993): 213-231.

29. H. Brody, *Placebos and the Philosophy of Medicine: Clinical, Conceptual, and Ethical Issues* (Chicago: University of Chicago Press, 1977).

30. A. M. Garber, "No Price Too High?" *New England Journal of Medicine* 327 (1992): 1676-1678.

31. J. F. Burnum, "Medical Practice *A la Mode*," *New England Journal of Medicine* 317 (1987): 1220-1222.

32. R. Weiss, "Medicine's Latest Miracle," *Hippocrates* 9, no. 1 (1995): 53-59.

33. *Wilk v. American Medical Association*, 895 F. 2d 352, 363 (7th Cir. 1990) (cert. denied 111 S. Ct. 513 (1990)).

34. *In re Guess*, 393 S. E. 833 (NC 1990). Interestingly, there is some scientific evidence that homeopathy is effective. See C. Bayley "Homeopathy," *Journal of Medicine and Philosophy* 18 (1993): 129-45. Similarly, an Indiana court issued an injunction against a woman practicing iridology. She examined eyes for clues and hints to detect physical conditions–unlawfully making a "diagnosis" without a medical license. *Indiana v. Stetina*, 477 N. E. 2d 322 (Ind. App. 1985).

35. D. M. Eisenberg, R. C. Kessler, C. Foster, F. E. Norlock, D. R. Calkins, T. L. Delbanco, "Unconventional Medicine in the United States: Prevalence, Costs, and Patterns of Use," *New England Journal of Medicine* 328 (1993): 246-252; E. W. Campion, "Why Unconventional Medicine?" *New England Journal of Medicine* 328 (1993): 282-283.

36. *Walker v. Superior Court (People)*, 763 P. 2d 852 (Cal. 1988); *State v. McKown* 461 N. W. 2d 720 (Minn. App. 1990); S. D. Robinson, "Commonwealth v. Twitchell: Who Owns the Child?" *Journal of Contemporary Health Law and Policy* 7 (1991): 413-31.

37. *Custody of a Minor*, 434 N. E. 601 (Mass 1982); *Matter of Hamilton*, 657 S. W. 2d 425 (Tenn. App. 1983).

38. V. E. B. Kolder, J. Gallagher, M. T. Parsons, "Court-Ordered Obstetrical Interventions," *New England Journal of Medicine* 316 (1987): 1192-96; G. J. Annas, "Protecting the Liberty of Pregnant Patients," *New England Journal of Medicine* 316 (1987): 1213-14; J. L. Nelson, N. Milliken, "Compelled Medical Treatment of Pregnant Women: Life, Liberty, and Law in Conflict," *Journal of the American Medical Association* 259 (1988): 1060-66. Note that the reciprocal does not occur: medical physicians are never prosecuted for failing to use spiritual approaches when their own remedies are clearly failing.

39. "The GUSTO Investigators. An International Randomized Trial Comparing Four Thrombolytic Strategies for Acute Myocardial Infarction," *The New England Journal of Medicine* 329 (1993): 673-682; "The GUSTO Investigators. The Effects of Tissue-Plasminogen Activator, Streptokinase, or Both on Coronary-Artery Patency, Ventricular Function, and Survival after Acute Myocardial Infarction," *The New England Journal of Medicine* 329 (1993): 1615-1622; K. L. Lee, R. M. Califf, J. Simes, F. Van de Weft, E. J. Topol, "Holding GUSTO up to the Light," *Annals of Internal Medicine* 120 (1994): 876-881.

40. F. A. Lederle, W. A. Applegate, R. H. Grimm Jr., "Reserpine and the Medical Marketplace," *Archives of Internal Medicine* 153 (1993): 705-706.

41. M. Chen, S. Landefeld, T. H. Murray, "Doctors, Drug Companies, and Gifts," *Journal of the American Medical Association* 262 (1989): 3448-51.

42. J. Avorn, M. Chen, R. Hartley, "Scientific Versus Commercial Sources of Influence on the Prescribing Behavior of Physicians," *American Journal of Medicine* 73 (1982): 4-8; R. I. Shorr, W. L. Greene, "A Food-Borne Outbreak of Expensive Antibiotic Use in a Community Teaching Hospital, *Journal of the American Medical Association* 273 (1995): 1908; R. K. Schwartz, S. B. Soumerai, J. Avorn, "Physician Motivations for Nonscientific Drug Prescribing," *Soc. Sci. Med.*

28 (1989): 577-582.

43. Havighurst, "The Changing Locus," 700.

44. As Donald Light has noted: "The best observers of American medicine have described in detail how the monopoly established by the medical profession earlier in this century has led to its promoting the most profitable lines of work, organizational arrangements, and financing schemes while denigrating public health, preventive medicine, primary care, prepaid programs, and other approaches that have contributed to better health in other advanced societies." Light, "Is Competition Bad?" 1316.

45. *Virginia Pharmacy Bd. v. Va. Consumer Council*, 425 U. S. 748 (1976).

46. *Virginia Pharmacy Bd. v. Va. Consumer Council*, 425 U. S. 748, 768-770 (1976).

47. *Virginia Pharmacy Bd. v. Va. Consumer Council*, 425 U. S. 748, 770 (1976).

48. *Bates v. State Bar of Arizona*, 433 U. S. 350 (1977).

49. *Bates v. State Bar of Arizona*, 433 U. S. 350m 368 (1977).

50. *Bates v. State Bar of Arizona*, 433 U. S. 350, 379 (1977). In *National Society of Professional Engineers v. United States*, 435 U. S. 679 (1978), engineers made a similar case on behalf of their rule forbidding engineers to engage in competitive bidding or in negotiating on price before a client had selected an engineer for a particular job. As in the pharmacy case, the engineers painted a dismal picture of their clients, as people who will almost invariably award contracts to the lowest bidder, regardless of quality or other factors. And they painted a dismal picture of themselves: if permitted to bid competitively, engineers may begin providing a poorer product, submit deceptively low bids, or the like (694, 696). Again, the Supreme Court rejected the arguments, favoring competition.

51. L. A. Weithorn, "Mental Hospitalization of Troublesome Youth: An Analysis of Skyrocketing Admission Rates," *Stanford Law Review* 40 (1988): 773-837.

52. A. J. Barsky, "The Paradox of Health," *New England Journal of Medicine* 318 (1988): 414-18; M. A. Rodwin, "Patient Accountability and Quality of Care: Lessons from Medical Consumerism and Patients' Rights, Women's Health and Disability Rights Movements," *American Journal of Law and Medicine* 20 (1994): 147-67.

53. Weithorn, "Mental Hospitalization," 785-798.

54. R. J. Bonnie, "Soviet Psychiatry and Human Rights," *Law, Medicine & Health Care* 18 (1990): 123-131.

55. D. Callahan, "The WHO Definition of 'Health'," in *Contemporary Issues in Bioethics*, ed., L. Walters (Belmont: Wadsworth, 1982, 2nd ed.), 51.

56. In Tennessee, for instance, misuse of drugs features in 5 of the 18 explicit reasons by which the state's Board of Medical Examiners can deny, suspend, or revoke a physician's license. T.C.A. §63-6-214. The Office of Inspector General in the federal Department of Health and Human Services has reported that "approximately 75 percent of all disciplinary actions were based on drug and alcohol abuse by the physician or for inappropriate prescription for drugs." Cited in Furrow *et. al., The Law of Health Care*, 53-54.

57. M. Angell, "Breast Implants: Protection or Paternalism?" *New England Journal of Medicine* 326 (1992): 1695-96.

58. M. J. Underwood, J. S. Bailey, "Coronary Bypass Surgery Should Not Be Offered to Smokers," *British Medical Journal* 306 (1993): 1047-1048.

59. A. Moss, M. Siegler, "Should Alcoholics Compete Equally for Liver Transplantation?" *Journal of the American Medical Association* (1991): 1295-98.

60. L. Stell, "The Noncompliant Substance Abuser," *Hastings Center Report* 21 no. 2 (1991): 31-32; J. LaPuma, C. K. Cassel, H. Humphrey, "Ethics, Economics, and Endocarditis," *Archives of Internal Medicine* 148 (1988): 1809-11.

61. P. D. Kramer, *Listening to Prozac*, (New York: Viking Press, 1993). The concept of "pharmacological Calvinism" is attributed to Richard Schwartz: See Chapter 9, 250 ff. Kramer notes that "Jean-Paul Sartre wrote his last books while on amphetamines, fully believing he was hastening his death but preferring his version of Achilles' choice: the short, productive life. In the United States, we do not grant the individual this option" (244-45). Because amphetamines cause addiction and paranoia, U. S. laws only allow them to be prescribed for very narrow indications. Hence, an "American doctor would have to say to Sartre, 'The choice is not yours: the book goes, you stay; we are caretakers for a whole society, not potentiators of your work'" (245).

62. E. H. Morreim, "Profoundly Diminished Life: The Casualties of Coercion," *Hastings Center Report* 24, no. 1 (1993): 33-42.

63. H. T. Engelhardt, Jr., *The Foundations of Bioethics* 2nd ed., (New York: Oxford University Press, 1996), 227.

64. *Foundations,* 375.

65. *Foundations,* 205.

66. For further discussion of these varying standards of care see E. H. Morreim, "At the Intersection of Medicine, Law, Economics, and Ethics: The Art of Intellectual Cross-dressing," in *Perspectives on Philosophy in Medicine*, eds., Ronald A. Carson and Chester R. Burns, Philosophy and Medicine Series 50 (Dordrecht: Kluwer Academic Publishers, 1996), forthcoming.

67. "How Do Non-physician Providers Function in HMOs?" *HMO Practice* 8, no. 4 (1994): 151-56.

68. J. P. Kassirer "What Role for Nurse Practitioners in Primary Care?" *New England Journal of Medicine* 330 (1994): 204-5; C. D. DeAngelis, "Nurse Practitioner *Redux,*" *Journal of the American Medical Association* 271 (1994): 868-71; E. S. Sekscenski, S. Sanson, C. Bazell, M. E. Salmon, F. Mullan, "State Practice Environments and the Supply of Physician Assistants, Nurse Practitioners, and Certified Nurse Midwives," *New England Journal of Medicine* 331 (1994): 1266-71.

69. Eisenberg *et. al.*, "Unconventional Medicine"; E. W. Campion, "Why Unconventional?"; R. Weiss, "Medicine's Latest Miracle," *Hippocrates* 9 no. 1 (1995): 53-59; P. Long, "The Naturals," *Hippocrates* 9 no. 5 (1995): 30-35; T. L. Delbanco, "Bitter Herbs: Mainstream, Magic, and Menace," *Archives of Internal Medicine* 121 (1994): 803-4.

70. Delbanco, "Bitter Herbs," 803-4.

71. H. T. Greely, "The Regulation of Private Health Insurance," in *Health Care Corporate Law: Formation and Regulation*, ed., H. A. Hall, (Boston: Little, Brown, and Company, 1993), 8-32.

72. Furrow *et. al.*, *The Law of Health Care*, 190.

73. J. C. Goodman, G. L. Musgrave, *Patient Power* (Washington DC: Cato Institute, 1992); P. DuPont, "The Free-market Health Proposal," *Wall Street Journal*, (July 1, 1994): A-10; P. Gramm "Why We Need Medical Saving Accounts," *New England Journal of Medicine* 330 (1994): 1752-53; M. S. Forbes, "Health Care: Trust the People," *Forbes* (May 23, 1994): 23-24;

J. C. Goodman, "A Plan to Empower Patients," *Wall Street Journal*, (May 2, 1995): A-20; E. H. Morreim, "Lifestyles of the Risky and Infamous: From Managed Care to Managed Lives," *Hastings Center Report* 25, no. 6 (1995): 5-12.

74. For further discussion, see E. H. Morreim, "Diverse and Perverse Incentives in Managed Care: Bringing Patients into Alignment," *Widener Law Symposium Journal* 1(1995): 89-139.

75. M. R. Gillick, "Common-sense Models of Health and Disease," *New England Journal of Medicine* 313 (1985): 700-703.

76. Roughly half of reported deaths in 1990 could be attributed to factors such as tobacco, diet and activity patterns, alcohol, microbial agents, toxic agents, firearms, sexual behavior, motor vehicles, and illicit drugs. J. M. McGinnis, W. H. Goege, "Actual Causes of Death in the United States," *Journal of the American Medical Association* 270 (1993): 2207-2212.

77. Morreim, "Lifestyles of the Risky," 5-12; A. J. Slomski, "Maybe Bigger Isn't Better After All," *Medical Economics* 72, no. 4 (1995): 55-58.

78. American College of Physicians, "Physician Assistants and Nurse Practitioners," *Annals of Internal Medicine* 121, (1994): 714-716, at 715.

79. For further discussion of the pros, cons, and consequences of managed care, see: K. Davis K. S. Collins, C. Schoen, C. Morris, "Choice Matters: Enrollees' Views of Their Health Plans," *Health Affairs* 14, no. 2 (1995): 99-112; D. G. Safran, A. R. Tarlov, W. H. Rogers, "Primary Care Performance in Fee-for-service and Prepaid Health Care Systems," *Journal of the American Medicine Association* 271 (1994): 1584; K. Grumbach, T. Bodenheimer, "The Organization of Health Care," *Journal of the American Medical Association* 273 (1995): 160-67; P. D. Gerber, D. S. Smith, J. M. Ross, "Generalist Physicians and the New Health Care System," *American Journal of Medicine* 97 (1994): 554-558; E. J. Emanuel, N. L. Dubler, "Preserving the Physician-Patient Relationship in the Era of Managed Care," *Journal of the American Medical Association* 273 (1995): 324-25.

80. For studies supporting the value of continuity of care, see, D. A. Barr, "The Effects of Organizational Structure on Primary Outcomes under Managed Care," *Annals of Internal Medicine* 122 (1995): 353-359; J. H. Wasson, A. E. Sauvigne, R. P. Mogielnicki, W. G. Frey, C. H. Sox, C. Gaudette, A. Rockwell, "Continuity of Outpatient Care in Elderly Men: A Randomized Trial," *Journal of the American Medical Association* 252 (1984) 2413-17; C. L. Shear, B. T. Give, J. K. Mattheis, M. R. Levy, "Provider Continuity and Quality of Medical Care: A Retrospective Analysis of Prenatal and Perinatal Outcome," *Medical Care* 21 (1983): 1204-1210; D. S. Rubsamen, "3 Scenarios that Spotlight the Malpractice Hazards Pervading Managed Care," *Physicians Financial News: Managed Care Report* (4/30/95), S-1, S-14, S-15.

81. E. L. Hannan, H. Kilburn Jr., M. Racz, E. Shields, M. R. Chassin, "Improving the Outcomes of Coronary Artery Bypass Surgery in New York State," *Journal of the American Medical Association* 271 (1994): 761-766.

82. Morreim, "Diverse and Perverse Incentives."

83. Havighurst, *Health Care Choices*.

84. Goodman, *et al.*, *Patient Power*.

85. Morreim, "Diverse and Perverse Incentives." Note that these changes would require courts to look quite differently on health care. In order to permit patients to contract for the level of care they want, courts would have to abandon their insistence that health plans are generally contracts of adhesion whose terms may be discarded any time they disadvantage the individual patient. If patients are to have the freedom to make contracts in the first place, those contracts must be

enforced. Havighurst, *Health Care Choices*; P. E. Kalb, "Controlling Health Care Costs by Controlling Technology: A Private Contractual Approach," *Yale Law Journal* 99 (1990): 1109-1126; E. H. Morreim, "Moral Justice and Legal Justice in Managed Care: The Ascent of Contributive Justice," *Journal of Law, Medicine & Ethics* 23 (1995): 247-265.

In like manner, increased access to alternate health care providers would require courts to place greater responsibility on these providers, and less on physicians. When nurses market their services directly to patients, physicians who no longer 'supervise' others should not be held legally accountable for what the latter do. In *Adams v. Krueger*, 856 P. 2d 887 (Idaho App. 1991), a physician was held vicariously liable for the acts of a nurse practitioner employee, even though the nurse practitioner was not herself found liable. Such holdings may need reevaluation if allied health care providers gain greater independence, as proposed here.

86. Although this chapter argues that medicine's monopoly should be mitigated, it is admittedly not clear just how far or how fast this should occur. One might argue, for instance, that it may be best to let physicians retain some control over prescription medications, if only for public health reasons. Instant public access to antibiotics, for instance, may contribute to the development of resistant organisms that pose a threat to everyone. On the other hand, perhaps physicians have contributed to the development of these resistant organisms as much or more than direct public availability might have. Physicians, wary of malpractice suits and sometimes concerned that they must please the demanding patient by writing a prescription, may have overprescribed common antibiotics over the years and thereby contributed to the rise of resistant organisms in conditions such as otitis media, for instance. See N. Joshi, D. Milfred, "The Use and Misuse of New Antibiotics," *Archives of Internal Medicine* 155 (1995): 569-577. The question is empirical, and cannot be settled by reason alone. Suffice it here to conclude that, at the very least, we need to reexamine the notion of permitting one particular group of healers exclusive control over all access to such a broad array of powerful healing tools.

87. As Blumenthal notes, patients not only recognize an asymmetry of information and skill between themselves and their physicians–they want their physicians to know more than they do. D. Blumenthal, "The Vital Role of Professionalism in Health Care Reform," *Health Affairs* 13 no. 1 (1994): 252-56.

88. E. Pellegrino, "Altruism, Self-interest, and Medical Ethics," *Journal of the American Medical Association* 258 (1987): 1939-1940; E. Pellegrino, D. C. Thomasma, *For The Patient's Good* (New York: Oxford University Press, 1988).

89. Blumenthal, "The Vital Role of Professionalism," 253.

4

ENGELHARDT'S COMMUNITARIAN ETHICS: THE HIDDEN ASSUMPTIONS

KEVIN WM. WILDES, S.J.

Few people would characterize H. Tristram Engelhardt's thought as "communitarian." For many in bioethics Engelhardt is widely regarded as a committed libertarian and secular humanist. This is not the case. This essay will argue that Engelhardt is not a libertarian by choice but by default. His libertarian conclusions can only be understood in light of his arguments about the failure of the modern philosophical enterprise in ethics and the implications of the postmodern dilemma. I think if one understands that the heart of his work is an assessment of the modern philosophical project in ethics then one can (1) bring together his libertarian views about the moral limits of the secular state with (2) his communitarian views of morality. The two conclusions flow from his argument about postmodernity.

I hope, however, to go further than demonstrating this tie. I want to argue that Engelhardt has a very particular view of moral community at work in *The Foundations*. After summarizing the broad outlines of Engelhardt's argument in the first two sections of this essay, the third section will lay out the model of community that is at work in Engelhardt's thought. One can say that his is a model of "strict community." In this model there is a strong definition of who is and is not a member of the community. There also is a strong sense of what members of the community should believe and how they should act as well as who has authority within the community. It is this model of community that leads to Engelhardt's negative conclusions about the possibilities for moral bonds with those outside the community and shapes his distinction between moral friends and moral strangers. It is this model of community that leads to his conclusions about the possibilities for morality in a secular society.

To understand this argument we must revisit his argument about the nature of secular moral thought and secular bioethics and postmodernity. The first section of this essay traces Engelhardt's own argument about the failure of reason to overcome the phenomenon of moral pluralism. This argument leads two conclusions. The first is Engelhardt's well known libertarian position that only a minimal, libertarian state can be justified in secular moral terms. The second conclusion is communitarian: substantive moral discourse can only take place in moral communities. These two conclusions are inextricably bound

B. P. Minogue et al. (eds.), Reading Engelhardt, 77–93.
© 1997 *Kluwer Academic Publishers. Printed in the Netherlands.*

together and they lead to the two tiers of morality which is the focus of the second section of this essay. It is from this argument that Engelhardt distinguishes the concepts of moral friends and moral strangers. This distinction gives further insight into Engelhardt's communitarianism. The third section of this essay argues that Engelhardt has a very particular view of moral community in his work. One needs to understand this view of community in order to understand the distinction of moral friends and strangers.

THE HOPE FOR UNIVERSAL AUTHORITY

Since antiquity the West has sought to articulate an understanding of the moral life grounded either in reason itself or in particular normative human affections. There has been an assumption that there is an accessible understanding of what it is to be human. Plato's account of creation in the *Timaeus* reflects a world which is harmonious, ordered, and open to reason (37a). This Greek view of an ordered, intelligible world influenced not only the development of Western science but the development of the Western understanding of the moral life. The West came to regard moral life as ordered and open to discovery. Cicero, reflecting Stoic influences, speaks of the *jus naturale* forming a basis for Roman law.[1] In an empire that spanned many cultures Cicero and the Stoics argued that there was a moral law that could guide the behavior of all citizens and subjects. The Romans adopted and developed a distinction, from the Greeks, between positive law and natural law.[2] In time, Western faith in reason was interwoven with the Faith of Latin Christianity.[3] Latin Christianity distinguished nature (which is known by reason) and faith (which is given by grace or revelation). The moral law was to be understood within the order of nature. Thus it could be known by appeal to natural reason. In Roman Catholicism the Stoic understanding of the Natural Law was rearticulated in an account of the Eternal Law of God.[4]

Engelhardt argues that the Reformation and the Wars of Religion radically transformed the medieval faith in Faith.[5] The Roman Catholic hegemony over the Christian faith shattered in the West and a complex reshaping of the Western understanding of religion and morality followed. The individual was addressed outside of what had been the traditional community of religious men and women. This anticipated the modern shift towards the individual as the source of justification in political, religious, and economic thought. Nonetheless faith in a common human nature, grounded in reason or in morally relevant affections, continued to be a hallmark of the Western culture. As reason was deployed to chart the world, the universe, and the evolution of species so too it was deployed to discover the character of the moral life. Reason became the principal source of the moral life and of moral justification.[6] The project of discovering a universal morality has also been played out by those who relied on appeals to moral sense, sympathy, or common fellow feeling.

Engelhardt argues that the fundamental conceptual difficulty for the project of resolving moral controversies on the basis of rational argument is that one needs a rational standard. Such standards have been sought in: (1) the very content of ethical claims, or in intuitions, as self-evidently right; (2) the consequences of actions; (3) the idea of an unbiased choice made by an ideal rational observer or group of rational contractors; (4) the idea of rational moral choice itself; or (5) the nature of reality. None of these strategies can, however, succeed because there is no way uncontroversially to select or discover the right or true moral content in reason, in intuitions, in consequences, or in the world.[7] The crisis of finding a common starting point is the postmodern dilemma for Engelhardt. If one understands modernity as the search for a common moral framework, postmodernity arises because there are too many narratives.[8] There are too many places from which moral discourse can begin.

The emergence of these many different moral voices articulates the postmodern dilemma for ethics. The modern age had, as one of its characteristics, the hope of discovery of a common, content-full moral view. The postmodern age, exemplified in intellectual movements like feminism, critical legal theory, and deconstructionism, recognizes that pluralism not only has to do with content but with one's understanding of "reason." There is a pluralism of moral theories and values, but no way to choose among the competing accounts. This moral diversity represents a challenge for the way bioethics understands itself. Rather than seeing itself as a unified field articulating a common morality bioethics might come to understand itself as a "field" with many voices. Different assumptions about moral justification lead to different accounts of bioethics. Indeed one might borrow a turn of phrase from Alasdair MacIntyre and ask: Whose Bioethics? Which Rationality?

Engelhardt argues that bioethics brings the postmodern condition into sharp relief. That is, in seeking to address the concrete moral problems of the clinic or health policy bioethics needs some particular moral content. Any ethical theory that addresses particular moral questions must presuppose a set of moral commitments and a view of moral justification. Without such commitments moral language can take on so many meanings as to become meaningless. For

Engelhardt bioethics needs a particular moral content if it is to address the concrete problems of health care. But how are we to choose the content?

In the last thirty years with the emergence of secular bioethics, many of the philosophical attempts to develop a content-full morality from reason have been replayed in bioethics. We find appeals to consequences[9] and hypothetical-contracts,[10] rational decision makers,[11] and natural law. But, these projects tend to be carried out without addressing the foundational questions of moral philosophy. In so far as that is the case, they still suffer from the same foundational and conceptual questions that have plagued moral philosophy in general. They incorporate a particular moral sense to choose accounts of consequences or to discern which account of hypothetical choosers should be endorsed. But, as has already been noted, the rational project of modern moral philosophy appears to have failed.

There have been two important attempts to offset the theoretical dilemmas faced in appeals to rationality in order still to be able to justify particular accounts of bioethics. One well known attempt is that of Beauchamp and Childress and their appeal to mid-level principles.[12] They acknowledge the reality of moral pluralism and the impossibility of deciding between moral theories. They try to meet the problem by developing four "mid-level" principles which persons from different moral frameworks can agree upon and use to resolve controversies. This effort, however, is freighted with difficulties.[13] There are, in general, two problems with this approach.

First, there is the difficulty of determining the meaning of any of the four principles. While Beauchamp and Childress agree on the principle of autonomy, "autonomy" in fact has several possible meanings. Just as Kant and Mill both speak of "autonomy" while having different meanings in mind, one suspects that others use the term in different ways. For a preference utilitarian, like Beauchamp, autonomy will be concerned with the liberty to pursue preferences. For a deontologist, autonomy is not concerned with the pursuit of heteronomous desires but with the demands of reason imposing the moral law. So while the two use the same words, Beauchamp and Childress speak two different languages and must in addition mean different things. The principles become so general that they can take on many meanings and nuances. The language of bioethics goes on holiday from moral practice.

Beauchamp and Childress could reply that the issue is not one of meaning but one of specification. That is, that the meanings of the principles are commonly shared and known. The difficulty is one of specifying the meaning to a particular situation. In their model the process of specification, weighing, and balancing, along with the criterion of coherence are what enables us to address moral issues. Engelhardt's view is that the meanings of the principles are far from clear. One might turn, for example, to the principle of justice which, even formally, can be defined in different ways. Engelhardt argues however, that even if there are common meanings they would be so general, so formal, as to make the principles useless. It is in the specification of the principle that the issues of bioethics are addressed.

There is a second problem with the principlism approach in that it is never clear how the principles are related one to another. Each of the principles is conceived to be *prima facie* binding. That is, they are all of equal weight. How, in conflict situations, are we then to decide rationally which principle to follow? Seeking to avoid the difficulties of theoretical accounts, Beauchamp and Childress have attempted to excise the secondary principles from any type of comprehensive structure. However, shorn of theoretical and contextual moorings the principles can become incomprehensible and incoherent.

A second attempt to offset the difficulties of moral theory has been to revive casuistry. For example, Jonsen and Toulmin provide an historical account of casuistry, and call for the use of casuistry in the postmodern world.[14] However, they never develop an account of how a secular casuistry would work. Traditional casuistry was built upon particular cases and their resolutions which were paradigmatic for moral dilemmas. The casuistry outlined by Jonsen and Toulmin depends on a taxonomy of paradigmatic cases. The obvious question, in a secular, morally pluralistic society, is how we are to identify the paradigmatic cases. Also, the problem exists of how the cases, paradigmatic and new, are to be interpreted in light of the particular moral questions at hand. For example, is physician-assisted suicide best understood under the paradigm of compassion or the paradigm of killing? The difficulty with a secular casuistry is that there is no way to decide which cases are to be the paradigmatic ones.[15] Again, like the appeal to middle level principles, casuistry, shorn of a moral viewpoint offers no way to select the central cases to make the machinery run. Furthermore, in the practice of casuistry the confessor had leeway in which to select the cases on which to model the case of a penitent. Even if a secular casuistry could develop a set of paradigm cases, outside of any particular theoretical and cultural framework, there is still no non-arbitrary way to choose which case should be the model for the dilemma before us outside of a particular moral or theoretical context.

Both the appeal to middle level principles and to casuistry presuppose a moral context not available in a general secular context that is morally pluralistic. Beauchamp and Childress, on the one hand, and Jonsen and Toulmin on the other, each in his own way has attempted to take moral strategies, which succeed within a content-full moral context, and to apply them in circumstances where a common canonical moral content is in fact not available. The general secular context is committed to no particular set of moral values or particular view of moral justification. To the degree that it is morally pluralistic there will be many different views of bioethics. The first part of Engelhardt's argument can be understood as a *via negativa*. He asks why, in principle, the different attempts to resolve moral controversies in bioethics fail. To address specific controversies, he argues, people must share enough in common by way of moral premises and rules of reasoning. Only then can they think through the moral dilemmas at hand. Since a secular society is committed to no particular view of the good (morally) the society is open to moral pluralism. This moral pluralism, while a sociological reality, poses a conceptual dilemma for secular ethics insofar as we have no way to know which is the best set of premises to use.

Engelhardt argues, in *Foundations*, that there is a way to talk about moral authority in the midst of this pluralism. He argues that we should move away, on a secular level, from talking about moral authority in light of a particular content, set of values, or ideas since there is no way to pick out the correct content. But we can know who has moral authority or who is in moral authority. Persons are the source of moral authority.

Insofar as men and women seek to resolve moral controversies, when they lack a common religion or moral vision, when reason cannot discover a rationally authoritative moral vision, and when they do not make a foundational appeal to force, the only source of moral authority is the authority of moral agents through consent and agreement. This appeal, for Engelhardt, is *procedural*. It allows moral strangers to contract with one another without substantive agreement on what is good or bad. It is an appeal that can be understood and shared without sharing a common understanding of the good life or a content-full understanding of the right. Moral strangers can understand whether permission has been given. Contemporary secular practices provide instructive examples of authority by mutual agreement. Limited democracies, with limited authority and enclaves of privacy, have their moral authority insofar as they are grounded in the consent of the governed. The exchanges of the free market provide innumerable examples of the authority, grounded in consent, that can be understood by moral strangers. The practice of free and informed consent in health care is another example of moral strangers collaborating with moral authority grounded in consent. Indeed many of the achievements of bioethics (informed consent, advance directives, prior notification, futility policies) are examples of procedural morality.

The root meaning of authority is the word for the producer of a work such as a writer, an author, or the founder of a family. Authority is drawn from those, who like an author, give rise to a work. Postmodern secular society requires this foundational sense of "authority" in that the only source of moral authority, intelligible to moral strangers, is the authority of moral agents. Justification of choices–whether or not one is praised or blamed–is limited to an account of proper moral authority. The lines of moral authority are traced to the consent of the moral agents rather than the content of a moral worldview.

Universal authority of agreement is content-poor. It is this poverty which allows it to be universal. It does, however, provide a minimal basis for procedures by which one can account for moral authority. This understanding of authority offers a way to justify moral authority without a foundational appeal to force while avoiding a nihilism. This appeal to procedural authority offers a way to understand when force can be morally justified: it can be used against those who use others without permission.

Some label this as simply one more liberal appeal to individualism. This is certainly one reading, perhaps the most widespread one, of the first edition of *The Foundations*. But such labels misunderstand Engelhardt's argument. It is not an argument that appeals to individualism or the value of freedom, or the value of autonomy. Such appeals would involve giving accent to some values over others, and thus be only one among numerous possible accounts. Rather, what is offered by Engelhardt is a transcendental argument that sets out a minimal grammar for moral discourse when men and women do not share the same substantive views of moral justification or content-full views of the moral life. This is a transcendental argument in the sense of setting out the necessary condition (i.e., what he now has rebaptized as the principle of permission) for the possibility of general secular morality. The conceptual problems of moral justification, in a morally pluralistic, secular society lead to a communal libertarianism but not to a community of libertarians. Robust, thick views of the moral life must be developed within moral communities that share common moral frameworks. In a political society that understands itself as secular, there will be limits on the moral vision, health care policy, and content-full conclusions of bioethics that can be imposed justifiably by the state. Such limits stem from the limits of our moral knowledge. We can only justify what is shared. What we can always share is agreement. Common projects, like health care, are possible insofar as they are freely undertaken.

FRIENDS AND STRANGERS

The communitarian conclusions of Engelhardt's argument are often lost in discussions of his work. And this is not surprising. The focus of his project, in both *Foundations* and *Secular Humanism*, is on *the possibility of general secular bioethics*, not on a communitarian ethics. The books set out the problems of moral pluralism, the limits of philosophy, and the justification of moral authority. The resolution of the postmodern condition that leads to his libertarian view of the state also leads to his communitarian thought. Furthermore, his communitarian views are also lost, in part, because by Engelhardt's own logic, one cannot write a communitarian bioethics except within a particular moral community. The moral pluralism that creates the postmodern condition is antithetical to a common communitarian ethics. A society is not a community. It is, however, important to understand Engelhardt's communitarian views because they directly influence his view about the extent to which a common morality is possible for a secular society.

One finds three elements in Engelhardt's work that identifies the broad spectrum of moral communities. Moral communities will have (1) some particular, content-full moral view, (2) some understanding of moral authority within a community and (3) some understanding of how the community should relate to other communities and views.

Some moral communities, most notably religious ones, provide thick backgrounds for understanding the meaning of life and the moral life. *The Foundations* begins with the recognition that there are concrete communities within which men and women can live coherent moral lives and pursue virtue. Each community possesses a concrete bioethics in some form or other. Some moral communities are able to give a full and substantial context for the moral life. He writes "[t]his book begins with the recognition that there are concrete communities within which men and women can live coherent moral lives and pursue virtue."[16] Communities often provide a thick context for moral and bioethical choices and practices. Other communities, by definition, may be much more eclectic and open. That is, they define themselves by a more ecumenical view of the world. Of course how communities define themselves shapes how they see themselves in relationship to the world. To investigate these elements in Engelhardt's work it is helpful to sort out the language of moral strangers and moral friends.

There seems to be an analogy at work in Engelhardt's writing. Just as friends and strangers are defined in relationship to one another, so too are communities and society. The terms moral friends and moral community rely on one another. Engelhardt writes that "...*community* is used to identify a body of men and women bound together by common moral traditions and/or practices around a shared vision of the good life, which allows them to collaborate as moral friends."[17] Later he writes that "[i]t is within communi- ties, not large-scale societies, that one is embedded in a full matrix of moral content and structures. It is within particular moral communities that one lives and finds full meaning in life and concrete moral direction."[18] Communities teach by way of example (e.g., saints, heroes, heroines) and stories (e.g., histories, literature). "Those who live in such a moral community will recog- nize their position as that which all *ought* morally to embrace."[19] Friends are those who share a common vision within particular moral communities.[20] It is the common moral vision that helps to constitute the community and identify moral friends. Engelhardt writes: "It is within particular moral communities that one lives and finds full meaning in life and concrete moral direction. It is within particular moral communities that one possesses a content-full bioethics."[21] Within such communities one learns the moral and non-moral good(s) that ought to be pursued and in what way. One learns what promises should be made, and the proper attitude toward death and suffering. Communi- ties teach morality through example. Role models of the virtues are important to the life of the community. Within the life of a community morality, Engelhardt argues, is not simply an aesthetic choice. Rather it is a truth to be lived.[22]

Moral discourse in a secular society is the discourse of moral strangers. For Engelhardt to be moral strangers requires "only that the other be seen as other because of differences in moral and/or metaphysical commitments. The recognition of moral strangers leads to the recognition of the limits of state authority."[23] At first glance one would think that moral strangers ought to be opaque to one another. But while this may be the case, it is not a necessary condition for people to be moral strangers. Engelhardt writes: "it is important to understand that moral strangers do not find each other morally inscrutable.

Moral strangers may share the same values, but only have different orderings of these values."[24] The discourse of bioethics in general, is in secular society a discourse that Engelhardt characterizes as an empty, procedural framework.[25] Yet, because it is empty, this framework provides a way that moral strangers can cooperate in health care.

Moral friends not only share a common content-full view of morality but they have common understandings of authority within a community. It would seem that almost any community will have figures who are considered as "experts" or moral "authorities." These may be wise women or men, holy people, saints, or theologians. A community may also have a juridical notion of authority: those *in* authority (e.g., Bishops, Pope, confessors). At times the two types of authority may even overlap. A community has beliefs about matters of proper behavior as well as regarding the boundaries of the community. A Roman Catholic who is involved in the procurement of an abortion knows that a sin is involved.[26] A Roman Catholic who publicly contends that the Church is wrong, that abortion is not a sin, commits an act so wrong as to be subject to excommunication. The authority of a community contrasts with authority in the secular state–between moral strangers–which is procedural. The secular state is libertarian because it lacks an authoritative, content-full moral vision. Its moral authority rests on consent and permission.

Matters of bioethics are not simply isolated principles or propositions but part of the actual life of real communities. How people respond to the issues of bioethics will indicate whether or not they are in or out of the community. Bioethical commitments can be integral to the moral boundaries of the communities. For communities of robust commitments and strict observances the strongest possible penalty that a community could use would be excommunication. Religious communities have deployed such penalties (excommunication, shunning) extensively. Even secular "religions," like Marxism or the Greens, expel from the party members judged heretical. Like the procedures for admission to a community, the forms of correction–even excommunication–are part of the community's ability to maintain its own identity. These procedures indicate the gravity of offenses and remind members of both the penalty and the reason for or justification of the punishment.

There is a third element that gives shape to the identity of a moral community: its understanding of its mission and relationship to other communities. As part of its self-understanding of mission each community will have to determine how it will relate to the other communities in a secular society. At one extreme is what can be termed the "Amish" option: a withdrawal from the world. This option does not always, however, represent a "clean" break with the secular world in that there will inevitably be some interaction.

If the Amish option represents one end of a spectrum of communal responses, the other end might be called the "Unitarian Option." Rather than strive to maintain moral integrity at all costs, a community with a moral vision can engage the world *in terms the world will understand.* That is, in terms that can bind moral strangers. This option involves a significant risk for the moral faith and integrity of a community. In the search for agreement with those outside the community, the content of that community can be evacuated. This evacuation of moral content, as the community attempts to avoid offending others, accommodates the character of the age. Communities which seek to engage in substantive moral compromise with moral strangers expose themselves to the risk of loosing their own moral identity. The drive to be ecumenical, to bridge differences and particularities, can suppress differences and devour content.[27] The Ecumenical Content Monster (ECM) threatens to destroy the particular content of any community in the search for common moral ground and agreement. In this way Christian communities have, for example, come to accept abortion, assisted suicide, mindless vitalism, or the ideology of equality.

The ECM is a particular danger for moral communities that want to address moral problems in the world in terms the world can easily understand.[28] The difficulty is to discover *how* to address such problems in common with others who do not share the same moral point of view or the same interpretation of human experience. To begin with, members of a particular community must recognize their own background assumptions (e.g., the "sacredness of life," "common good") as well as those of others. In an effort to reach those outside the boundaries of a particular community, the community may try to express its own moral vision through the moral languages and concerns of the moral strangers and acquaintances they confront. In the process moral meaning may be attenuated and the guidance of traditions lost. The result can be that the moral community blends without border into the larger society and loses its particular moral commitments and its moral integrity. Such loss of content can occur in what appears to be an innocent moral dialogue which simply forgoes strong reminders of moral differences and of the need for morally condemning what one must also tolerate.

In exploring the relationship of the distinctions of moral friends and strangers, community and society, one can find the broad outlines of Engelhardt's communitarian thought. Each community will have its own content-full moral vision, its own understanding of moral authority, and its own view of how to relate to other communities. Engelhardt does not propose a communitarian ethic. By his own argument about postmodernity, there cannot be a communitarian bioethics. There will be many.

ENGELHARDT'S SECTARIAN MODEL OF COMMUNITY

In spite of his views of the varieties of moral communities there is reason to suspect that Engelhardt has a particular, sectarian view of community in mind in his writing. This suspicion is fostered because of Engelhardt's strong distinction between moral friends and moral strangers and his view of the minimal possibilities for moral discourse in a secular society. His view of moral strangers indicates that he presumes a strong, sectarian model of community. Moral strangers are any who have "differences in moral and/or metaphysical commitments."[29] Friends, presumably, share the same moral and/or metaphysical commitments. However, on Engelhardt's view men and women within a religious community who have different commitments would be strangers. Antiochean Catholics and Roman Catholics surely are moral strangers. However, even Franciscans and Dominicans are moral strangers on this account because they have different metaphysical views. While they are members of different religious communities, with different metaphysics and spiritualities, Franciscans and Dominicans still see themselves as part of the larger community of Roman Catholics. The only way to account for Engelhardt's claim about moral strangers is to understand that he has a particular model of community and he fails to take seriously other models. I want to argue that this view fails to take seriously that it is possible for a community to understand itself, *qua* community, as diverse and ecumenical. Roman Catholicism has been able to endure the different metaphysics of Franciscans (nominalism) and Dominicans (realism) and still see itself as a community. Engelhardt's view of community does not seem to allow for communities that define themselves around overlapping values or overlapping projects with other communities. If Engelhardt holds that they can't see themselves as part of a larger community, then he is importing his own view of community, something he cannot do by his own postmodern argument.

In addition to Engelhardt's claims about metaphysical differences and community, one also finds a second clue to Engelhardt's ideas about community is his discussion and references to ecumenism in the second edition of *Foundations*. Engelhardt uses the term *cosmopolitan ecumenist* "to identify those individuals who hold that, given sufficient discussion, individuals will come to see that they share a common content-full morality, however sparse."[30] Throughout the text he uses the term pejoratively. The ecumenist, on Engelhardt's view, seeks bonds of unity that are not there or minimizes differences that are. Engelhardt uses the term in the same way that MacIntyre uses the term "cosmopolitan" in *After Virtue*. That is, the ecumenist is seen as the rootless individual who eclectically builds his/her identity from bits and pieces of traditions but who is unable to claim any tradition. In linking the term "ecumenism" with "cosmopolitan" Engelhardt dismisses communities that define themselves, *qua* community, as ecumenical.

Out of these different clues one finds a view that sees moral communities as very particularized and separated one from another. It is a view that assumes that communities will have strong definitions of themselves, of who is in and who is out, and of the boundaries with other communities. Yet, by his own postmodern lights we know that Engelhardt cannot philosophically hold that this is the only vision of community. Absent a canonical framework he will have to allow that there are other, less strict, models. Yet, his account of moral friends and strangers seems to rely on a particular vision of moral community.

One can surmise that this view of community is influenced by his reflection on the project of modernity and the project of reason. In acknowledging the limits of reason Engelhardt not only turned away from the Enlightenment project, but turned toward moral fideism. One can agree with Engelhardt that there is no rational argument that will lead one to "faith" (a basic moral world view). Yet one does not have to hold that this precludes "faith seeking understanding."

It is this fideistic stance that leads to Engelhardt's implicit view of moral communities and their incommensurable relationship. However, there is no reason to think, in principle, that moral communities cannot understand and express themselves in ways that others can understand and agree with. They may not see one another in the light of day but they can see through the glass darkly. There seems to be no room for those who share overlapping commitments and, thus, the possibility for a weaker sense of community. One can think for a moment of different moral communities opposed to abortion.

Members of different moral communities can find common points of agreement around specific issues. We should not make more of this agreement than is warranted. Real differences remain. That is why different communities remain distinct. Nonetheless, in the differences there are possibilities of agreement and understanding. There can be moral acquaintanceship as well as moral friendship and moral strangeness.

Again, by his own lights, we know that there is more overlapping of communities than Engelhardt seems to allow. If procedures, such as the free market, are to succeed, then there must be overlapping commitments to moral values such as honesty, and consent. It is possible for a secular society to find within itself moral agreements reached by diverse moral communities. This does not mean that the state can impose a particular moral view but it does mean that there can be a moral culture in the society. Certainly there must be some basic agreements that underlie the procedures of a secular society. It seems that it is also possible for communities to understand themselves in such a way that they define themselves, in part, by their relationship to other communities. They need not exist as isolated monads incapable of discussion and argument.

MORAL ACQUAINTANCES

In a postmodern era, with many moralities, there will be, potentially, a variety of moral communities. It is possible to envision a whole spectrum of voluntary moral communities reflecting the degree of commitment required to form a community. At one end, there are communities that require a person to volunteer his or her whole life (e.g., religious communities) while at the other end there are communities that are focused on a particular service (e.g., Kiwanis, Rotary). Another way to understand the spectrum of possibilities is to see at one end what could be described as "laxist" moral communities. Here "laxist" refers to the entrance and maintenance requirements of the community. The other end of the spectrum is marked by communities of "strict observance." Candidates are screened and they go through a rigorous process of admission. Christian rituals of the catechumenate, continued to this day, exemplify this. In the process one is schooled in the beliefs and ways of the community. In this process the community renews its identity not only in the new members, but also in repeating its own narrative. The extent to which bioethical accounts have both a theoretical and material coherence will depend not only on the possibility of authoritatively resolving moral controversies but as well on the extent to which bioethical commitments are supported in a community with an integral wholeness.

There is no reason to think that members of different communities will only have differences. They may have moral similarities as well. They may be different enough so as not to be moral friends but still share enough in common so as not to be moral strangers. Insofar as they could share certain moral commitments so as to understand one another and work together (e.g., those in the prolife movement), they could be called moral acquaintances. Engelhardt's view of community, focused on moral differences, leads to a view of the moral world as made up of strangers and friends.

Yet even the procedural relationship of moral strangers reflects the reality of moral acquaintanceship. Procedures, like all method, can be distinguished from content, but they cannot be separated. Much of modern philosophy has followed Descartes' search for a pure method. Yet, as thinkers such as Wittgenstein have argued, establishing a rule, method, or procedure reflects a particular point of view (or content, in Engelhardt's language). While Engelhardt has understood part of the postmodern challenge he still stands with one foot in the Enlightenment tradition insofar as he thinks he can find a procedure that is content-free. Yet, for the procedures of consent to work there are necessary commitments to particular views of rationality, the value of peace, and the value of persons. Engelhardt's procedures point us in the direction of common moral commitments that are shared across communal boundaries.

CONCLUSION

This essay has argued that Engelhardt must be understood as both a libertarian and a communitarian. His argument about the postmodern condition leads to both conclusions. One must look through this argument to find its communitarian conclusions and implications. If one looks through the argument one can see the dim outlines and implications for communitarian bioethics. There are three central elements of a moral community: content, authority, relationship to other communities. These elements provide a way to understand a wide range of moral communities that give us communitarian bioethics. The essay has further argued that Engelhardt does have a particular model of community in mind in *The Foundations* and this model leads to his view of the emptiness of secular society. However, if one examines the practices of a secular society one finds an area of moral acquaintanceship.

NOTES

1. M. T. Cicero, *De Res Publica*, trans. C. W. Keyes, (Cambridge: Loeb Classical Library, 1928).

2. *Dikaion nomikon* (positive law) and *dikaion physikon* (natural law). See Francis de Zulueta, *The Institutes of Gaius* (Oxford: Clarendon Press, 1976), Vol. 2, p. 13.

3. One can trace this movement by the shift of the center of theological reflection from the monastery to the cathedral schools. The scholastic methodology led to the systematic and comprehensive study of theology as an *academic* discipline (See Jean Leclercq, "From St. Gregory to St. Bernard" in *The Spirituality of the Middle Ages*, vol. 2 of *A History of Christian Spirituality* by J. Leclercq, F. Vandenbrouche, and L. Bouyer (New York: The Seabury Press, 1968). Scholastic theology was not rationalistic. Indeed one finds in St. Thomas Aquinas a careful exploration of the relationship of faith and reason. He writes: "Therefore it is useful that besides philosophical science there should be other knowledge...[I]t was necessary that there should be a knowledge revealed by God, besides philosophical science built up by human reason...Hence it was necessary for the salvation of man that certain truths which exceed human reason should be made known by divine revelation" (*Summa Theologica* [Westminster, MD: Christian Classics, 1948], I, Q.1, art.1). Yet scholasticism was often tempted by rationalism (See, Chrysostom Frank, "St. Bernard of Clairvaux and the Eastern Christian Tradition," *St. Vladimir's Theological Quarterly* 36, 315-328). One can trace the centrality of natural, philosophical reason through the Middle Ages into the Renaissance and find that theologians in the 17th century responded to atheism with a defense of Christianity "without appeal to anything Christian" (See, Michael Buckley, *At The Origins of Modern Atheism* (New Haven: Yale University Press, 1987), 67. The first Vatican Council officially promulgated the Church's position that the existence of God could be known by natural reason ("*Si quis dixerit, Deum unum et verum, creatorem et Dominum Nostrum, per ea, quae facta sunt, naturalit rationis humanae lumine certo cognosci no posse: anathema sit*," Canones 2, *De Revelatione*, #1, cited in H. Denzinger & A. Schonmetzer, *Enchiridion Symbolorum* (Freiburg: Herder, 1963), #3026. See also, Jaroslav Pelikan, *Christianity and Classical Culture: The Metamorphosis of Natural Theology in the Christian Encounter with Hellenism* (New Haven: Yale University Press, 1993).

4. T. Aquinas, *Summa Theologica*, I-II, Q. 93.

5. H. Tristram Engelhardt, Jr., *Bioethics and Secular Humanism: The Search for a Common Morality* (London: SCM Press, 1991).

6. See I. Kant, *The Fundamental Principles of the Metaphysics of Morals* (Indianapolis: The Liberal Arts Press, 1949); T. Nagel, *The View From Nowhere* (New York: Oxford University Press, 1986); J. Rawls, *A Theory of Justice* (Cambridge: Harvard University Press, 1971).

7. H. Tristram Engelhardt, Jr., *The Foundations of Bioethics* (New York: Oxford University Press, 1996), especially Chapters One and Two.

8. See J.-F. Lyotard, *The Postmodern Condition*, trans. G. Bennington and B. Massumi, (Manchester: Manchester University Press, 1984), and Engelhardt, *Foundations*.

9. P. Singer, *Practical Ethics* (Cambridge: Cambridge University Press, 1979).

10. R. Veatch, *A Theory of Medical Ethics* (New York: Basic Books, 1981).

11. N. Daniels, *Just Health Care* (Cambridge: Cambridge University Press, 1985).

12. Tom L. Beauchamp and James F. Childress, *Principles of Biomedical Ethics*, 4th Ed., (New York: Oxford University Press, 1995).

13. See B. A. Brody, "Quality of Scholarship in Bioethics," *Journal of Medicine and Philosophy* 15 (1990); R. Green, "Method in Bioethics," *Journal of Medicine and Philosophy* 15 (1990); K. D. Clouser and B. Gert, "A Critique of Principlism," *Journal of Medicine and Philosophy* 15 (1990); B. A. Lustig, "Principles: A Critique of the Critique," *Journal of Medicine and Philosophy* 15 (1990); D. De Grazia, "Moving Forward in Bioethical Theory: Theories, Cases, and Specified Principlism," *Journal of Medicine and Philosophy* 15 (1990).

14. Albert Jonsen and Stephen Toulmin, *The Abuse of Casuistry* (Berkeley: University of California Press, 1988).

15. K. W. Wildes, "The Priesthood of Bioethics and the Return of Casuistry," *Journal of Medicine and Philosophy* 18 (1993): 33-49.

16. Engelhardt, *Foundations*, viii.

17. Engelhardt, *Foundations*, 7.

18. Engelhardt, *Foundations*, 74.

19. Engelhardt, *Foundations*, 74.

20. Engelhardt, *Foundations*, 76.

21. Engelhardt, *Foundations*, 74.

22. Engelhardt, *Foundations*, 77.

23. Engelhardt, *Foundations*, 81.

24. Engelhardt, *Foundations*, 24 n.13.

25. Engelhardt, *Foundations*, 78.

26. The penalty is as follows: "A person who procures a successful abortion incurs an automatic (*latae sententiae*) excommunication." (A *latae sententiae* penalty is a penalty inflicted by the law itself upon commission of the offense. It is distinguished from a *ferendae sententiae* penalty which is imposed by the action of a judge or superior.) See, *Code of Canon Law* (Washington, D.C.: Canon Law Society of America, 1983), c. #1398.

27. See George Marsden, *The Soul of the American University: From Protestant Establishment to Established Non Belief* (New York: Oxford University Press, 1994). Marsden argues the Protestant universalism became the very ideology that undermined strong Christian beliefs in Protestant universities.

28. L. S. Cahill, "Theology and Bioethics: Should Religious Traditions Have a Public Voice?" *Journal of Medicine and Philosophy*, 17: 263-272.

29. Engelhardt, *Foundations*, 80.

30. Engelhardt, *Foundations*, 27 n.17; *Bioethics and Secular Humanism*, 33-40.

5

MONOPOLY WITH SICK MORAL STRANGERS

WADE L. ROBISON

Engelhardt believes that with the loss of firm foundations for moral theory, the only morally proper ground for public policy can be what we agree to when we meet as moral strangers. The result for health care, he thinks, is at best a multi-tier system with what is minimally adequate health care being contestable.

Individuals may agree to enter into richer forms of moral relations–loving, caring, helping–but these fuller relations are fragile, the more difficult to sustain the more they demand of participants and the greater the number of participants. Yet it is not just the difficulties of sustaining richer forms of moral life that prevent their widespread application for public policy matters. It is that in a pluralistic society such as ours, citizens meet only as moral strangers and will not agree to share rich moral lives. What can be agreed to gains its moral legitimacy from the process itself and is thus, he says, immanently grounded. As the results for health care show, what he thinks we can agree to is thin indeed.

We should be skeptical. Nothing contingent is unconditioned, and so when moral strangers meet to work out how to engage in a common enterprise, such as health care, there are conditions for their negotiations with each other. Some of these, as we shall see, are morally loaded and subject to the same sorts of skeptical concerns Engelhardt directs against other supposed moral bases such as utilitarianism or deontology. His enterprise fails in the same way he thinks they fail, by "presupposing what they set out to establish: canonical moral guidance."[1]

In addition, at least some of the conditions Engelhardt presumes for negotiation are themselves subject to negotiation–and would be negotiated, were it possible, by self-interested individuals concerned with the stability of the system. We could have, following his principles, a very different system than he thinks possible. Engelhardt thus cannot only not justify morality, he cannot justify the particular conception of our health care system he hawks.

I begin with a situation which captures some essentials of what occurs between moral strangers engaged in a common enterprise. I am concerned to illustrate Engelhardt's remark that "even if one does not attain transcendental rationality, one obtains an immanent, transcendental grounding for this decision

B. P. Minogue et al. (eds.), Reading Engelhardt, 95–112.
© 1997 *Kluwer Academic Publishers. Printed in the Netherlands.*

of...[free] will: a game, a grammatical possibility that cannot be avoided and which comes with inescapable rules but no content (69)."

THE LANGUAGE-GAME OF *MONOPOLY* [2]

Monopoly is a game in which wealth is distributed, and so we may ask, "Is it just?" Indeed, the way the game begins emphasizes its deep concern with justice.

First, everyone is equally situated with respect to the goods of the game. The end of the game is the accumulation of as much money and property as the limits of the game permit. At the beginning, no one has any property, and everyone has the same amount of money.

Second, since only with property is it possible to retain any money we accumulate and since we can only purchase property by landing on it, it is an advantage to land first on any property and so an advantage to go first. The determination of the order of play has consequences for the final distribution of wealth. The rules ensure that no player begins with an unfair advantage:

(a) Everyone is to toss a die, the player with the highest number to go first and then each in order around the board. This is an instance of pure procedural justice:[3] the order of play is determined by a procedure free of any defect that could bias the result.[4]

(b) In some versions of the game the players must round the board once, or even twice, before being entitled to make a purchase. The aim is to ensure that any disadvantages created by the initial determination of order of play be mitigated by subsequent tosses.[5] The presumption apparently is that the luck of further tosses will mitigate the bad luck of an initial toss.

One reason to take such pains to ensure that the players begin equally situated is that by the end of the game, if it is played to the end, they are normally situated very unequally, with one having all the wealth of the game and the rest having none. But this inequality is produced by a pure procedure that maximizes freedom of choice while holding everyone to the same rules.

As the players roll the dice in turn, they are required to move the number of squares shown on the dice. If they land on property, they have three choices–pay the owner rent or, if it is unowned, buy it from the bank or pass it by. Each choice causes a redistribution of the goods of the game. Money passes to another player for rent or to the bank for the property, or an opportunity to purchase passes to other players.

As the game proceeds in this way, money and property are distributed and then redistributed, but each transaction is subject to the rules common to all the players and, where possible, to the control of the player affected. A player has no choice about getting $200 for passing GO, but can choose to purchase property or not if it is available.

Players may make poor choices, refraining from buying a crucial piece of property when they could have, or spending their resources on poor properties at the beginning and not having enough left to purchase more valuable property as the game progresses. But these are their choices, not anyone else's, and as someone, such as Engelhardt, articulating the implications of this game must say, "They can have no just complaint because the game allows poor choices."[6]

What would justify a complaint within the game is something that skews the procedure by which the game operates–some irregularity in the determination of order of play or in the process of play. We all know what can go wrong in such games. Someone cheats by turning over mortgaged cards without paying off the mortgage. Or an older sibling may tell a younger, "You better not buy B&O! That's mine!" To the extent that the final results of the game reflect a player's being coerced, or cheating that occurs, they are as unfair as if the player stole the B&O. Yet if the transactions of the game are uncoerced and in accord with the rules, the final results, whatever they may be, are just. No player has any proper ground of complaint even if everything is lost. Or so the argument must run.

As Engelhardt would put it, we can meet as moral strangers when we play *Monopoly*. We need not even know each other, let alone share any richer moral life. Yet the structure of the cooperative enterprise that is *Monopoly* provides for a moral result as long as the players act, without coercion or cheating, in accord with the rules by which they effectively agreed to abide in agreeing to play the game. Indeed, the structure respects the players, putting them in positions where they must make choices that make significant differences to their lives in the game and to the lives of the other players as well. The result of the game is a negotiated solution, on Engelhardt's view, created by the choices of participants as they pursue the ends of the game.[7]

Monopoly is Engelhardt's view of society writ small.[8] In competition in the marketplace, the argument runs, no one is entitled to complain when, at the end of the day, the farmer ends up with less produce and more money and various customers have less money, but more produce. As long as no one cheated, and no one was coerced, the exchanges of money for produce are just, the distribution at the end of the day is as just as the distribution at the beginning. This is true even if a customer paid too much for rutabaga or the farmer sold endive for too little. As long as the procedure according to which the transactions took place is itself pure, as long, that is, as the transactions are agreed to by the parties, however ill-conceived or stupid or faulty in any other way we or they may come to think the transactions to be, the end results, however unequal they may be, are just, and no party to the process can have any moral ground for complaint (69).

With cooperative enterprises such as *Monopoly*, or the marketplace, we can "reach to individuals across moral communities" and rely only on their permissions to achieve whatever results occur (5). Trying to found public policy on such ethical theories as utilitarianism or intuitionism fails, Engelhardt argues, because these theories impose the grounds of agreement: they have content and are not just procedural (46). But appealing "to permission as the source of authority involves no particular moral vision or understanding. It gives no value to permission" (69). Such an appeal provides "moral authority" (71), and that authority has powerful moral consequences. It makes morally right the outcomes not only of such cooperative enterprises as *Monopoly* where individuals agree to start out with equal shares and, though a series of voluntary transactions, end up with unequal shares.[9] It makes right the outcomes of any cooperative enterprise in which we distribute benefits and burdens–provided only that the procedure for producing the distribution rests upon the agreements of the parties involved.

Or such is the story Engelhardt tells. The question is whether such outcomes are legitimate, whether we obtain "an immanent, transcendental grounding" through the procedures of the game–where the only content is presumably provided by the rules that create the conditions for play and by the play of the participants. Does the game smuggle in values somehow, or is the grounding untainted by moral presuppositions?

CONDITIONS OF PLAY

Monopoly is a form of cooperative enterprise that makes prominent certain features of the players, accentuating the value of some and depressing the value of others. A willingness to acquiesce in what we judge to be the interests of others will not serve us well in *Monopoly*, for we will pass over property we should purchase to maintain our competitive position. Indeed, someone who always willingly refuses to purchase property others say they might want would soon be invited to play only whenever everyone wanted a patsy. There are, in short, conditions of play for *Monopoly*–including features individuals must have if they are to play the game or play it well.

For instance, players need to comprehend the strategic ends of the game and how features of the game are connected to those ends–how purchasing houses and hotels furthers their chances of winning.[10] They need a capacity to judge what best advances those ends–when purchasing hotels most advances their cause or best sets back the position of some other player.[11] They need the competitive drive to act when it is most advantageous to act–purchasing valuable property when they can and giving less weight to whatever interests another player may have in, say, having all the railroads. In short, players need a game-sense and a competitive spirit–as well as such features as patience and a willingness to continue to play even when the chances of winning begin to approach zero.[12]

Monopoly is thus no more value-free than commerce. The commercialization of tomatoes has produced tomatoes with a longer shelf life that ripen only off the vine and are less juicy–a natural consequence of retailers wanting tomatoes that will withstand the rigors of being squeezed by various potential customers and yet remain relatively attractive for some time afterwards.[13] And just as some consumers do not value such tomatoes, so some do not want to play *Monopoly*. The values it accentuates need not be shared. Someone of a cooperative and generous nature may be ill-disposed towards the competitive atmosphere *Monopoly* engenders and prefer playing a different game that makes competitive features deficits and cooperative features assets. *Monopoly* is no more value-neutral than value-free.

Monopoly does not smuggle in values. They are of its essence. The conditions of play are as value-laden as anything predicated on such moral theories as utilitarianism or intuitionism. Any game shares these features, accentuating the value of certain characteristics over others, some, such as soccer, or doubles in tennis, requiring cooperation among the players, others, such as *Monopoly* or poker, requiring an intensely individualistic competitive spirit within the cooperative structure created by the rules of the game. And each has its conditions of play, each requiring, as with poker, such capacities as knowing "when to hold them and when to fold them."[14]

Just so, Engelhardt does not smuggle in values. Values are of the essence in understanding how permissions can function in producing public policy. We would not choose to have those negotiate for us who are psychologically unwilling to press others. Such individuals are not well positioned to further their own ends, or any ends, when they negotiate to achieve some public policy objective. Engelhardt's conception makes other sorts of individuals prime players–those who are adept at negotiation because they understand the significance of making demands that cannot be met in order to get more than they might otherwise obtain, because they are willing to stand fast by their demands way past the time compromise seems appropriate in order to pressure the other parties to accede to their wishes, because they are willing to bluster, feign anger, and cause scenes, because they understand the limits of such behavior, because they can use their emotional responses to the ends in question and not get so caught up in them that they cannot discard them when they become counterproductive, and so on. Getting permission is sometimes not easy, and since Engelhardt objects only to coercion, those able to push what he calls "peaceable manipulation" to the limits are better positioned to win their ends than those who are not (308).[15]

Manipulating others, even peaceably, seems *prima facie* at odds with the sort of respect for others that one might think would underpin any theory of morality which relies upon getting permissions of the parties involved for any joint project. What may come to mind when we think of an instance of what Engelhardt considers the basis of morality are individuals, fully rational and fully informed, negotiating with each other, in respectful ways, to find some solution to a common problem. We may picture two individuals listening to each other's positions, each trying to understand fully what the other wants and jointly committed to working out some solution to a common problem that would be mutually acceptable–about what to do for an evening, or what to have for dinner, or how to proceed regarding some difficulty with a child.

This conception is not value-free, of course. To listen respectfully to those with whom one disagrees is to have an attitude towards those others, and an attitude towards the point of mutual discussions, which is rich with moral value, but the picture Engelhardt is willing to accept is different. So long as I do not coerce the person whose permission I am trying to obtain, I may do what I wish–so construct the choice situation that those I am negotiating with will think they have put one over on me when, in fact, I have gotten just what I want, so construct it that they will feel guilty about thinking they are putting one over on me and so will choose what I want, and so on. I am not permitted to force my views on others involved in a common enterprise, but am permitted to manipulate them in any way "as long as the individual being manipulated can still act, that is, choose, and be held responsible" (308).

Working out the details of the limits of such manipulation would be essential for a fully articulated theory of morality based on permissions, but we need not know the details to know that such a theory is not value-free or value-neutral–and to wonder whether we should wish to encourage a moral theory which accentuates the value of manipulating others. The rules of his game create a procedure that is morally loaded, that is, in ways we may lament since it encourages what some may consider disreputable character traits. In any event, requiring that public policy be based on the permissions of individuals accentuates some features of individuals and depresses others, makes some assets and others deficits for the ends in question. Engelhardt's theory is thus neither value-free nor value-neutral. It remains to be shown, however, that its lack of neutrality affects the substantive moral conclusions Engelhardt draws.

CONSTITUTIVE CONDITIONS

The dependence of *Monopoly* on those aspects of individuals which emphasize their competitive spirit is an artifact of the game, and we could choose to play a game in which helping others was a crucial determinant to whether we won or lost, for instance. But we would then change games. The conditions of play we have articulated for *Monopoly* are expressive of its constitutive features, the rules and conditions that give it an essentially competitive nature.[16]

It is, for instance, a constitutive condition of *Monopoly* that players are subject to the same rules. A variant of *Monopoly* might allow inexperienced players to borrow from the bank to make purchases so that early bad judgments about what to purchase would not quickly end the game. It is another constitutive condition that all the players be able to play. Infants cannot play *Monopoly*.

That claim has the ring of analyticity to it that we should expect from articulating the constitutive conditions of a cooperative enterprise such as *Monopoly*. That such propositions seem obvious might seem so obvious as not to be worth mentioning except that Engelhardt's substantive moral views consist primarily of articulating the implications of the constitutive conditions he imposes for permissions.

A moral stranger for Engelhardt is someone who is self-conscious and rational, with at least a minimal moral sense and the capacity to make decisions

(139). Fetuses and infants lack these characteristics, he says, and so he concludes that abortion is morally permissible, fetuses having only extrinsic value "for [the] actual persons" who are players in his moral game (143). The appropriate stance Engelhardt thinks we should take towards infants is more complicated, but since they are not persons, they have no claim on those of us who are (150). At most, we can agree to accord them value because of value they have to us.

Engelhardt makes these moral claims about fetuses and infants as though they were patently obvious, and they are if we accept certain constitutive conditions of his position. An entity who (or which) is not entitled to participate in the moral process that underpins for Engelhardt our minimal common moral life can, at most, hope that those who are entitled to participate will consider their interests. Not being players in Engelhardt's game, they can have no more claim on what moves participants make than a *Monopoly* kibitzer has that his or her preferred moves be made by one of the players.

Similarly, Engelhardt says, there is no "defensible basis to forbid the rich from purchasing health care not available to the poor" (78). This too is obvious–provided at least that health care is treated as a commodity and that the system is so arranged that moral strangers making decisions about health care need not be similarly situated with respect to their capacity to purchase health care. Again, Engelhardt says that physicians have the right to refuse to provide abortions (82). Their right follows from their being moral strangers. They cannot be coerced into providing something they do not agree to provide.

It is as with *Monopoly*. Just as no one can prevent the rich from buying more health care than the poor, as the health care system is currently configured, so no one can properly prevent players in *Monopoly* from purchasing whatever unowned property they land on, and as the game proceeds, players will become differently positioned with respect to their capacity to purchase. Similarly, just as the current health care system is configured in a way that makes requiring physicians to provide abortion coercion, *Monopoly* is so configured that players cannot be coerced into purchasing unowned property.

We can imagine a variety of different versions of *Monopoly* where the particular configuration of choices and relations is changed because we have changed the constitutive conditions of the game. We can imagine a version where the property is allocated along with the order of play so that everyone starts equally situated with respect to property. There would be no unowned property. So purchasing property would not be an option in the game, and players could never be differently situated with respect to their capacity to purchase property. In such a version shrewd purchasing of property could not be valued, and coercion regarding purchasing could not exist.

The "could not" in that last proposition is meant to signal that it follows from constitutive features of the game. We are laying out logical implications here. And, of course, such propositions are *obvious*–as obvious as it is for Engelhardt, given the constitutive features he imposes on morality, that abortion is morally permissible or that physicians cannot be coerced into providing abortions or that a two-tier health care system is morally permissible.

These implications have moral content and follow from constitutive conditions of Engelhardt's conception. If fetuses and infants do not have standing as moral strangers, their only value can be the extrinsic value they have to those who do have standing in a system which creates value through the permissions of moral strangers. If moral strangers are unequally situated with regard to their capacity to purchase a commodity, and health care is a commodity, nothing can prevent some from purchasing more than others.[17]

Whether we agree with these implications is not the issue. What is at issue is that they follow from constitutive features of the structure Engelhardt articulates. But just as we can readily imagine changing the constitutive conditions of *Monopoly* to create completely different sets of possibilities for players and so completely different configurations of values, so we can readily imagine changing the constitutive conditions Engelhardt supposes exist for public policy matters. We would then have completely different possibilities and moral relations, not the ones he thinks obvious.

Engelhardt thus fails in his bid to provide "an immanent, transcendental grounding" for morality by providing "a game...with inescapable rules but no content" (69). The constitutive conditions Engelhardt presumes in trying to found public policy on the permissions of moral strangers are morally loaded in ways that affect the substantive moral implications Engelhardt draws. He is thus no better positioned morally to restructure our health-care system than those he attacks. His appeal to permissions presupposes "what it sets out to establish: canonical moral guidance" (42). It is not just a procedural device to obtain agreement, without substantive moral content, but a procedural device to impose agreement because its constitutive conditions have moral substance.

COOPERATIVE ENTERPRISES

Monopoly captures nicely one odd feature of Engelhardt's conception. He envisages individuals meeting one-on-one, or in combinations of one-on-one, to work out their relations with one another. He thus urges physicians opposed to abortion to inform patients of their unwillingness to provide that service–as though our capacities to accommodate competing interests morally were exhausted by such exchanges between one party and another. As in *Monopoly*, all that is morally relevant occurs within the confines of the rules of the game. The game is not itself an object of negotiation–presumably because, to be as charitable as we can be, the market economy replicated by the conditions of the game is just what would be agreed to by moral strangers concerned to exchange without any coercive regulation what, Engelhardt would argue, morally must belong to them, namely, their goods and services.

But the framework within which these exchanges between, say, physicians and patients are to occur is itself subject to negotiation. If the basis of morality is agreement between moral strangers, and there are no further constraints upon what can be an object of agreement, anything can be an object of negotiation.[18] Nothing about the nature of permissions prevents turning Engelhardt's conception upon the conditions he presupposes for such exchanges. That would be like asking whether players could agree to alternative conceptions of *Monopoly*. They could, of course, and if moral strangers are self-interested and concerned about the long-term stability of the health-care system, they will query some of the conditions Engelhardt assumes. We could opt, from within the constraints of his own system, for a very different form of health-care than the system he envisages.

Consider his claim that physicians need not provide abortions. Nothing could seem more obvious, I presume, given our health-care system or Engelhardt's view that the only foundation for morality comes from the permissions of moral strangers. Forcing a physician to provide an abortion seems paradigmatically coercive. It looks necessary that they cannot be forced to provide abortions because physicians are moral strangers for Engelhardt, and by his view no one can morally coerce moral strangers to do anything they do not agree to do.

But it is not difficult to imagine a very different configuration of relations in which that inference could not be drawn. One reason we get the result Engelhardt draws is that we imagine ourselves in the current situation, with physicians who already practice being forced to provide abortions when they are morally opposed to them. But suppose none are permitted to become physicians unless they are willing to provide all medical care that is legally permissible. By changing the conditions of entry into the health-care professions, we would change the configuration of moral relations between physicians and patients and among physicians. We would in effect be denying permission for moral strangers to become physicians. Since no individual has a right to be a physician, no one's rights will be violated by our agreeing to this condition for entry into the profession–any more than anyone's rights are denied by our requiring that physicians have a certain sort of education or that they be licensed by the state before they practice.

Indeed, it is arguable that we would have agreed to a morally better world. Physicians would be members of a single moral community, defined by the professional ethics of the discipline, including an obligation to provide all legal medical services they are competent to provide.[19] Under such a conception it would sound as obvious, and be as obvious, to say that physicians must provide abortions as it sounds, under Engelhardt's conception, to say the opposite.

The form of this argument can be repeated for every condition Engelhardt's conception presupposes.[20] Consider that in *Monopoly* each player is subject to the same set of rules, but in the health-care system Engelhardt envisages, and to a large extent in ours, we subsidize some players by paying part of their educational costs and then permit them a monopoly over the odd commercial transaction of both telling other players what they must purchase if they are to be healthy and then setting the price.

What we have for our health-care system is like a variant of *Monopoly* in which one player controls when property can be purchased, telling the other players what property they must purchase to remain healthy in the game, and then setting the price, whether they can afford it or not. In such a variant, some players will be squeezed out of the game because, for instance, no one can force the privileged player to sell anything to anybody at any particular price. Agreeing to play this game would be odd since one's surviving as a player would depend wholly upon the player with the special privilege deciding one's fate. This variant with *Monopoly* makes it clear just how odd the position of physicians is within our current health-care system. It is hard to suppose their position the result of any agreement of ours.

Some of the inequality they have with the rest of us comes from their having an expertise we do not have and from our needing to appeal to them to use their expertise when we are most vulnerable and least able to assert our interests. So some of the inequality of our situations is built into the system–as it would be in any relationship between a professional and a client. But all of it need not be.

For instance, the variant of *Monopoly* just elaborated makes clear how contingent it is for us to have a system that requires insurance. Insurance would become essential in such a version of *Monopoly* since no one can predict when they would be told they need to purchase what property at what cost and no one can protect themselves adequately against such an eventuality without insurance. Without the capacity to purchase insurance they could be squeezed out of the game as quickly as many are squeezed out of the health-care system. In 1993 "40.9 million citizens under the age of 65 lacked health insurance, along with several hundred thousand older Americans who did not qualify for Medicare for various reasons." 1.2 million a year more are being squeezed out, and so in 1995 43.4 million did not have insurance. That is "18.7 percent of those under 65."[21] Not to have insurance is not to have the cards necessary to play the health-care game. That is not to say we cannot get health-care without insurance, but that we can get it only on sufferance, in emergencies. It is to say that we have a health-care system so structured as to accentuate the need for insurance and that the most burdened by that need are those too poor to purchase insurance on their own and too rich or too young to qualify for governmental health insurance in the form of Medicare and Medicaid.

We could choose to have a system in which everyone who needed health care received it, whether they had the ability to pay or not. Nothing about the nature of health-care and nothing about the nature of Engelhardt's conception of how we are to found morality requires that health care be a commodity, subject to market forces. Nothing about the nature of health-care, or morality, requires that anyone be without it. We could choose to have a system without insurance companies, knowing that the inexorable commercial logic of providing insurance is that those who are healthy enough not to need insurance will be the preferred customers and those who need insurance will be weeded out. We could choose to have a system in which those health-care profession-als who are subsidized by our current system must provide some compensation for the subsidy. We might require them to provide a set percentage of *pro bono* work for a set percentage of their working lives, for instance.

We can, in short, change the conditions of play Engelhardt presumes. From within the conception Engelhardt hawks, the conclusions he draws are inescapable. "Of course," one wants to say, "the rich can purchase more health-care services than the poor." "Of course," one wants to say, "physicians cannot be obligated to provide services they do not want to provide." But we can and should question the conditions of Engelhardt's conception. For by that conception sick moral strangers are forced to play the health-care equivalent of *Monopoly*, and many would lose out even were they not ill-positioned to play it well.

ON THE WAY TO A NEW BEGINNING

We have not quite returned to where we began. We know that Engelhardt not only fails to provide a basis for morality which does not beg moral questions, but fails to show that the particular moral conclusions he draws need be drawn. We should not adopt his vision, at least on the grounds he demands, and even if we did, we need not accept his conclusions. We know this without exploring the whole range and depth of problems Engelhardt's vision entails–the difficulties with a theory of justice that precludes many from achieving what *prima facie* seems a fair share of a public good,[22] the difficulties we should expect regarding any theory that relies upon permissions without understanding how it is that permission is achieved in an on-going social system where many are never asked and ought to be presumed to refuse consent if they were asked, and so on. One or two fatal flaws can do a theory in, even if it is subject to other problems as well.

But it may be unclear what lessons we are to draw from all this except that we should not try to refashion our health-care system, or any on-going social institution, on the grounds Engelhardt proposes. Indeed, the way I have argued may mislead. There is a suggestion that if we were to turn Engelhardt's critical stance on the conditions he thinks hold for negotiations between moral strangers, we would find far richer possibilities for our health-care system, from within his conception, than he allows–as though nothing were wrong with what he is suggesting except a lack of thoroughness; as though I agree that since no other moral theory is without its problems, the only appeal we can have is to what we would agree to; as though the concept of "what we would agree to," though not clear enough to support Engelhardt's conception, is clear enough to support alternatives; as though the alternatives were themselves clear and appropriate.

But these questions presuppose what I think is a fundamental mistake Engelhardt (and others) make in regard to public policy matters, namely, that they are objects of choice in the way, for instance, playing *Monopoly* is an object of choice. Our health-care system is what I call a natural social artifact–"natural" because some form of health-care system will exist given that we are humans subject to ills and faults; "social" because whatever form is created will be normative for those operating within it; and an "artifact" because it is the result of human decisions and acceptance.[23] It is a cooperative enterprise, but more like language than *Monopoly*.

Thus, just as an individual's decision about what to say has little effect on our ever-changing language, an individual's decision about health care is equally inefficacious. In our personal relations, we permit a great deal we would not agree to. Someone has done something we would not have agreed to; it or its consequences are somewhat harmful to our interests; but now, after the fact, it is so much trouble to go back to try to make what has happened an object of negotiation that it is not worth the effort. The harm of trying to rectify the situation outweighs the harm already done. It would thus be a mistake even in our personal relations to suppose that whatever we accept we would have agreed to. It is far more unlikely a claim to suppose regarding our health-care system that what we acquiesce to we would have agreed to permit.

To suppose that we consent to what we have regarding health care, merely because we acquiesce, is to misunderstand the nature of the entity we find ourselves enmeshed in. It is a complex social structure, with a myriad of causes and a multitude of effects, some intended, many not, and neither it nor its elements are, or can be, in any simple manner an object of choice. So besides Engelhardt's begging the question and there being no necessity about the particular implications he draws, the idea that we could refashion our health-care system in terms of people's permissions is like the French Academy supposing it can keep French pure. The hubris is charming, but stems from a fundamental misconception of the nature of natural social artifacts.

NOTES

1. H. Tristram Engelhardt, Jr., *The Foundations of Bioethics,* 2nd edition (New York: Oxford University Press, 1996), 42. All further references will be in the text, with only a page number.

2. I am trying to lay bare the essential features of Engelhardt's view in the ways in which I think Wittgenstein in the *Philosophical Investigations* lays bare Augustine's view of language or in which H. L. A. Hart in *The Concept of Law* lays bare John Austin's view of the nature of law. Wittgenstein attempts to provide a language, language-game (2), that exactly fits the conception of language implied by Augustine's description of how he learned language, and Hart provides an example of someone's being obliged in the way in which Austin thinks sovereigns oblige. One tries to construct a perfect example of the view articulated, without resorting to any change

in the usual meaning of the terms used, and uses that example both to contrast with what is supposed to be described, and thus show its failure, and to tease out the bases for its failures. Austin's description, Hart claims, actually fits the situation of a gunman mugging someone where the gunman is part of a gang, and Augustine's description, Wittgenstein claims, among other things, applies to the learning of a foreign language, not one's original language, and then only to a foreign language of nouns.

Just so, in providing *Monopoly* as an instance of how we provide a morally acceptable justification for a system and its outcomes, I mean to both indicate and undermine its essential features. Being in a health-care system, I suggest, ought to be nothing like playing *Monopoly*.

3. For an explanation of pure procedural justice, see John Rawls, *A Theory of Justice* (Cambridge, Mass.: Harvard University Press, 1971), 85ff.

4. Two obvious ways in which we could influence what otherwise would be an instance of pure procedural justice would be to skew the die or the toss. The toss might bias the result if someone had so mastered the art of rolling the die as to affect the outcome. Much more often than not I can produce a heads over a tails, or vice versa, when I toss a coin I catch in my hand. Making use of such a skill would make the procedure impure.

5. The more chance has of determining the order of play, on this view of justice, the more just that order will supposedly be and the less any player will be entitled to complain. (b) is meant to protect both against someone skewing the initial toss (on the assumption, presumably, that skewing cannot be sustained) and against a single appeal to luck determining the order of play (on the assumption, presumably, that a single appeal to luck is insufficient to ensure the purity of the procedure).

6. These implications are internal to the game. The game so defines what constitutes just playing that making poor choices, for instance, is not a matter of injustice. Whether it is (really) just to create a game where one's life prospects can be determined by poor choices is an issue I do not address in this paper.

7. I should emphasize that this is the world according to Engelhardt. One source of difficulty with his views we shall briefly remark on later concerns the status of the permissions that are to be the basis of moral authority. Deciding not to purchase a piece of property is not obviously a matter of negotiation between one player and another, for instance. In fact, to be honest to the game, we rarely negotiate or give our permissions for any particular play. We just let things go on without complaining, unless we see cheating or coercion. Engelhardt would presumably say that because the procedure is pure, and because we have agreed to play in accord with the procedure defined by the rules, letting things go on is all that is needed to constitute permission. The question we shall consider is whether that description, which may seem to work for *Monopoly*, works at all for our health-care system.

8. *Monopoly* is also an instance of Nozick's theory of justice writ small. The question of whether the distribution at any particular time is just or unjust is a question of its history: was it achieved through uncoerced transactions, without anyone cheating? If so, then it is just, despite whatever inequalities, however vast, may result.

One basis of criticism that producing this miniature of a just Nozickian state makes clear is that it is only if we start equally situated in regard to our social position (our wealth, income, and so on) that a pure procedure could produce a just result. But we never start equally situated in life. The distribution of advantages and disadvantages at any particular time is the result of a complex history, filled with coercion and cheating. So it is not possible ever to begin instituting Nozick's theory without simply further entrenching the injustices with which the process must begin. Rectification is required before the process can properly proceed, and even if we could provide such a principle, it is not practically possible to apply it in a world of constant and unjust changes.

There are other objections, obviously, but this one is of especial importance given that we are concerned with our health-care system and that the terms of entry into it are dependent upon our having enough money to purchase insurance.

9. At least that is the way Engelhardt apparently thinks about this game. Engelhardt seems to think only coercion is impermissible, but I have assumed, in elaborating the *Monopoly* example, that cheating is impermissible as well.

It is another question whether these are the only two ways in which one can cause moral harm in giving permissions. There are certainly a richer set of conditions that informed consent requires than Engelhardt's view supposes.

10. Such an example may seem such an obvious feature of the game to those of us who are competent at it that we may think such things should go without saying, but anyone who has played with smaller children knows how much learning is involved in explaining to them that though they may not want "all that stuff" on their property, they are better off, in terms of achieving the ends of the game, having it there than not.

11. This is a complex and compound capacity. Among other things, we need to know how different purchases will make significant differences in the outcome of the game (Boardwalk and Park Place being more valuable than all the railroads); how intimidation in a game matters and what form of intimidation is appropriate and effective for *Monopoly*, if any; the ability to take advantage of unforeseen opportunities (someone not purchasing a piece of property you thought they would); how not to feel set back by small defeats; how to squeeze as much out of a situation as we can to achieve the ends of the game; and so on.

12. Assessing the value of these features is another matter entirely. How much competitive spirit is a good thing in competitive games is no easy matter, for instance. Being overly competitive can harm one's own interests as well as the pleasure others take in the game. Again, the capacity to play on despite knowing one will lose may also be counter-productive for the pleasure of other players, forcing the clear winner and everyone else to continue play long past the time when any competitive pleasure is derivable from the game.

Indeed, this capacity is seemingly at odds with the competitive spirit essential for playing. Perhaps this is one reason why it is so hard sometimes to find others to play. Once we know we are going to lose, the residual pleasure may not be enough, and the great likelihood for most is that they are going to lose.

In addition, someone poorly provided with features the game makes valuable, or overly endowed with features the game makes deficits, may find it unenticing to play. Arguably the game is doubly flawed. It first defines what count as assets and deficits, making winning and losing depend upon them, and then fails to compensate those who, through no fault of their own, have a wrong mix. Put another way, those with a disadvantageous mix of what the game makes assets and deficits do not begin on an equal footing, through no fault of their own, and yet the game fails to provide any compensation except what comes from playing with others who are far more likely to win.

13. See my "Management and Ethical Decision-Making," *Journal of Business Ethics* 3 (1984): 287-291.

14. From "The Gambler," sung by Kenny Rogers.

15. I have played with social work students a game in which tokens are distributed randomly among small groups of students. Those with two gold tokens are entitled to advance to the next stage of the game, and since there are few gold tokens, one player must negotiate with others in the small group to obtain two. I have found that the following form of argument is success-

ful–incredible as this seems to me. I simply say to the social work students that it is obvious that if no one has two tokens, no one will advance to the next stage. So someone ought to have two tokens to achieve that end. Otherwise our small group will fail to have a representative. But since we are all equal with each other, I continue, there is no reason why one should be chosen rather than another. So, I conclude, it might as well be me. If anyone objects, I say, "You are all social work students, and you are supposed to be concerned to further the interests of others, not yourself. I am not a social work student," I continue, "and so you should give all your gold tokens to me." The first time I did this I presumed that it would not be effective, but it was, and I have found that it works almost all the time. I am amazed, but Engelhardt is right: "peaceable manipulation" can get you what you want.

16. It is no easy matter providing a criterion of what counts as a constitutive condition. Examples are easy. It is a constitutive condition of being a State in the United States that it have powers equal to those of the original states. It was this condition that was used in the Dred Scott decision to declare the Missouri Compromise unconstitutional since it denied to any states coming from the Louisiana Territory the power to determine for themselves whether to be slave or free, a power the original states had. But clearly what is constitutive can be, and is likely to be, contentious since appealing to the constitutive conditions of a practice to justify anything is to make the highest appeal within the practice one can. It will trump any other but another appeal to constitutive conditions. Thus the criterion for determining what counts as constitutive is as likely to be contentious. I think the examples I provide are clear instances of constitutive features of *Monopoly* or of Engelhardt's conception of the proper basis for public policy, and that will have to suffice for the purposes of this argument.

17. I isolate these two premises because they are crucial conditions: changing them will significantly alter the structure of moral relations in the system.

18. The only constraint is that coercion and cheating are prohibited, both in the process of negotiation and regarding what we agree to. But nothing I will suggest that we could change about the health-care system requires that we coerce or cheat anyone.

19. The general premise of this argument is generalizable to all the professions. It is that we can create moral communities, of the sort Engelhardt envisages, through conditioning the licensing of various professionals. We are both benefitted and burdened by such monopolies, burdened if only because we generally subsidize the education of many professionals, and we are both permitted and, I would argue, obligated to ensure that practitioners in the monopoly do well by us.

20. For instance, our current system is weighed towards crisis management. The full force of our health-care system is brought to bear only after someone has fallen ill. That is one reason so many of our health-care resources are spent towards the end of one's life. But suppose we agreed to take as the primary objects of concern not ourselves, but infants. Nothing about our being moral persons–self-conscious and rational, with at least a minimal moral sense and the capacity to make decisions–precludes a decision to consider as the primary objects of the health-care system those who still have most of their lives to lead. It is true that *we* would be agreeing to this, but nothing about Engelhardt's view requires that we always be completely absorbed in our own self-interests, and, besides, such a stance would benefit us since the subsequent change in the stance of the system towards crisis-prevention would arguably produce better health for all of us.

21. These figures are derived from Keith Bradsher, "As 1 Million Leave Ranks Of Insured, Debate Heats Up," *New York Times* (August 27, 1995): A1 & 20.

22. There are two problems that the theory Engelhardt proposes must overcome to have even a minimal claim on us to consider it. First, as I suggested in note 8, the theory he proposes about how to distribute such a good as health care must presuppose, as *Monopoly* makes explicit, that those within the system start equally situated. How this could be achieved in our on-going health care system, where we would have to discount for all past coercions and cheatings, boggles the imagination.

Second, the end result of the theory of justice Engelhardt assumes is, as with *Monopoly*, that some have much and many have nothing. It is not obvious that this is just when, as is often the case, the blessed and the unblessed by his theory hold the positions they do through no fault of their own. It is even less obvious when the conditions of the distribution, as I have remarked at length, require traits of character that are not distributed evenly across the population and are in themselves less than fully desirable.

23. For a more thorough, but still truncated discussion of this concept and its importance for public policy decisions, see my *Decisions in Doubt: The Environment and Public Policy* (Hanover, NH: University Press of New England, 1994), Chapter 2.

6

BEYOND FORBEARANCE AS THE MORAL FOUNDATION FOR A HEALTH CARE SYSTEM: ANALYSIS OF ENGELHARDT'S PRINCIPLES OF BIO- ETHICS

RORY B. WEINER

H. Tristram Engelhardt, Jr., in his *The Foundations of Bioethics*, constructs what he calls the foundations of a "general secular morality"[1] of bioethics. "This account," he explains, "can be regarded as a transcendental argument to justify a principle of freedom as a side constraint, as a source of [moral] authority" (70).[2] This principle, which he calls the principle of permission (or forbearance), justifies a *basic* moral right against the use of unconsented-to force against the innocent (15). But it does not justify a basic moral right to assistance, including access to basic health care. "A basic human secular moral right to health care," Engelhardt explains, "does not exist–not even to a decent minimum of health care" (375). However, he argues, if a moral community chooses to do so, it may *create* a right to basic health care by establishing at least a two-tiered health care system: an upper tier where persons use private funds to purchase whatever medical care they wish, and a bottom tier where persons have access regardless of their ability to pay. The principle of permission and its derivative principle of private ownership justify the upper tier, which is universally required as a basic right, while a principle of beneficence justifies a bottom tier, which is always optional.

This chapter argues that Engelhardt's concept of secular morality would go beyond the principle of forbearance and include a principle of cooperative beneficence, which prescribes a basic duty of beneficence to cooperate in collective efforts to benefit the least well-off members of a moral community. This principle would require all moral communities to have a health care system that includes a tier that guarantees access to medical care regardless of one's ability to pay. The structure of the argument (and how the chapter proceeds) is this: (1) The chapter outlines and critically comments on Engel- hardt's principles of bioethics; in particular, how they converge to support his two-tiered health care system. (2) It argues that Engelhardt incorrectly assumes that moral strangers can collaborate with moral authority, i.e., accept mutual consent as the means for resolving moral disputes, despite relevant inequalities among participants. To collaborate with moral authority, I will argue, moral

B. P. Minogue et al. (eds.), Reading Engelhardt, 113–138.
© 1997 *Kluwer Academic Publishers. Printed in the Netherlands.*

strangers must go beyond the principle of forbearance and accept a principle that helps the least well-off members of their community. Moreover, I argue that this principle is not just a way to connect Engelhardt's theory with Daniels's theory of justice in health care. This principle requires each moral stranger to cooperate in guaranteeing universal access to health care not because the unequal distribution of disease and disability is unfair, but because a universal commitment to mitigating relevant inequalities, like disease and disability, is a necessary condition for collaborating with moral authority, i.e., for obtaining universal permission to use mutual consent as the procedure for determining the framework of rights and duties that would subsequently resolve moral disputes among moral strangers. (3) The chapter concludes by outlining this principle of cooperative beneficence and explaining how to apply it to health care policy.

THE FOUNDATIONS OF BIOETHICS

This section outlines what Engelhardt calls his "transcendental argument" to justify a foundational principle for a "general secular bioethics" (70). He seeks this foundation in response to the myriad of moral views current in bioethics and the need for moral guidance that does not presuppose any particular one. He seeks, in other words, "*a neutral [moral] framework* to address moral problems in biomedicine [where] individuals generally hold a diversity of moral views" (6, 16, emphasis added). "It is an ethic," he explains, "that aspires to provide a logic or grammar for speaking across a plurality of ideologies, beliefs, and bioethics" (35).

Engelhardt locates the foundations of bioethics in the necessary condition for moral discourse among moral strangers. "Moral strangers," according to Engelhardt, "are persons who do not share sufficient moral premises, or rules of evidence and inference to solve moral controversies by sound rational argument, or who do not have a common commitment to individuals or institutions in authority to solve moral controversies" (7). If we assume, he argues, that "secular ethics and bioethics are at the very least *means* for resolving controversies regarding proper conduct on bases *other than appeals to force* as the fundamental basis for the resolution," then finding the necessary condition for this means or procedure (which does not itself presuppose any substantive moral view) will reveal the necessary, objective moral criterion to guide it (67, emphasis added). It will reveal, in other words, "the morality that should guide individuals when they meet as moral strangers" (11).

The following summarizes Engelhardt's overall argument:

1. Ethics and bioethics contain a plurality of ideologies, beliefs, moral visions, etc., none of which can be shown to be the correct one (6, 35, 59).

2. If there is no correct moral view, then no one can claim to have (moral) authority for resolving controversies in ethics and bioethics (65ff.).

3. If no moral authority exists, then people will use some form of direct or indirect force or coercion to resolve moral controversies.

4. But force, even subtle force, has no moral authority, since it "will not answer the ethical question, such as intellectual queries as to why a controversy ought to be resolved in a particular fashion...Brute force, unless it is justified, is simply brute force. Subtle force remains force. *A goal of ethics is to determine when force can be justified.* Force by itself carries no moral authority." (67, my emphasis)

5. "Secular bioethics" seeks a procedure that provides secular moral authority for resolving moral disagreements among moral strangers without a fundamental recourse to force (67).

6. "If one is interested in collaborating with moral authority in the face of moral disagreements without fundamental recourse to force, then *one must accept agreement among members of the controversy or peaceable negotiations as the means for resolving concrete moral controversies*" (68, my emphasis).

7. If one accepts mutual agreement for resolving moral controversies, then "one can account for the moral authority of this common endeavor: mutual consent," i.e., "the permission of those who choose to collaborate" (69, 83).

8. If secular bioethics is an enterprise for resolving moral controversies among moral strangers without recourse to force, but with the moral authority of mutual consent, then the principle of permission, which forbids using the "innocent"[3] without their consent (70, 83), is the defining (or necessary) condition for the very possibility of this enterprise.

9. Thus, the principle of permission is a transcendental condition, a necessary condition for the possibility of a general secular bioethics; it is the moral foundation of secular ethics and bioethics, since it does not presuppose any particular moral view.

For Engelhardt, then, the principle of permission, or the morality of mutual respect, is necessary for the possibility of secular bioethics as an enterprise for peaceable negotiations among moral strangers. Importantly, he believes that his account of ethics and bioethics requires *only* a decision to solve moral controversies and "commits one to no concrete moral view of the good life... or of content-full obligations" (68-69).[4] Yet, presumably, it does commit one to the "absolute and universal secular moral [content-less] conclusion," "[d]o not use unconsented-to force against the innocent," i.e., a duty of forbearance (78). In other words, when one collaborates with moral authority, when one seeks mutual consent, one must accept, according to Engelhardt, a prior commitment to the duty of forbearance. Thus, secular morality provides the framework of individual rights and duties of forbearance within which in-dividuals may pursue their own conceptions of the good life, of virtue, etc., depending on which moral community they choose to belong (102). I will now turn to how the principle of permission generates what Engelhardt calls the principles of bioethics.

THE PRINCIPLES OF BIOETHICS

This section briefly summarizes and critically comments on Engelhardt's principles of bioethics: the principle of permission, of beneficence, of owner-ship, and of political authority. It also aims to explain how these principles converge to justify a fifth principle, a principle of health care allocation, which justifies his two-tiered health care system.[5]

The principle of permission. The principle of permission derives from the formal property of secular morality, i.e., the necessary condition for its practice. It forbids using force against the innocent without their consent. "[P]ermission or consent," Engelhardt explains, "is the origin of authority, and respect of the right of participants to consent is the necessary condition for the possibility of a moral community" (123). The principle is expressed by the maxim: "Do not do to others that which they would not have done unto them, and do for them that which one has contracted to do" (123). It provides, for policy purposes, "moral grounding for public policies aimed at defending the innocent" (123). It is a basic right, then, not to be used without one's consent provided that one does not use others without their consent.

Importantly, according to Engelhardt, this principle "justifies the *process* for generating [moral] content" (108). In other words, it justifies using mutual agreement or an agreement procedure as the only authority (or means) for resolving moral disputes in a secular, pluralist society, and thus for determining all subsequent rights and duties that govern public life. Thus, according to Engelhardt, the principle of permission is basic: it justifies agreement as the process of generating moral content, but it is not itself the result of that agreement.

The commitment to the principle of permission results from moral strangers *accepting* agreement as the means for resolving subsequent moral disputes. It is, according to Engelhardt, a necessary condition for collaborating with moral authority, i.e., for obtaining the consent of all moral strangers. But this raises a potential problem: Is the principle of permission the only necessary condition for collaborating with moral authority? In other words, would moral strangers "accept" agreement as the means for resolving subsequent moral disputes despite inequalities in education, power, health, information, etc., which would place some moral strangers at a disadvantage in the subsequent negotiations? Or, must moral strangers commit to ameliorating these inequalities as a necessary condition for collaborating with moral authority? If Engelhardt believes that moral strangers will "accept" agreement as the source of controversy resolution despite relevant inequalities, then he is presuming norms for the "acceptance" of agreement. Can he justify these norms across all moral communities? If not, must moral strangers go beyond forbearance when they collaborate with moral authority? Must they commit to a principle that would require ameliorating relevant inequalities prior to using mutual consent to resolve moral disputes? I will return to these questions in the next section.

The principle of beneficence. Unlike the principle of permission, the principle of beneficence, according to Engelhardt, identifies the content of morality; it aims to promote good and to avoid harm. Since, however, "no particular ordering of goods and harms can be established" across all moral communities, not every moral agent will agree to the content for duties of beneficence. Thus, explains Engelhardt, we cannot justify any universal, absolute duties of beneficence (123, 124, 128). We may justify duties of beneficence only when an implicit or explicit agreement exists between the giver and the receiver (123). In other words, in general secular ethics, any application of the principle of beneficence requires the permission of all the benefactors and beneficiaries. Thus, the principle of beneficence "provides the moral grounding for *refusable* welfare rights drawn from common holdings" and is expressed by the maxim: "Do to others their good [provided that they consent]" (124, emphasis added).[6]

The principle of ownership. The principle of ownership is derived from the principle of permission (164). Engelhardt provides an account of the right to ownership that, he says, relies only "on persons as the source of permission *and* on objects as possessions in so far as they are extensions of persons" (163, emphasis added). Following Locke and Nozick ("but in a Hegelian reinterpretation"), Engelhardt claims that a person possesses a thing if she "enters into a thing, refashions it, remolds it...and mingles labor with it," or if she receives a thing from another through a legitimate transfer such as a gift or in trade (157).

For Engelhardt, the principle of permission, which permits one to do as one wishes with oneself, extends to objects one transforms or refashions "in the images and likeness of one's ideas and according to one's will" (157). "In this fashion," writes Engelhardt, "one increases the sphere of one's embodiment and extends the border of one's rights to the forbearance of others" (157). Thus we may extend our right of self-ownership, and the forbearance right that protects it, to any other object that we transform by our will. Once we have marked some object by our will we have a property right to it and may freely sell it or transfer it as we would with ourselves.

Engelhardt distinguishes private ownership from what he calls "communal" and "general" (or common) ownership. "Communal ownership" is the product of moral friends, or moral strangers who universally consent, pooling their resources for creating communal funds and using these funds for projects they agree to establish (160). "General ownership" expresses the fact persons, although they may own products that they transform by their will, may never own "the brute matter itself, the stuff out of which the products are fashioned" (157-8). Engelhardt argues that the "thing" or matter that one transforms, or mingles his labor with, *is not completely* that person's—some is always left for everyone else. "Matter itself, the dimension of things that remains after the things are transformed into products, remains in common ownership," he explains (158). In other words, when one marks off a thing by one's will, transforming it into something new, one merely owns the form, but not the matter itself. As such, he claims, "it would appear possible to speak of the rights of all to have equal access to that matter" (158). This notion of "general ownership," he believes, justifies collecting taxes, where such a tax "would need to reflect a fair rent on such material, apart from considerations of its status as a product" (158). For example, it is permissible to tax private or governmental ownership of freshwater lakes but not expensive or rare drugs made from common and readily available materials (164). When distributed, this tax could also provide some with funds to purchase health insurance, if the community chooses to do so.[7]

Apart from any limit to ownership associated with the notions of communal or general ownership, for Engelhardt the rights to and exchange of private property are extensive. One can own animals (provided one is beneficent to them), young children (provided one produced them), and persons generally (provided they agreed to it) (156). Moreover, he claims, "Since the principle of permission holds precedent, one should be moved to respect property rights *even under such conditions of tension within the principle of beneficence (i.e., between giving individuals their property and giving to others what is necessary for life)*" (165, emphasis added). Finally, he argues, the right to ownership includes "a fundamental moral right...to participate in the black market. No secular polity has the right to forbid free individuals from exchanging their services or property for the services or property of other free individuals" (166).

Unfortunately, Engelhardt never specifies under what conditions a person is "free" or makes "free" exchanges of goods or services. Is a person who sells crack cocaine to raise money to supply his habit a "free individual," "freely exchanging" his or her services with other "free individuals"? Presumably that person would not have a basic right to the cocaine market, if he or she were not "free." These questions underscore the importance of determining under what conditions we can accurately attribute "free" to a person's exchanges. The paucity of analysis to this issue is a major disappointment of this book. It leaves the reader with a principle of permission that resembles an empty platitude rather than a moral requirement.

Still, other problems exist for Engelhardt's principle of ownership. Does the principle of ownership derive directly from the principle of permission? Or does this derivation require an additional moral premise? According to Engelhardt, the right to ownership is a conjunction of two claims: (1) the principle of permission, *and* (2) a theory of how we come to own objects (163). Even if, as he claims, (1) is neutral with respect to all moral communities, (2) is not. How a person may or may not come to own an object requires a theory of private ownership that is not neutral among all moral strangers.

Recall that Engelhardt claims that a person may extend self-ownership into an object by mingling his labor with it and thus transforming the object through his will, which makes it his own. Although he admits that some of what a person fashions will always be left behind—we may own the form but not the matter itself—must all moral strangers accept the claim that we may privately own the form? Some moral strangers could defend an equally plausible view that no one may privately own anything, that private ownership is a conventional arrangement that different communities but not all communities may or may not decide to adopt. Others might deny the possibility of self-ownership, arguing that everyone is God's property. In other words, the claim that ownership of ourselves extends into private ownership of other things does not follow directly from the principle of permission. This extension thesis is one of a number of equally plausible theories of ownership, none of which could be established as the correct one. Even if the principle of permission is basic, the principle of ownership is not.

Thus Engelhardt cannot successfully defend a basic right to private property, but only a conventional one. At one point in his discussion he complains that Rawls's theory is inadequate because some cultures (BaMbuti pygmies) would not rank liberty more highly than other societal goods. Yet Engelhardt never considers whether all cultures would rank acquiring private property so highly, or whether some cultures even recognize a concept of self-ownership. In fact, in his own example of BaMbuti pygmies he describes them as people who do not invest their energies in accumulating goods. Moreover, he admits, "Any particular system for speaking of possessors and possessions appears to be culturally relative" and compares the way European immigrants and various native American Indian tribes would differ in their ranking of the importance of property ownership (155). Thus, he cannot claim all moral communities must accept his principle of ownership, since not all moral strangers must accept *his assumptions* about ownership: "I side with Locke," he explains, "but in a Hegelian reinterpretation" (155).

Finally, Engelhardt's concept of "general ownership" requires some very dubious assumptions. Recall that he says "general property" is "*matter itself*...[which] remains in common ownership of persons generally" (131, emphasis added). Moreover, he claims, because of common property, "not all property is privately owned. Nations and other social organizations may invest their common resources in insuring their members against losses in the natural and social lotteries" (399). However, questions remain: What is this "matter" that remains after things are transformed into products? Suppose I am athletic and transform *myself* into a marketable baseball player; what is the "matter" left over? My body? My skills? (is a skill "matter"?) Or something else? If parents own the children they produce (as he says they do), does everyone partly own these children? Given the controversial nature of these questions,

I do not believe everyone will accept his notion of "general ownership" or its use for some taxation.

Since the principle of ownership requires controversial assumptions not necessarily accepted across all moral communities, the principle of ownership does not derive directly from the principle of permission, but it is one of possibly many plausible extensions of the principle of permission. Thus not all moral strangers must accept Engelhardt's argument for an *unlimited* right to private property. As a result, this weakens his use of the principle of ownership to justify requiring the free market tier of his health care system. Even if everyone accepts his principle of permission, everyone need not accept an unlimited right to private property, or the corollary thesis that governments have no authority to redistribute goods and services because of that right. Since the right to private property is not basic–it is not a necessary condition for the possibility of a moral community–we must not impose the legal institutions that protect and nurture it upon all moral strangers without their consent. We may permit these institutions if communities choose to have them. Yet it would be wrong, according to secular morality, to use governments (or any other means) to force people to participate in or support institutions of private property if they did not wish to do so.

The principle of political authority. Morally justified political authority, Engelhardt claims, derives from the principle of permission, i.e., "from the *actual* consent" of the governed (171, my emphasis). Political authority, he argues, is limited to protecting the innocent from unconsented-to force. For example, a government may enact and enforce laws that protect the innocent from murder, rape, robbery, fraud, coercion or breech of a contract (171). A government may also provide health care "as a welfare right out of commonly held resources" if everyone in that community consents (171). Thus the government's authority is very limited and should not be used to restrict, for example, the sale of human organs, or the use of contracts for commercial surrogate mothers. Moreover, the state has no authority to interfere with a person's basic right to the black market. Therefore, according to Engelhardt, the state must tolerate "victimless" crimes in which all those involved have freely agreed to participate, e.g., the "sale of pornography, the conduct of prostitution, the sale of heroin and marijuana" (173).[8]

In cases where explicit agreement cannot be secured, Engelhardt claims that "one will need to do *the best one can and resolve controversies by means that involve the least coercion and the greatest amount of consent*" (171, emphasis added). The best means, says Engelhardt, for providing the least amount of coercion and the greatest amount of consent are market mechanisms, because "these reflect the results of numerous acts of consent and *do not incorporate a particular moral vision* but the result of individuals acting with each other out of divergent moral understandings" (171-172, emphasis added). The next best procedure, he says, is "limited democratic mechanisms" (172).[9] Given the superiority of markets to secure consent and reduce coercion, Engelhardt argues that the general moral authority of governments is not as strong as corporations, assuming employees have joined freely. Governments, he says, traditionally use force to coerce "those in their territory to accept their authority" (174). "There is no evidence, for example, that Dow Chemical has ever drafted individuals to serve in its security forces," he writes (174).

But such a comparison is odd. When an employee freely joins a corporation, it does not, as democracies in theory do, seek to secure her permission in all future decisions that affect her. For example, must a corporation, in theory, get the employee's permission if it plans to reduce safety standards to save costs? Corporations make these decisions privately without employee input or public scrutiny; thus, in theory, they do not seek to gain prior consent from all employees. Although corporations do not draft employees into their security force, theoretically they can do much to them without their consent.

Thus, Engelhardt's comparison between the free market and democracy is flawed. It is my guess that if we were actually to compare market mechanisms with the democratic process as means for controversy resolution to determine which produces the lowest amount of coercion and the greatest amount of consent, then we would find the democratic procedure is better. Theoretically, the reason is this. Assuming one freely joins a democracy, its subsequent decisions continue to be democratic; it continues to seek permission from its constituents. In a democracy, decisions are open to public scrutiny and in theory require the consent of all the people they affect. Moreover, because it is in theory open–it cannot keep its records closed from public scrutiny–participants can attack its decisions and inform other participants about problems that exist in it. This kind of public scrutiny of records and decision making is not typical for corporations.

Even Engelhardt admits that public scrutiny makes a moral difference. Engelhardt at one point criticizes the Clinton proposal for health care reform because it was initially fashioned "without public hearings" (410, see also 401). Public hearings make a moral difference because they increase the amount of consent and decrease the amount of coercion. But how is the public to debate and scrutinize the way corporations fashion the distribution of health care services? Will corporations hold public hearings? How much information will consumers have about how Health Maintenance Organizations (HMOs) decide when to allow referrals to specialists, or when to allow the use of expensive medical equipment? Can consumers rely on physicians for this information? Not likely since physicians are increasingly becoming employees of health care corporations, which now are requiring physicians to sign loyalty contracts forbidding them to discuss corporate allocation decisions to their patients.[10] Without the proper information, patients cannot freely choose which provider to use.

Thus it seems odd that Engelhardt endorses corporations and markets as having more moral authority than a constitutional democracy and democratic principles. On the face of it, if one were to compare the amount of consent and the level of coercion between an employee of a corporation such as IBM, Dow Chemical, or Exxon, and a citizen of a constitutional democracy such as the United States, surely all told the citizen has greater levels of consent and is coerced less than a corporate employee. Engelhardt merely assumes that governments as such will be oppressive and corporations and markets will not. There is no doubt that both can be oppressive, but determining whether they actually are is an empirical matter that Engelhardt does not explore; he merely assumes that everyone in a market chooses from equal positions of knowledge and power and thus what they buy they consent to. Yet in *real life* participating in the market is more complicated; and because Engelhardt refuses to address its complications, he overlooks the moral problems the market contains.

The Principle of Health Care Allocation. Engelhardt claims that his "analysis of the principles of permission and beneficence and of entitlements to property support a multi-tier system of health care" (399). In particular, a two-tiered system, he says, is inevitable and "in many respects a compromise. On the one hand," he says, "[this system] provides some amount of health care for all, while on the other hand allowing those with resources to purchase additional or better services. It can endorse the use of communal resources for the provision of a decent minimal or basic amount of health care for all, while acknowledging the existence of private resources at the disposal of some individuals to purchase better basic as well as luxury care" (399). Moreover, he writes, a two-tiered system "allows for the expression of individual love and the pursuit of private advantage, though still supporting a general social sympathy for those in need" (399).

What is important to note here is that communities are never required to provide a tier of universal basic health care. According to Engelhardt's principle of ownership and its application to the principle of health care allocation, a community can agree to create a universal bottom tier, but no requirement exists–no *basic* right to health care exists. Governments, according to his principle of political authority, do not have the moral authority to force a community to create such a right. Communities, following his principle of beneficence, may express their social sympathies to others by pooling their resources and investing them into a system that guarantees a basic minimum of health care to anyone who needs it. Thus, Engelhardt provides us with the following health care allocation maxim: "Give to those who need or desire health care that which they, you, or others are willing to pay for or provide gratis" (403).

Engelhardt's principles of bioethics, then, converge to support a two-tiered health care system. A mandatory upper tier, which forbids any interference with individuals from using their private money to purchase whatever health care they are willing to pay for, and an optional bottom tier, which makes health care available to those unable to pay. Although some problems with Engelhardt's principles have been identified above, the following will specifically attack Engelhardt's assumption about the necessary conditions for collaborating with moral authority. I will argue that his theory of secular morality, to be plausible, must go beyond forbearance and include a principle that requires helping the least well-off members of society.

BEYOND COOPERATIVE RESTRAINT

In this section, I will argue that Engelhardt incorrectly assumes that moral strangers can collaborate *with moral authority* by only granting forbearance rights, or cooperative restraint. To collaborate with moral authority, moral strangers must also grant a principle that prescribes a duty to help the least well-off members of society. A more careful analysis of what Engelhardt means by collaborating with moral authority reveals that moral strangers must have a prior commitment to guaranteeing some level of well-being (a level of education, power, wealth, health) to all persons. This commitment is as necessary (as defining, as basic) as some level of forbearance for practicing secular morality.

To analyze Engelhardt's assumption–that forbearance is sufficient for collaborating with moral authority–let us look at what he means by "collaborating with moral authority." He writes:

> If one is interested in collaborating *with moral authority* in the face of moral disagreements without fundamental recourse to force, then one *must accept agreement* among members of the controversy...as the means for resolving concrete moral controversies (68, my emphasis).

For Engelhardt, "collaborating with moral authority" means accepting mutual consent, or an agreement procedure, as the alternative to force for deciding rights and obligations that will direct subsequent public life. In other words, to collaborate with moral authority is to secure universal permission by *accepting* mutual consent as the sole means for generating all subsequent moral content.

The question I will explore is this: When moral strangers *accept mutual consent* as the means for resolving moral controversies–as the "neutral" procedure for generating moral content–*must they also accept* the existing relevant background conditions that might place some moral strangers at a disadvantage in subsequent decision making, i.e., in deciding the rights and duties that will subsequently guide their lives? In other words, can moral strangers collaborate with moral authority *despite* significant differences in levels of education, of health, of wealth, of security, of access to information, of power, etc., which give some moral strangers an advantage over others when resolving subsequent moral disputes?

According to Engelhardt the answer is, "Yes." He assumes that moral strangers can collaborate with moral authority and accept mutual consent as the source of all subsequent moral decisions despite any relevant background differences. He writes:

> In summary, *all persons* can envisage the *notion of the peaceable (moral) community.* Insofar as they act in accord with this notion, *despite inequalities in intelligence, power, and wealth,* they *participate with others in the peaceable (moral) community* (i.e., defined by general secular pluralist morality) (137, emphasis added).

Because Engelhardt assumes that moral strangers can accept mutual consent despite relevant background inequalities, he also assumes that they only have a commitment to forbearance (restraint) as basic, i.e., as prior to any actual agreement. He assumes that forbearance is *the* only antecedent condition necessary for the possibility of mutual consent, for the possibility, that is, of obtaining universal permission.

But is this assumption correct? To answer this, we must discover whether or not all moral strangers would accept mutual consent as the means for resolving moral disputes despite inequalities that place some at a disadvantage during moral deliberations. If they would not, then Engelhardt cannot assume that moral strangers can collaborate with moral authority with only a prior commitment to forbearance. Instead, I will argue, moral strangers must also accept a prior commitment to softening relevant inequalities, since without this commitment some moral strangers would not accept mutual consent as the "neutral" decision procedure. In other words, a commitment to ameliorating relevant inequalities is also necessary for obtaining universal permission.

Would moral strangers "accept" mutual consent as the source for resolving subsequent moral disputes despite relevant inequalities? Some would, e.g., moral strangers who have sufficient education, wealth, power, etc. These inequalities would not put them at a disadvantage in subsequent resolutions of controversies. These inequalities would not jeopardize their ability genuinely to consent in subsequent agreement procedures. Thus, these moral strangers would grant a prior commitment only to forbearance rights, since those rights would be sufficient to secure their consent or permission.

However, other moral strangers would not accept mutual consent despite relevant inequalities, e.g., those who have no or little education, wealth, power, or health insurance. These inequalities place them at a disadvantage in subsequent agreement procedures. They would jeopardize their ability to give genuine consent. Although forbearance is essential for them, it is not sufficient. For these moral strangers, then, a prior commitment to ameliorating relevant inequalities is also a necessary condition for "accepting" mutual consent as the means for determining rights and obligations that govern subsequent public life. They require a level of well-being that helps secure their ability to consent, to give permission, when participating in peaceable negotiations.

Thus, if Engelhardt's aim is to disclose the necessary conditions for secular ethics among *all moral strangers*, and not just among the elite, well-off ones, then he cannot assume that all moral strangers would "accept" mutual consent as the means for resolving moral disputes despite relevant inequalities. Some moral strangers will not accept mutual consent unless there is a prior commitment to reducing relevant inequalities. In other words, for *all moral strangers* to collaborate with moral authority there must be a commitment not only to a principle of forbearance but also to a principle of beneficence, namely, a principle that requires each moral stranger to help soften relevant inequalities. I will say more about this principle of beneficence below.

Engelhardt might argue that any moral requirement beyond forbearance is wrong because it coerces the innocent. Since most people living today, he would argue, did not cause the inequalities that place some at a disadvantage–those inequalities resulted from unfortunate accidents of natural or social circumstances–we should not force some to help reduce these inequalities. To do so would risk punishing the innocent (382). If we could identify those responsible for the inequalities, he would argue, then it would be permissible to force them to redress the inequalities. But, he would argue, since most inequalities are the result of bad luck in the social and natural lotteries, it is wrong to correct these inequalities without everyone's consent. Besides, he might add, even if some people did cause them it would be difficult, if not impossible, to identify those who are responsible.

One response to this argument is to simply challenge the empirical assumption underlying it. Surely many people today played some role in creating these inequalities, although obtaining the historical information is difficult. These people and their descendants helped to marginalize others, denying them basic education, political participation and economic opportunity. Consider what the indigenous populations of the United States might have had today if their land had not been forced from them. Consider the possible economic and political power that women might have had today if they had not been oppressed and marginalized for so long.

But who is to blame? Who are the guilty? Who are innocent? Who can we point to now and say, "Your actions caused current inequalities and you (and all like you) should correct them"? To answer these questions Engelhardt might borrow Robert Nozick's solution. Nozick faces a similar problem when applying his principle of rectification. For Nozick, the principle of rectification permits a government to correct any current or past injustices that result (or resulted) from *using another without his or her consent.* As we have seen, Engelhardt also argues that a government's power is limited to this domain. Yet Nozick admits that although we lack the sufficient information to apply this principle in individual cases, we can, and should, apply it to society at large. He writes:

Perhaps it is best to view *some patterned principles of distributive justice as rough rules of thumb* meant to approximate the general results of applying the principle of rectification of injustice. For example, lacking much historical information, and assuming (1) that victims of injustice generally do worse than they otherwise would and (2) that *those from the least well-off group in the society have the highest probabilities of being the (descendants of) victims of the most serious injustices* who are owed compensation by those who benefited from the injustices (assumed to be those better off, though sometimes the perpetrators will be others in the worst-off group), then a rough rule of thumb for rectifying injustices might seem to be the following: *organize society so as to maximize the position of whatever group ends up least well-off in society*...Although to introduce socialism as the punishment for our sins would be to go to far, past injustices might be so great as to make necessary in the short run *a more extensive state* in order to rectify them.[11]

Would Engelhardt accept Nozick's solution? Nozick's principle of rectification justifies a patterned principle of justice for correcting inequalities based on correcting past injustices, which resulted from the actions of others. Such a principle would justify a more extensive government that would require, among other things, universal basic health care rights across all moral communities. Moreover, such a requirement would be within the context of Engelhardt's secular morality.

But I do not believe that Engelhardt would not accept Nozick's solution. He would want to err on the side of the innocent. He might argue that by adopting Nozick's solution, we risk punishing the innocent. Although he could admit many "guilty" exist, he would argue that a principle that requires everyone to help the worst off sweeps inappropriately across too many moral communities, indiscriminately punishing the innocent, i.e., those who played no role in current inequalities.

Perhaps one should help the worst-off irrespective of whether one actually caused the relevant inequalities. But, Engelhardt would argue, such a principle of beneficence, which required everyone to help the worst-off in society, is not necessary for the coherence of the moral world. Since it is not necessary, it is not basic, and so it must not be adopted across all moral communities. He writes:

Obligations to act with beneficence are more difficult to justify across particular moral communities than the principle to refrain from unauthorized force, in that *one can have the possibility of coherent resolution of moral disputes by agreement without granting the principle of beneficence.* The principle of beneficence is not required for the very coherence of the moral world, or of bioethics. It is in this sense that this principle is not as basic as what I will term the principle of permission. The principle of beneficence is not as inescapable. One can act in nonbeneficent ways without being in conflict with the minimal notion of morality (105, emphasis added).

For Engelhardt, any principle of beneficence is not as basic as the principle of forbearance. Consequently, a principle of beneficence is limited in its use in redistributive policies. Governments cannot use it to justify forcing anyone to help others, even if their lives are in danger. For instance, he says, "Since the principle of permission holds precedent, one should be moved to respect property rights even under such conditions of tension within the principles of beneficence (i.e., between giving individuals their property and giving to others what is necessary for life)" (165).

But this response is not open to Engelhardt. If the above argument is correct, Engelhardt mistakenly assumes that only forbearance is necessary among moral strangers "for the possibility of coherent resolution of moral disputes by agreement" (105). Contrary to Engelhardt, it is simply not true that moral strangers can collaborate with moral authority (in secular bioethics) without granting a principle of beneficence, i.e., a principle that requires moral strangers to help soften the inequalities that undermine mutual consent. It is not true that "one can act in nonbeneficent ways without being in conflict with the minimal notion of morality" (105), *since without a prior commitment to reduce relevant inequalities, not all moral strangers would accept mutual consent as the basis for resolving moral disputes.* And without universal acceptance, universal permission, moral strangers cannot collaborate with moral authority. Thus, contrary to Engelhardt, some kind of beneficence is required for the coherence of the moral world.

Moral strangers, then, would universally "accept" mutual consent as a neutral decision procedure only if there is a prior commitment to ameliorating relevant inequalities among moral strangers. Without such a commitment, secular morality cannot secure universal permission; moral strangers could not collaborate with moral authority when participating in peaceable negotiations. Thus, the only way moral strangers can collaborate *with moral authority* to resolve moral disputes–the only way they can accept mutual consent as an alternative to force–is if they have a prior commitment to both a principle of forbearance (or cooperative restraint) *and* a principle of beneficence, which requires helping the worst-off in society. Since some level of beneficence is necessary for collaborating with moral authority, requiring it does not risk punishing the innocent. The principle would prescribe a basic requirement that all moral communities must adopt, because it is what all moral strangers must accept as necessary for peaceable negotiations.

SECULAR MORALITY AND FAIR EQUALITY OF OPPORTUNITY

Is my argument that Engelhardt's moral theory includes a principle that requires benefiting the worst-off just another way of arguing that Engelhardt's theory, or my extension of it, is similar to Norman Daniels's theory of justice in health care, which also requires that society help the worst-off? I will briefly explain Daniels's theory and say why it is different from my extension of Engelhardt's.

Daniels, following John Rawls,[12] believes that justice requires society to arrange its background institutions to help the worst-off members in terms of liberty, opportunity, income and wealth by correcting for undeserved natural and social differences, which are arbitrary from a moral point of view. According to Daniels, this would include health care institutions, since having access to health care is necessary to mitigate the misfortunes of disease and disability, which adversely affect one's fair share of equal opportunity for his or her society.[13]

Following Rawls, Daniels distinguishes between protecting *formal* equality of opportunity and *fair* equality of opportunity and argues that society ought to go beyond the former and secure the latter as well. The former requires society to eliminate barriers to opportunity (i.e., it requires equal protection under the law), while the latter requires society to take positive steps to help its citizens, those disadvantaged at no fault of their own, to compete better for jobs and offices open to all.[14] For example, Rawlsian justice defends social programs like affirmative action and Head Start, given their role in protecting fair equality of opportunity. The point is, stresses Daniels, "none of us *deserves* the advantages conferred by accidents of birth–either genetic or social advantages. These advantages," he continues, "are morally arbitrary, because they are not deserved, and to let them determine individual opportunity–and reward and success in life–is to confer arbitrariness on the outcomes."[15] Daniels believes, like Rawls, that justice includes a principle of fair equality of opportunity that requires society to arrange institutions, including health care institutions, for protecting opportunity in the face of different starting points resulting from the arbitrariness of the natural and social lotteries.

But Daniels goes further than Rawls by using the fair equality of opportunity principle to justify mitigating the effects of disease on opportunity.

"Doing so," he argues, "required broadening Rawls's principle so that it protected individual shares of the normal opportunity range and *not merely access to jobs and offices.*"[16] The extension of this principle, he says, is natural and compatible with the central aim of protecting opportunity. "It is equally important," he explains, "to use resources to counter the natural disadvantages induced by disease. (Since social conditions, which differ by class, contribute significantly to the etiology of disease, we are reminded that disease is not just a product of the natural component of the lottery.)"[17] However, he warns, his approach does not require "leveling" all natural differences. "Health care has normal functioning as its goal: it concentrates on a specific class of obvious disadvantages and tries to eliminate them. That is its limited contribution to guaranteeing fair equality of opportunity."[18]

So, Daniels argues, if justice guarantees fair equality of opportunity, and if disease and disability impair an individual's fair share of opportunity he would have had if healthy, then, according to Daniels, "health-care institutions should have the limited–but important–task of protecting people against a serious impediment to opportunity. On this view," he continues, "shares of the opportunity range will be *fair* when positive steps have been taken to make sure that individuals maintain normal functioning, where possible."[19] "Moreover," he says, "my account is not equivocal...The social obligation I discuss is rooted in the considerations of justice...[and] such obligations will correspond to the rights of individuals."[20]

But Engelhardt would argue that despite the fact that the natural and social lotteries might cause some diseases and disabilities that would adversely affect a person's equal opportunity, these conditions and their effects are not unfair or unjust, but simply unfortunate. "Life in general," Engelhardt explains,

> and health care in particular, reveal circumstances of enormous tragedy, suffering, and deprivation. The pains and sufferings of illness, disability and disease, as well as the limitations of deformity, *call on the sympathy of all to provide aid and give comfort.* Injuries, disabilities, and diseases due to the forces of nature are unfortunate. Injuries, disabilities, and diseases due to the unconsented-to actions of others are unfair. Still, outcomes of the unfair actions of others are not necessarily society's fault and are in this sense unfortunate (382).

According to Engelhardt, then, justice does not require society to help the diseased and disabled since society, for the most part, is not (causally) responsible for their unfortunate conditions. It is up to communities to call upon individual sympathies to help them. Helping those less fortunate, in other words, is not a matter of justice, according to Engelhardt, but a matter of charity–a voluntary, not a required practice. Although people ought to be charitable or sympathetic to those less fortunate, society may not force people to act charitably, since losses in the natural and social lotteries do not generate rights to health care (383).

SECULAR MORALITY AND COOPERATIVE BENEFICENCE

Yet although individuals, according to Engelhardt, are not required to correct for diseases and disabilities that they did not cause, if my extension of his theory is correct, they are required to correct for relevant inequalities that are necessary to achieve moral collaboration among all moral strangers, which would include inequalities associated with disease and disability. A prior commitment to some level of beneficence (in addition to forbearance) is required for the very possibility of secular morality, namely, peaceable nego-tiations among *all* moral strangers. Unlike Daniels, the requirement to act beneficently to the worst-off members of society does not derive from the assumption that disease and disability are unfair, but from the assumption that without a prior commitment to reducing some of their adverse effects, moral strangers cannot collaborate with moral authority; they cannot obtain universal permission to use mutual consent as the procedure for determining the framework of rights and liberties that would subsequently guide their lives. Engelhardt, I argued, mistakenly assumes that secular bioethics does not contain a principle of beneficence as basic as the principle of forbearance because he mistakenly assumes that it is not necessary for collaborating with moral authority, which it is. Some level of beneficence is as necessary (as defining) for the possibility of secular morality as the principle of forbearance, since moral strangers would not "accept" peaceable negotiations without a prior commitment to both. Since it is as basic as the principle of permission, we may use coercive power to assure its compliance.

However, a principle of beneficence that requires individuals to help the conditions of the worst-off requires collective efforts for its success. Thus each moral stranger who collaborates with moral authority must accept a prior commitment to a duty to cooperate in collective efforts that benefit the worst-off members of society. This final section will attempt to formulate what I call a principle of cooperative beneficence as prescribing a basic duty of benefi-cence for secular morality.

A Principle of Cooperative Beneficence. If the above argument is correct, then secular morality would include a principle of cooperative beneficence that prescribes a basic duty of beneficence. This principle would prescribe some cooperative behavior as obligatory, namely behavior that helps the worst-off members of society. For example, the principle would prescribe for each of us a role in collective efforts that guarantees universal access to medical care in the United States. Importantly, this principle would require, not merely permit, a health care system to include a tier that guarantees access to everyone regardless of his or her ability to pay.

A principle that benefits the worst-off members of society, however, requires collective efforts for its success. Unlike most instances of forbearance, benefiting the worst-off requires the efforts of many people.[21] An individual, or even a small group, cannot significantly help alleviate relevant inequalities that affect the worst-off, e.g., the disadvantages that befall the millions of people without any or adequate health insurance.[22] Helping to alleviate these disadvantages requires the cooperation of millions of people. Thus, the principle of cooperative beneficence would direct each person to perform a beneficent act *together with others* as part of a cooperative beneficent effort.[23]

Yet Engelhardt would complain that such a collective effort is too demanding for individual participants, which undermines its obligatoriness across all moral communities. Each participant could always do more to reduce inequalities and different communities would have different standards for the demands it required its members to perform. For example, each participant, together with others, could always give one more hour, or spend one more dollar, to prevent or ameliorate relevant inequalities. Thus, Engelhardt might complain, requiring moral strangers, even collectively, to alleviate inequality, although praiseworthy, cannot be a moral requirement, since such an effort would require endless giving, which is too demanding for many moral communities (111).[24]

There are two responses to this criticism. First, it does not follow that from the fact we cannot determine specifically how much inequality to eliminate (how much beneficence to give) that we ought to do nothing to eliminate inequalities, that we ought to help no one. In fact, Engelhardt does not allow indeterminacy of the principle of permission to undermine its obligatoriness. For example, he writes: "Since the web of explicit and implicit consent is usually very intricate, it will often be difficult to chart exactly when consent has occurred. It will frequently not be at all clear what one ought to do, or where and when secular moral obligations exist. However, one should do the best that one can under prevailing circumstances" (74). Engelhardt admits that just because one cannot know exactly when another has given permission it does not follow that we ought to ignore obtaining permission as a fundamental moral requirement. Thus, if Engelhardt does not allow indeterminacy to undermine the obligatoriness of the principle of permission, he should not allow it to undermine the obligatoriness of a principle of beneficence.

Second, we can begin to overcome the demandingness problem if we stipulate that one's duty to cooperate only includes fulfilling a reasonable, well-defined equitable role. In other words, each person's duty to cooperate in beneficent efforts for alleviating relevant inequalities would be limited, in part, by the weight of other duties that a particular moral community requires its members to fulfill, e.g., legitimate parental and professional duties, or other legitimate contractual duties. This point merely reminds us that the duty the principle prescribes is one of many moral duties that a particular community will have; and although it deserves a prominent place among a community's set of moral duties, it should not necessarily override other duties in that set, as no duty should, *ceteris paribus*.[25] The reason it should not be so overriding is that this would essentially undermine the very principle itself, for community members would rarely, if ever, follow such a requirement.

Thus, one's duty (of beneficence) to cooperate in collective beneficent efforts does not require endless giving, but fulfilling a reasonable, well-defined equitable role. One "fulfills" one's role by contributing positively towards cooperative success, which usually involves merely complying with the effort. Although for some, it may involve initiating the effort, e.g., those with special skills and knowledge. A "reasonable" role is one that does not force a person to compromise his (or her) other (legitimate) *prima facie* duties of equal or greater weight. A "well-defined" role is one that a person can easily understand and completely discharge. And finally, an "equitable" role is one whose demands are similar to others with relevantly similar capacities and existing social roles. Moreover, it is one whose demands will not increase because some people refuse to cooperate.[26]

Of course moral communities can and will disagree over what is reasonable and equitable, but that will not undermine the basic requirement that the principle prescribes. After all, communities disagree over what is a reasonable level of forbearance to preserve agreements, or what is a reasonable level of competence to preserve free and informed consent. Nonetheless, although we should expect differences in the level of beneficence to vary among moral communities, there must be a standard of beneficence that no community should fall below.

Cooperative Beneficence and Health Care Policy. What kind of health care system would the principle of cooperative beneficence require for a pluralistic society? First, it would require that the system contain a tier where everyone has access to medical care regardless of his or her ability to pay. This tier may not be left to the discretion of communities. Second, since the duty to cooperate would not override other duties we have, e.g., familial duties, it would not forbid communities to allow anyone to use their income to buy extra medical care. But since, as discussed above, the principle of ownership does not prescribe a universal unlimited right to private property across all moral communities, moral communities may not allow this privilege to undermine the tier that guarantees universal coverage.

Nevertheless, since the system must have a universal tier, we must design the system such that this tier is successful and effective in the long run. Moreover, it must only require a person to contribute a reasonable, well-defined and equitable role toward that success. Since an adequate discussion of how to design this health care system, especially its universal tier, requires extensive empirical debates that I cannot accommodate here, for purposes of this chapter I will provide only very general features that this system should include if it is to comply properly with a principle of cooperative beneficence. For example, the system's design should include universal eligibility for a standard package of comprehensive medical benefits; it should be simple enough for a typical cooperator to understand his or her role; and its design should facilitate broad-based participation in using that standard benefit package. A design can facilitate broad-based participation if its benefits are attractive enough so that most (say at least 60 percent) community members use it as their primary source of medical care. In this way, the tier is stable in the long run, since such broad-based participation will command political respect.

The universal tier might resemble a kind of single payer system, since the evidence suggests that such a system would better achieve universal coverage, is simpler, fairer, and better facilitates broad-based participation than market-driven approaches.[27] But I cannot here make a detailed comparison.[28] Nonetheless, using a single-payer design for the universal tier would not forbid communities from also using a market-based tier for supplemental insurance. However, other tiers may not undermine a commitment to the universal tier.

Conclusion

Let me summarize and conclude. First, I explained how Engelhardt's foundations of bioethics support a two-tier health care system: one tier requires access to whatever medical care a person is willing to pay for, and a bottom tier permits, but does not require, access to medical care for those unable to pay. Second, I argued that Engelhardt incorrectly assumes that moral strangers can collaborate with moral authority by only granting a principle of forbearance, when in fact they would also have to grant a principle of beneficence that requires that we cooperate to help the worst-off members of society. Moreover, I pointed out that this principle is a requirement independently of any similarity to Daniels use of Rawlsian justice to defend a principle of justice for health care institutions. Finally, I argued that a principle of beneficence to help the worst-off, to be effective, would require the collective efforts of all moral strangers. Thus, to collaborate with moral authority moral strangers must grant a principle of cooperative beneficence, which prescribes a duty of beneficence to cooperate in collective efforts that benefit the worst-off members of society. This principle would require that a health care system include a tier that guaranteed everyone access to medical care regardless of his or her ability to pay, but it would not forbid other tiers, provided they did not undermine the universal one. This tier, I concluded, should have a universal, simple and stable design. But most importantly, secular morality would require it across all moral communities as basic.

Notes

1. H. Tristram Engelhardt, Jr., *The Foundations of Bioethics*, 2nd ed. (New York: Oxford University Press, 1996). All further references will be in the text with only a page number.

2. Engelhardt believes he is providing a transcendental argument for Robert Nozick's principle of freedom as a side constraint (97). See Robert Nozick, *Anarchy, State, and Utopia* (New York: Basic Books, 1974). Although others still defend Nozick's libertarianism, he now believes his views in *Anarchy, State, and Utopia* were inadequate and has revised them. See Robert Nozick, *The Examined Life* (New York: Simon and Schuster, 1989), 286-292; also, *The Nature of Rationality* (New Jersey: Princeton University Press, 1993), 32. For example, he writes, "The libertarian position I once propounded *now seems to me seriously inadequate*, in part because it did not fully knit the humane considerations and *joint cooperative activities it left room for* more closely into its fabric" (1989: 286-7, emphasis added).

3. In the context of "general secular morality" the "innocent," according to Engelhardt, "are those who have not used moral agents without their permission" (85).

4. See also, H. Tristram Engelhardt, Jr., *Bioethics and Secular Humanism: The Search for a Common Morality* (Philadelphia: Trinity Press International, 1991); H. Tristram Engelhardt, Jr., "The Four Principles of Health Care Ethics and Post-modernity: Why a Libertarian Interpretation is Unavoidable," in *Principles of Health Care Ethics*, ed., Raanon Gillon (John Wiley and Sons, 1994), 135-147.

5. Engelhardt also formulates a sixth principle, "the principle for intervention of the behalf of a ward," which I will not analyze here.

6. Engelhardt recognizes an exception in the case of emergency medical help. In emergency cases, one may benefit another without his permission because one can presume that the other would have consented to the help (see *Foundations*, 127).

7. H. Tristram Engelhardt, Jr., *The Foundations of Bioethics* (New York: Oxford University Press, 1986), 131.

8. It is not at all clear that these practices are "victimless." However, I cannot discuss this here.

9. Since, as we argued above, private ownership presupposes a particular moral assumption, Engelhardt's claim that the market presupposes no moral vision appears problematic.

10. Paul Gray, "Gagging the Doctors," *Time* (January 8, 1996): 50.

11. Nozick, *Anarchy*, 231, emphasis added.

12. John Rawls, *A Theory of Justice* (Cambridge, Mass.: Harvard University Press, 1971).

13. Norman Daniels, *Just Health Care* (Cambridge, Mass.: Cambridge University Press, 1985).

14. Daniels, *Just Health Care*, 46.

15. Daniels, *Just Health Care*, 46.

16. Daniels *Just Health Care*, 57, emphasis added.

17. Daniels, *Just Health Care*, 46.

18. Daniels, *Just Health Care*, 46.

19. Daniels, *Just Health Care*, 57.

20. Daniels, *Just Health Care*, 54.

21. Of course there are many instances where forbearance requires the efforts of millions of people, e.g., for preventing foreseeable pollution.

22. For an in-depth study of the connection between health insurance and accessing and receiving adequate health care services, see Office of Technological Assessment, "Does Health Insurance Make a Difference?–Background Paper," OTA-BP-H-99 (Washington D. C.: U. S. Government Printing Office, September, 1992). The report concludes that "[r]esearch conducted in the last decade supports the common-sense notion that having or lacking health insurance coverage is related to gaining access to services, to the types, quality and intensity of the care delivered, and *logically, to patient health*" (2, emphasis added).

23. Rory B. Weiner, "Cooperative Beneficence and Professional Obligations," *Professional Ethics: A Multidisciplinary Journal* 3, nos. 3 & 4 (1994): 83-115; Donald Regan, *Utilitarianism and Co-operation* (New York: Oxford University Press, 1980); Derek Parfit, *Reasons and Persons* (Oxford: Oxford University Press, 1984), esp. pp. 70ff.; Liam Murphy, "The Demands of Beneficence," *Philosophy and Public Affairs* 22 (1993): 267-292.

24. See also James Fishkin, *The Limits of Obligation* (New York: Yale University Press, 1982). For a nice overview of this "demandingness problem" see Murphy, "The Demands."

25. Although see Shelly Kagan, *The Limits of Morality* (Oxford: Oxford University Press, 1989), who argues that a principle of beneficence does, and should, override all other moral "requirements."

26. See Murphy, "The Demands"; Weiner, "Cooperative Beneficence."

27. Congressional Budget Office, "Estimates of Health Care Proposals from the 102nd Congress," *CBO Papers* (Washington D. C.: Congressional Budget Office, 1993). For a more comprehensive analysis of these types of proposals see Office of Technology Assessment, "An Inconsistent Picture: A Compilation of Analyses of Economic Impacts of Competing Approaches to Health Care Reform by Experts and Stakeholders," OTA-H-540 (Washington D. C.: U. S. Government Printing Office, June, 1993).

28. For a more detailed comparison see Weiner, "Cooperative Beneficence."

7

ENGELHARDT'S ANALYSIS OF DISEASE: IMPLICATIONS FOR A FEMINIST CLINICAL EPISTEMOLOGY

MARY ANN GARDELL CUTTER

In the *Foundations of Bioethics* and elsewhere,[1] Engelhardt develops a contextual account of disease. As this essay illustrates, Engelhardt's account can be employed in framing a feminist clinical epistemology. Feminists[2] claim that medicine, with its authority to define what is normal and pathological and to command compliance to its norms, tends to strengthen patterns of stereotyping and reinforce existing unjustified power inequalities. As a consequence, ageism, gender bias, and racism occur as various ways of accounting for the structure of and procedural character of contexts in medicine. This essay focuses its attention on gender bias in clinical medicine and argues that a gender-neutral account of clinical reality (and the diagnosis and treatment of disease) is *not* the response one can or should give to current concerns regarding gender bias in clinical medicine. Rather, the essay establishes that a feminist clinical epistemology is worth considering in order explicitly to incorporate gender into our accounts of clinical reality. Moreover, a feminist clinical epistemology is what is needed if we are to develop scientific research projects, medical care, and public health policies that more accurately reflect biological and psychosocial gender differences. This analysis is to extend Engelhardt's work in ways that carry special implications for our discussions concerning how we are to understand clinical reality, which in turn fuel our dialogues in biomedical ethics and public health policymaking.

ENGELHARDT'S ANALYSIS OF DISEASE

Engelhardt provides a three-fold analysis of disease. First, Engelhardt understands disease in terms of languages of medicine:[3] the descriptive, explanatory, evaluative, and social. As he says:

> Medical reality is the result of a complex interplay of evaluative, descriptive, explanatory, and social labeling interests. The ways in which we speak of, react to, and experience medical reality are shaped and directed by these interests. These form clusters of concerns I will synoptically call the languages of medicine. However, they are more than languages. They represent four conceptual dimensions, within which clinical problems are regarded. They are modes of medicalization.[4]

139

B. P. Minogue et al. (eds.), Reading Engelhardt, 139–148.

For Engelhardt, facts available within the spheres of medicine are seen as problems of certain kinds in terms of particular webs of descriptive conventions, explanatory models, values, and social roles. These four different clusters of constraints shape the ways we speak of, understand, and experience clinical reality and the disease and illness encountered therein. On the one hand, the clusters account for similarities among interpretations of disease. The accidentally constant descriptions and values given to certain widespread physiologic phenomena (e.g., coronary artery disease and myocardial ischemia) and the sensations they evoke (e.g., pain) illustrate agreements about certain states that interfere with whatever goals one might have interest in. That is, in almost any conceivable human context, the pain and disability of angina will be perceived as dysfunctional and as biologically improper. On the other hand, the modes of medicalization account for differences among understandings of particular diseases. Whether something is a sickness or poor training (e.g., stuttering), a defect or decay (e.g., presbyopia), a habit or disease (e.g., alcoholism), a disease or way of life (e.g., homosexuality), or a disorder or way of life (e.g., attention deficit disorder [ADD]) are decisions that health care professionals in conjunction with patients and related parties explicitly or implicitly make in particular cultures and contexts.

Second, Engelhardt understands disease in terms of a traditional philosophical distinction between 'ontological' and 'physiological' conceptions. He says:

> I wish to introduce the physiological and ontological concepts of disease from a primarily topological, not historical, point of view. They represent two general ways of talking about disease. Historically, they developed out of disputes whether disease was the result of the malmixing of humors, or was due to the entrance of a disease entity. The dispute roughly was whether diseases were primarily relational and contextual in character, or in some sense substantial things.[5]

Engelhardt supports the former position, i.e., the view that disease is a relational concept. He says: "...the concept of disease is in one respect pragmatic [i.e., functions as a treatment warrant], and in many respects influenced by issues of value [which tells us what limitations on human actions will be considered significant]. Particular diseases border on questions of moral and political significance."[6]

Third, Engelhardt understands disease in terms of "epistemological and ontological presuppositions concerning the levels of abstraction involved in disease theory."[7] Three distinct levels of abstraction may be distinguished: (1) *syndrome identification*, in which a pattern of observables (i.e., signs and symptoms) is recognized and identified; (2) *cause identification*, in which a cause, involving a level of theoretical explanation, is imputed to a syndrome and the pattern of observables are taken to be the effects of a cause; and (3) *relation identification* or *pattern-relation analysis*, in which a relation of variables is organized in a model of explanation with a nomological structure (i.e., according to the laws of pathology) to account for the pattern of signs and symptoms constituting a syndrome.[8]

Consider, for example, AIDS.[9] The year 1981 marks the emergence of a medical consensus that a pattern of observable signs and symptoms forecasting nearly inevitable death was occurring in isolated groups in the U.S. *Signs*, such as skin lesions, lymphadenopathy, and unusual infections, and *symptoms*, such as fatigue, recurrent fevers, unintended weight loss, and uncontrollable diarrhea, were brought together in an organized pattern, or *syndrome*. Syndromes provide the basis for the development of *etiological* accounts that allow signs and symptoms to be related in causal terms. Between April 1983 and August 1984, *a transmissible agent* was shown to be responsible for the manifestation and spread of AIDS. In May 1986, and after much debate among members of a consensus group, the transmissible agent is given a name, HIV. The search for a complete understanding of HIV as the causative agent of AIDS and for a magic bullet is inaugurated. Soon after, the recognition sets in that the etiological mechanism of AIDS is more complex. A *multi-factorial analysis or model* of AIDS is needed and allows the possibility of various understandings of AIDS, depending on whether one is a geneticist, an oncologist, a lung specialist, a social worker, or a feminist. In addition, *a clinical model* allows the possibility of a broad spectrum of treatments. It may be that in certain circumstances social variables (e.g., behavior), which presuppose the least technological advances, are easiest to alter. (Then again, behavior may not be the easiest to alter and one would consider other avenues of intervention.) By allowing the emphasis to fall upon relations, rather than objects or isolated causal agents, medicine conceives of disease in terms that are open to a wide range of cognitive and practical perspectives. As Engelhardt says, "In knowing a disease, one knows a relation, not a thing... Understanding disease as a relation of multiple factors accounts better for the peculiar entrance of normative judgements into disease theory."[10]

This brief overview illustrates the richness and complexity of Engelhardt's analysis of disease. Three distinct, but inseparable, accounts may be isolated. A first focuses on intersecting modes of medicalization; a second highlights the epistemological distinction and tensions between discovery and invention in disease concepts; and a third makes explicit levels of explanation that evolve in medicine. The accounts are distinct insofar as each brings attention to certain and diverse dimensions of disease concepts. They are inseparable insofar as each addresses the contextual character of such concepts. In short, disease is a descriptive, explanatory, evaluative, and social concept that is contextual and evolves in terms of levels of concretizations and abstractions.

TOWARD A FEMINIST CLINICAL EPISTEMOLOGY

Engelhardt gives us the basis for a clinical epistemology–for a study of knowing in clinical medicine. He does this through detailed analyses of concepts of disease. Disease concepts reflect how basic features of clinical reality are framed, classified, and explained. Moreover, and *without* his urging, Engelhardt provides us a basis for visioning a *feminist* clinical epistemology. His analysis of the interplay among facts, values, and socio-political contexts is shared by current feminist thought.

Women, Medicine, and Feminist Perspectives. As keepers of the home, as preeminent gatherers and then propagators of plants, and as caretakers of children until puberty, women traditionally cared for the sick, creating the earliest form of medicine, i.e., herbal medicine. Many deities of healing and reports of their attributes survive, from Isis and Gula in the Middle East to Panacea in Greece and Brigit in Ireland. Minerva Medica parallels Athena Hygeia–Great Goddesses worshiped for their healing powers.[11]

More recently, the rise of the women's health movement in the 1970s encouraged women to question established medical authority, to take responsibility for their own bodies,[12] and to express new demands for clinical research and access to health care. Between 1974 and 1983, the National Commission for the Protection of Human Subjects of Biomedical and Behavioral Research, and the President's Commission for the Study of Ethical Problems in Medicine and Biomedical and Behavioral Research[13] developed guidelines that require any research project that is federally funded to ensure humane treatment of (female and male) human subjects, including the acquisition of informed consent. In 1985, a Task Force on Women's Health Issues began work to aid the Public Health Service (PHS) "to improve the health and well-being of women in the United States."[14] In 1993, the U.S. Food and Drug Administration[15] issued guidelines concerning the participation of women in studies of medical products. Guidelines state that scientists must formulate research hypotheses so as not to exclude gender as a crucial part of the research question being asked. For example, when exploring the metabolism of a particular drug, one must routinely run tests on both males and females. And, in 1995, as reports from the Fourth World Conference on Women in Beijing and a recent issue of *Science*[16] illustrate, women's health and disease emerge as foci of concern for many researchers, health care practitioners, and public and private institutions.

Contributing to recent developments involving interest in women's health and well-being is the recognition that, among females and males, many diseases have different frequencies (e.g., heart disease, lupus, certain types of cancer), different symptoms (e.g., heart disease, gonorrhea), and different complications (e.g., most sexually transmitted diseases, and especially AIDS). Differences in manifestations call for different understandings of particular diseases and for different responses or treatments. Given that women have traditionally been excluded from clinical research but not from the clinical applications of research,[17] there emerges growing consensus that women need to be included in research projects, require their own special studies, and should be listened to in order to establish new lines of research. Such would bring about a broader view of women's health, one that would go beyond the con-fines of the reproductive system and would lead to more comprehensive definitions of women's health and disease. Such is needed for the development of scientific research projects, medical care, and public health policies that more accurately reflect biological and psychosocial gender differences. Such is important given that women constitute a greater proportion of caretakers of young children and needy offspring and of the elderly in developing and developed countries.

Claims regarding the lack of women's access to clinical research projects and proper medical care carry important implications in discussions in ethics and social and political philosophy–or social ethics, as Alison Jaggar[18] calls the intersection. Feminists, such as Susan Sherwin and Sue Rosser,[19] assert that the exclusion of women in research is a form of (continued) oppression and that such oppression must be voiced, criticized, resisted, and responded to with alternatives that promote women's emancipation. This may be the case but there is something more fundamental going on prior to the assertion of widespread oppression of women. This something is that modern medicine has sought to achieve a gender-neutral account of clinical reality, including disease, and feminists (along with others such as Engelhardt, albeit indirectly) show us that this goal has failed. What feminism offers is a gender-biased or gender-dependent account of clinical reality that uncovers the implicit bias of clinical reality offered by traditional medicine.

And so, and I admit that this is broad, "feminist" in this analysis means an ontological, axiological, and socio-political approach by and from the perspectives of women. Ontological in that it accepts differences between and among human organisms in terms of biological and psychosexual character. Axiological in that it accepts the role values play in epistemological endeavors and seeks to articulate such values–particularly as they have to do with the designification of women. Socio-political in that it sees that the social and political order is structured in a certain way that influences the experience of women and men–positively and negatively, beneficially and harmfully, happily and sadly.

The feminist literature that comments on medicine is primarily in feminist medical ethics with the predominant portion focusing on reproductive issues. Little is done in feminist philosophy of medicine and its subspecialty, feminist clinical epistemology. An account of feminist clinical epistemology contributes to what may be seen to be a crucial area of research for feminist thought and especially for the success of feminist medical ethics. This is the case because feminist clinical epistemology offers analyses of concepts, such as female and feminine, and underlying presumptions, such as gender-neutrality and gender-dependency, that illuminate the ways in which women and men examine, understand, and intervene in their world. One notes here that the phrase "feminist clinical epistemology" designates diverse and perhaps competing accounts of knowing in medicine.

Interplay Among Facts, Values, and Socio-Political Contexts–or Lessons from Engelhardt, Revised. I come to the view that a feminist clinical epistemology is worth considering from the standpoint that medicine and the disease concepts it fashions are not and cannot be gender-neutral (or neutral in any way for that matter). How is it, then, that medicine is gender-biased or gender-dependent? Let us begin with some "facts" or descriptions. At the start, we need to recognize that the distinction between and among *sex* differences is neither exhaustive nor exclusive. Human beings display a range of sexual diversity. There are those who fall in exclusive genetic classes (e.g., a "normal" homologous XX [female] or nonhomologous XY [male]). There are those who do not fall within either class (e.g., those with Turner's syndrome or Klinefelter's syndrome) and those who fall in both (e.g., a transverse or lateral hermaphrodite).

Nevertheless, there is something that we can say about sex differences or distinct expressions of sexuality. Anything does not go. There are currently limited expressions of genetic sexuality (e.g., XX, XY, XO, XXX, XXY, and XXXY), gonadal sexuality (e.g., ovaries, testes), hormonal sexuality (e.g., absence or presence of testosterone), genital sexuality (e.g., clitoris, penis), sex assignment (e.g., It's female!) and sex identity (e.g., "I am female!"). These limitations and expressions of sexuality come about through various theoretical assumptions including judgements concerning the simplicity, orderliness, and predictability of explanations. They give rise to a long-standing division in medicine between females and males and to the development and endurance of medical specialties such as obstetrics, gynecology, urology, and proctology. Clinical medicine and the classifications it designs presuppose and make empirically explicit sexuality and gender in various and complex ways.

Furthermore, classifications of sexuality give rise to the development of norms and particularly to gender-norms. In contexts where sexual or gender roles are well entrenched, the corresponding norms function *prescriptively*: they serve as the basis for judgments about how individuals *ought to be*, act, and so on. Furthermore, we decide how to act, what to strive for, and what to resist in light of such norms. Gender-norms of femininity and masculinity are clusters of characteristics and abilities that function as standards by which individuals are judged to be "good" instances of their gender. On one prominent model, to be "good" at being female (that is to be feminine), one should be nurturing, emotional, cooperative, sexually restrained, pretty, etc.; to be good at being a man, one should be strong, active, independent, rational, sexually aggressive, handsome, etc.[20] Nevertheless, it is important to recognize the absence of any single gender-norm cross-culturally and even within a given culture.

As seen here, the descriptive level of analysis in discussions of sexuality and gender is inextricably tied to the prescriptive level. Facts and values, as Engelhardt[21] teaches us, interweave in complex ways. Observations in medicine are always ordered around theoretical assumptions, including judgments concerning how to select evidence and to organize evidence into an explanation and, if appropriate, theory. Observations are always ordered around evaluative assumptions, including those concerning what objects are assigned significance and what actions are appropriate in order to achieve certain goals.

Moreover, the prescriptive force is backed by *social* sanctions fashioned in light of what goals are seen as worthy of achievement. If one aspires to conform to such norms, one is complemented. This is a message, for example, forwarded by cosmetic surgeons and health care professionals who prescribe hormone therapies and cosmetic surgeries. If one does not conform, one is censured, sometimes weakly and sometimes severely. For example, if a woman's behavior violates expected gender-role norms, her behavior is frequently attributed to various physical or mental illnesses and in turn is treated in a variety of ways, including pharmaceutical agents (e.g., anti-depressants[22]) and gynecological surgeries (e.g., hysterectomies and clitoridectomies[23]).

On this analysis, the quest to develop a gender-neutral clinical medicine is bound for failure. Given this, I reject a conclusion drawn by the Council of Ethical and Judicial Affairs of the American Medical Association (AMA) which asserts that "[p]rocedures and techniques that *preclude* or minimize the possibility of gender bias should be developed and implemented."[24] The Council goes on more specifically to address kidney transplant eligibility and states that "A gender neutral determination for kidney transplant eligibility should be used."[25] While I agree with the AMA that "[m]ore medical research on women's health and women's health problems should be pursued," I disagree that it is possible for clinical medicine to take a gender-neutral perspective, or any "neutral" perspective for that matter. Furthermore, I am concerned about the dangers of *not* taking gender and sex seriously in clinical diagnosis, prognosis, and treatment.

CONCLUSION

This essay has argued that a feminist clinical epistemology is worth considering on conceptual and practical grounds. Conceptually speaking, medicine has been shown to be a non-neutral, or more specifically non-gender-neutral, endeavor. Practically speaking, the current search to understand and to aid women's health and disease in developed and developing countries requires a reformulation of the presumptions and approaches provided by medicine. Feminist clinical epistemology is offered as one step in the direction of reformulating a traditional approach offered by medicine. I caution that such an epistemology must be done carefully, informed by studies and discussions involving those whose patient population is primarily women and those who are themselves women. The goal in my view is to bring about a future in which gender is not the focus but rather is seen as an influencing factor in arriving at the appropriate diagnosis, prognosis, and treatment of conditions suffered by women and men, girls and boys, infants, toddlers, children, adolescents, and adults.

NOTES

1. H. Tristram Engelhardt, Jr., "The Concepts of Health and Disease," in A. L. Caplan, H. T. Engelhardt, Jr., and J. J. McCartney eds., *Concepts of Health and Disease* (Massachusetts: Addison-Wesley Publishing Co., 1981): 31-45. See also, Engelhardt's "Explanatory Models in Medicine: Facts, Theories, and Values," *Texas Reports on Biology and Medicine* 32, no. 1 (1974): 225-239.

2. Helen Bequaert Holmes, and Laura M. Purdy, eds., *Feminist Perspectives in Medical Ethics,* (Indiana: Indiana University Press, 1992); Susan Sherwin, "Feminist and Medical Ethics: Two Different Approaches to Contextual Ethics," in H. B. Holmes and L. M. Purdy, eds., *Feminist Perspectives in Medical Ethics* (Indiana: Indiana University Press, 1992): 17-31.

3. Engelhardt, *The Foundations of Bioethics*, 2nd Ed. (Oxford and New York: Oxford University Press, 1996), see especially, Chapter 5, "The Languages of Medicalization."

4. See *Foundations*, 195.

5. Engelhardt, "The Concepts of Health and Disease," 33.

6. Engelhardt, "The Concepts of Health and Disease," 43.

7. Engelhardt, "Explanatory Models in Medicine," 237.

8. Engelhardt, "Explanatory Models in Medicine," 233.

9. Mary Ann Gardell Cutter, "Negotiating Criteria and Setting Limits: The Case of AIDS," *Theoretical Medicine* 11 (1990): 193-200.

10. Engelhardt, "Explanatory Models in Medicine," 237.

11. Autumn Stanley,"Women Hold Up Two-Thirds of the Sky: Notes for a Revised History of Technology," in Larry A. Hickman, ed., *Technology as a Human Affair* (New York: McGraw Hill Publishing Co., 1990), 308-323.

12. Boston Women's Health Book Collective, *Our Bodies, Ourselves* (New York: Simon and Schuster, 1973). Second edition appeared in 1984 under the title *The New Our Bodies, Ourselves.*

13. National Commission for the Protection of Human Subjects of Biomedical and Behavioral Research, *The Belmont Report* (Washington, D.C.: Department of Health, Education, and Welfare, 1978 [No. 78-0012]). See also, President's Commission for the Study of Ethical Problems in Medicine and Biomedical and Behavioral Research, *Making Health Care Decisions* (Washington, D.C.: U.S. Government Printing Office, 1983).

14. U. S. Department of Heath and Human Services, *Women's Health: Report of the Public Health Service Task Force on Women's Issues* 2 (Washington, D.C.: Public Health Service, 1985).

15. U. S. Food and Drug Administration, *Guidelines for the Study and Evaluation of Gender Differences in the Clinical Evaluation of Drugs* (Washington D.C.: FDA, 1993).

16. *Science*, Special Issue on "Women's Health Research," 269 (August 11, 1995): 765-801.

17. *Science,* "Women's Health Research."

18. Alison Jaggar, ed., *Living with Contradictions: Controversies in Feminist Social Ethics* (Colorado: Westview, 1994).

19. See S. Sherwin, "Feminist and Medical Ethics," 17-31, and Sue V. Rosser, "Re-Visioning Clinical Research: Gender and the Ethics of Experimental Design," 127-139; Holmes and Purdy, *Feminist Perspectives in Medical Ethics.*

20. Carroll Smith-Rosenberg, and Charles Rosenberg, "The Female Animal: Medical and Biological Views of Women and Her Role in Nineteenth-Century America," in A. L. Caplan, *et al.*, eds., *Concepts of Health and Disease*, 281-303.

21. Engelhardt, "Explanatory Models in Medicine."

22. Miriam Greenspan, *A New Approach to Women and Therapy* (Summit, Pennsylvania: TAB Books, 1993).

23. J. Waisberg and P. Page, "Gender Role Nonconformity and Perception of Mental Illness," *Women Health* 14 (1988): 3-16, and I. K. Broverman, *et al.,* "Sex-role Stereotypes and Clinical Judgements of Mental Health," *Journal of Consulting Clinical Psychology,* 34 (1970): 1-7.

24. Council on Ethical and Judicial Affairs, American Medical Association, "Gender Disparities in Clinical Decision Making," *Journal of the American Medical Association* 266 (1991): 560.

25. Council on Ethical and Judicial Affairs, AMA, "Gender Disparities," 561.

8

THE MAGIC MOUNTAIN: A PRELUDE TO ENGELHARDT'S PHENOMENOLOGY OF ILLNESS

RICHARD M. OWSLEY

Phenomenology as a philosophical method appears in many guises. In this paper, I shall use Edmund Husserl's basic position and the novel *The Magic Mountain* by Thomas Mann to suggest a *phenomenology of illness*, and throughout the analysis I will dialogue with Engelhardt's account of illness. Such a phenomenology should entail (1) a description of the essence or essences of disease as such essences appear to and within consciousness; (2) a lived experience of disease to an embodied subject; and/or (3) a noting and analysis of the structures and textures of the disease experience. In each of these areas, Husserl's admonition to consider things-in-themselves is presupposed. Illness is an experiential configuration in the lived-world both for those who undergo illness and for those professional health-workers who attempt to diagnose and treat such infirmities. A full disclosure of what it means to be ill involves a consideration of the possible social roles which result from the ill condition.

In an essay "Illnesses, Diseases, and Sicknesses," H. Tristram Engelhardt, Jr. erects a scaffold upon which a phenomenology of illness can be built.[1] One of his starting points is the question, "How does one experience him/herself as ill?" The answer to this question has many ramifications and subsequent questions: What changes of attitude toward oneself emerge with the onset of a temporary or chronic illness? What alterations appear in the relationships with the members of one's family, with friends, or with strangers? Finally, how does the world of things and of situations show itself to the ill? The presented answers satisfy theoretical curiosities, but they also provide guides for those who maintain, care for, and/or cure the sick. Engelhardt warns that this is not a simple task:

> In undertaking a phenomenology of disease, one will need, therefore, to take into account the complexity of the phenomena called illnesses, diseases, and sicknesses, as well as the fact that these phenomena are not necessarily all of one kind. Rather, what we call illnesses, diseases, or sicknesses are bound together in great part by family resemblances, not by the possession of a general disease property.[2]

B. P. Minogue et al. (eds.), Reading Engelhardt, 149–162.
© 1997 *Kluwer Academic Publishers. Printed in the Netherlands.*

Other authors whose work parallels that of Engelhardt can supply content for this framework. J. H. Van den Berg, in a book *The Psychology of the Sickbed,* is one such author.[3] Van den Berg sets the stage for the description of a routine, minor illness:

> Normally I am not aware of my body; it performs its task like an instrument. Now that I am ill, I have become acutely aware of my body's existence which makes itself felt in general malaise, in a dull headache, and in a vague nausea. The body which used to be a condition becomes the sole content of the moment. The present, while always serving the future, and therefore often being an effect of the past, becomes saturated with itself. As a patient, I live with a useless body in a disconnected present.[4]

Erwin Straus in *Event and Experience*[5] analyzes "traumatic occurrences," feigned or actual. Illnesses, disfunctions, and incapacities result in trauma for which there may be legal and medical compensation. In *The Psychology of Medicine,*[6] Medard Boss supplies descriptions of first-person "accounts" from those who are physically and psychologically ill. In *The Humanity of the Ill: Phenomenological Perspectives*, edited by Victor Kastenbaum, in which Engelhardt's aforementioned essay appears, Calvin Schrag, John O'Neil, and Edmund Pellegrino pursue similar themes.

Case histories of symptoms, suffering, and deliberations of mental illness appear in the work of psychiatrists Karl Jaspers and Ludwig Binswanger. Jaspers' *Strindberg and Van Gogh*[7] and Binswanger's *Being-in-the-World*[8] are replete with rich and detailed psycho-histories. Thomas Mann's *The Magic Mountain* provides a fictional parallel. Mann's novel is one of a long line of narratives preoccupied with disease and death. In the last two hundred years, writers such as Dostoyevsky, Tolstoy, Hemingway, and Kafka have explored the consequences to human beings of physical and mental malfunctioning. *The Idiot*, "The Death of Ivan Illych," *The Snows of Kilimanjaro*, "The Hunger Artist," and many others focus upon the illness motif.[9]

Ill health is an abiding theme in the work of Thomas Mann. Mann's morbid fascination for this subject is a prominent feature of *Buddenbrooks* (1900), "Death in Venice" (1911), *Doctor Faustus* (1947), and *The Black Swan* (1953). In each of these volumes, the disease examined varies. Cholera, tuberculosis, syphilis, and cancer are the occasions for clinical description and analysis. *The Magic Mountain*, begun in 1912, was finally published in 1924. This nine hundred page, two volume work presents a scientific and aesthetic picture of tuberculosis and the effects of this disease upon the character and outlook of its victims.

To label Mann's approach as phenomenological is not a new assertion. In an article, "The Philosophy of Thomas Mann," which appears in *Philosophy and Phenomenological Research* in 1943,[10] Fritz Kaufmann makes an excellent case for this designation. To Kaufmann Mann's efforts in *The Magic Mountain* and elsewhere exemplify Edmund Husserl's admonition to the philosopher: Pursue the "deepest meditation upon oneself."[11] Kaufmann continues, "this parallel [between Mann and Husserl] should at least be pointed out and the aims of both poet and thinker thus mutually corroborated."[12] Mann anticipates in *The Magic Mountain* Engelhardt's outline of a phenomenology of illness. In doing so, he utilizes Husserl's techniques of reduction, intentional analysis, constitution, and imaginative variation. Mann, unlike the philosopher, neither labels nor discusses such techniques. Instead, he illustrates them. In addition to the theme of illness, Mann's *Magic Mountain* contains distinctions between order and disorder, peace and conflict, the comic and the tragic, and the clear and the ambiguous. These distinctions are examined dialectically. The processes are described, but few conclusions are given. Embedded in the dialectic is a clear description of the essence of the disease tuberculosis as it appears within the consciousness of many characters. It becomes a unit of experience within a narrative which explores the mentality of tubercular victims.

The events of *The Magic Mountain* are framed within a specific time period and a definite geographical locale. The story takes place in an isolated region in and around Davos, Switzerland, during the years 1907–1914. In this place and at this time, Mann himself witnessed first-hand the challenges of tuberculosis. He recounts in *A Sketch of My Life*:

> In 1912, my wife had been attacked by a catarrh of the tip of the lung. She was obliged to stay for several months in the Swiss Alps. In May and June of 1912, I spent three weeks with her in Davos, and accumulated...fantastic impressions.[13]

The reader is slowly introduced to the atmosphere of the isolated sanatorium. Some seventy patients are undergoing treatments for lung disorders. All of the major countries of Europe and North America are represented. The interrelations between and among the various characters become a microcosm for Europe in the period which immediately precedes World War I. Conflicts and alliances among individuals and small groups are analogous to the political, diplomatic, and military confrontations between and among nation-states.

Mann's novel is paradoxically both simple and complex in narrative, character, and thought. Mann is aware of this ambiguity. He states, "The subject matter of *The Magic Mountain* was not by its nature suitable for the masses, but with the bulk of the educated classes, these were burning questions."[14] The strange, "magical" world of the mountain is refracted in the consciousness of a twenty-three year old naval engineer, Hans Castorp. Castorp is described as "a simple minded hero, a droll conflict between a macabre adventure and a bourgeois sense of duty."[15] The narrative alternates a direct articulation of Hans' stream of consciousness with a third person, objective discussion. Where dialogue is present, it is mostly presented from Hans' point of view. *The Magic Mountain* begins with an account of Castorp's journey to the sanatorium. He intends to visit his cousin, Joachim, who is a resident there. Upon his arrival, Joachim introduces Hans to the rituals, conventions, and practices of the therapeutic institution. Castorp, a "civilian," who has just accepted a position as a ship designer, is struck by the differences between himself and his cousin, a military officer of the same age. The opening chapters are an account of their re-acquaintance. The cousin, Joachim, has interrupted a promising military career to undergo a cure for lung disorder. In contrast to Joachim's supposed illness, Hans rejoices that he himself is healthy and vigorous. He is both amused and horrified by what he considers to be physical, moral, and emotional deformities within his "temporary" environment. Hans plans to stay three weeks: he remains seven years. During this time he learns to accept in others and even adopt for himself "bizarre" and "strange" attitudes, opinions, and behaviors. The character Hans Castorp anticipates Engelhardt's description: "To be seen as ill, to experience oneself as ill, is to have a lived experience of a state of deficiency or abnormality likely to be due to medical causes and warranting a sick role."[16] Hans does this. Initially, vicariously through his cousin and finally, directly in himself.

Hans' "learning" is on many levels. He apprehends the distinction between "apparent" and the "actual." Despite Joachim's radiance and healthful glow, Joachim continues to show symptoms of a serious disorder. Acceptance often masks rejection. Hans observes that seeming friendships among the patients disguise enmity. Solicitations concerning the health of individuals are a form of *schadenfreude*. The climax of Castorp's "learning" takes place when his own health and vigor becomes questionable. Soon after his arrival, Hans becomes ill. Upon examination he is discovered to be suffering from a lung infection, the seriousness of which is never definitively ascertained. Castorp is vaguely aware and Mann the author suggests that the character's discomfort and disfunction is an emotional upheaval masquerading as symptoms of medical difficulties.[17] Castorp meets each of his new experiences in a confusion of attraction and repulsion. As his supposed disease progresses, Castorp's feelings undergo fluctuations, cycles, and reversals. Mann's account of Hans' "adventures" anticipates Engelhardt's assertion:

> The experience of illness comes with social portent as well. To have a disease is to have
> an excuse from work, a right to sympathy, a need to see a physician, a right to disability
> pay. An experience of an illness state is thus many-layered.[18]

The encroaching illness colors the flat-lander's responses to the Mountain's mysteries. Landscape, weather, architecture, botany and other people contribute to a sense of strangeness and alienation. The reader of *The Magic Mountain* shares with Hans the food, the lodgings, the grounds, and the personal encounters. As Castorp becomes aware of the world-views, the motives and the responses of his co-inhabitants, what would have been trivial in the ordinary world becomes unexpectedly momentous. The overall mood of pessimism is gradually adopted by the central character of the novel. The initial frivolity, amusement, and fantasy steadily erodes. Most of the tubercular patients expect to remain chronic and uncured. Escape from the institution is always inadvisable and often futile. As Castorp witnesses the demise of many and as he is told of the sad endings of others, he becomes more depressed. The modes of death, suicide, murder, or acute infection all result in the survivor's forfeiture of the will to live.

Interspersed with a first hand account of Hans Castorp's external and internal adventures within the novel are Mann's third person accounts of illness in general and the tubercular illness in particular. The novel illustrates what Engelhardt has called "the state of affairs given to the experiencing person that would not have been given prior to the establishment of our prevailing medical scientific views."[19] Mann's account of tuberculosis is accurate for the first decades of the twentieth century. At that time there was no reliable cure. (Although the tubercular bacillus had been isolated by Robert Koch in 1882, it was only with the discovery of streptomycin in the 1940s that an effective remedy was found.) In 1912, a tubercular diagnosis was an indeterminate death sentence. The visit of Mann, of Castorp, and of the reader to a tubercular sanatorium, however short, is an *ascent* into an inferno whose inhabitants are damned. Nonetheless, the author, the hero, and the reader learn to accept damnation. Denials, escapes, and subterfuges are abandoned. Hans Castorp, with brutal honesty, catalogs these self-deceptions. He has much difficulty assimilating the disease which invades his body and conquers his soul. The wisdom accumulated by Hans during his sojourn on the Mountain is always fragile.

Mann notes the special characteristics of tuberculosis. In comparison to other disorders, it is glamorous, dramatic, and deceptive. Unlike conventional malfunctions of the heart, the liver, and the muscular system tuberculosis attacks the lungs of the prosperous, the young, and the seemingly healthy. The clinical features (pain, emaciation, coughing, and hemorrhaging) demand a psychological price. It is these psychological responses which have attracted Mann's attention. The various types of chemical, surgical, and dietary cures threaten security and self-esteem in a way that few other events produce. Mann dissects the temperaments of the victims extensively, ruthlessly, and honestly. As a detached author, he explores this subject matter with scientific detachment. As Hans Castorp the character acquires knowledge by research, observation, conversation, and reflection, Mann comments upon the significance, reliability, and usefulness of Castorp's knowledge.

Hans asks himself, the authorities, and others who have contracted tuberculosis the same question, "How does one justify the diseased life?" Disease has both pleasurable and painful aspects, but the pleasurable ones seem dubious, tentative, and unreliable. Hans is ambiguous about whether disease is uplifting or degrading; whether it is a mark of distinction, or simply a series of unfortunate events. He enquires as to whether natural or supernatural causes are involved. He is particularly intrigued by the possibility of disease as an aberration rather than the normal condition. Hans, who has previously assumed that a good citizen in an orderly society cannot and should not be ill, is forced to revise this view. Illness can and does strike in the most unexpected ways. The *bourgeois* places disease victims in a special category. The sick are excused from such requirements as maintaining a home, rearing a family, performing civic duties, or making a living. Since all of these tasks are thought to be "normal," illness releases one from responsibility. The infirm are not expected to fulfill the duties of others in work, play, love, or worship. They need not feel guilty at being unable to perform tasks which the healthy see as routine. Castorp realizes that he is tempted to use illness and death as an escape. The reader is not expected to accept all of Castorp's views of disease. Indeed, this is impossible: many are mutually contradictory.

In his stay at the sanatorium, Hans encounters others who have opposing views. Many attempt to "educate" him. Particularly crucial is his encounter with an impoverished Italian humanist who presents well-formulated views about character and bodily disfunction. Ludovico Settembrini, a man in his thirties, is a teacher and an advocate of the European enlightenment. In most areas of living, he espouses rationality, deliberate planning, and progress. He is opposed to romantic indulgence in feelings, gratuitous assertions of the will, and frivolous or incomplete thinking. Settembrini rejects the view that disease is inevitably associated with nobility, creativity, or refinement. A chronic tubercular himself, Settembrini sees his own disease as a curse which interferes with his aspirations and achievements.

> [S]o disease, far from being something too refined, too worthy of reverence, to be associated with dullness is, in itself, a degradation of mankind, a degradation painful and offensive to conceive. It may, in the individual case, be treated with consideration; but to pay it homages is—mark my words—an aberration, and the beginning of intellectual confusion.[20]

Settembrini rejects as a mark of decadence the tendency to welcome pain without relief and the wish for death. Human beings should be unembarrassed and unashamed of their striving for health. They should hold in contempt those who have ceased to struggle for a sane mind and a healthy body in an orderly society. Castorp assimilates Settembrini's teachings gradually. He initially rejects them, but later he accepts most of them. Hans, who is self-consciously prejudiced against Italians, learns to overcome his biases. At first he refers to Settembrini as an organ grinder, a windbag, and a phony. Later, however, when confronted by other viewpoints, Hans vigorously defends Settembrini's position. He affirms Settembrini's outburst:

> Do not, for heaven's sake, speak to me of the ennobling effects of physical suffering! A soul without a body is as inhuman and horrible as a body without a soul—though the latter is the rule and the former the exception. It is the body, as a rule, which flourishes exceedingly, which draws everything to itself, which usurps the predominant place and lives repulsively emancipated from the soul. A human being who is first of all an invalid is all body; therein lies his inhumanity and his debasement. In most cases he is little better than a carcass.[21]

Hans remains fascinated by instincts toward symptoms of, and conditions for, *dis-comforts*, *dis-eases*, and *mal-functions*. Hans' morbid interest parallels those of Mann the essayist. In a tract published just prior to the novel, Mann asserts, "if one is interested in life, one must be particularly interested in death. It is death and only death through which life becomes precious and meaning-ful."[22] Mann admits to this interest which he has and describes *The Magic Mountain* as "the fascination of death, the triumph of extreme disorder over a life founded upon order and consecrated to it."[23] The character Settembrini continues to protest "the only religious way to think of death is as part and parcel of life; to regard it, with the understanding and with the emotions, as the inviolable condition of life. It is the very opposite of sane...reasonable, or religious to divorce it in any way from life, or to play it off against it."[24]

A second character in the novel, Leo Naptha, opposes Settembrini in thought and action. He also adds to Castorp's insights. Of Jewish origin, Naptha has become a Catholic convert. As such, he accepts humanity's fallen condition as obvious and inevitable. It is this fallen state which explains why each human being is subject to sin, disease, death, and judgment. Such *dark* experiences are abiding, unavoidable, and unconquerable. The only worthy disposition for this condition is an enthusiastic but perverse defiance. For Naptha, the human being "is a sick animal" unsusceptible to rational analysis or scientific cure. He asserts, "disease is very human indeed, for to be man is to be ailing; man is essentially ailing. One's sick state, that is the state of un-healthiness, is what makes him man."[25]

To Naptha, pride in suffering distinguishes human beings from plants, animals, stones, and angels. It is Christ-like to appreciate, to celebrate, and even to enjoy infirmity. A life devoid of passion, in the literal sense, is un-Christian. The result is indifference and a life of humdrum, frivolity, and boredom. The agony of a suffering savior requires the agony of a suffering believer. Although Hans is unable to accept Naptha's conclusions, he acknow-ledges them as a corrective to Settembrini's humanism.

Unable to view suffering and disease as curse or divine opportunity, Hans remains ambiguous. He stands by as a duel, with weapons not with words, climaxes the Settembrini and Naptha conflict. For Hans the duel resolves nothing. His enquiries of the physician/custodians of the hospital likewise leave the issue unresolved. Hans acquires from the resident physicians a pretended neutrality concerning the metaphysical meaning of disease. Dr. Behrens, the superintendent, wears proudly the white coat of science, and he espouses antiseptic views. Both his opinions and his behavior are those of a detached, uncommitted spectator of diseased lives. Hans later discovers that

Behrens is himself a tubercular and that the doctor's detachment is a pose. Hans is shocked to learn that Behrens frequently becomes erotically involved with his female patients. The physician has even succumbed to the "animal glow" of the woman with whom Hans has fallen in love. The physician has painted her portrait, and he uses skills not only of an amateur painter but also of a scientist to ingratiate himself with the object of his passion. Hans thus suspects Dr. Behrens comments upon what constitutes life and living. "Life...is principally oxidation of the cellular *albuman* which gives us that beautiful animal warmth of which we sometimes have more than we need."[26]

A second physician, Krokowski, dresses in black and also presents the mild curiosity of a medical scientist. This also proves to be inaccurate. Hans learns that Krokowski is directly and emotionally involved with disease and diseased people. Exhibiting a superficial knowledge of Freudian psychoanalysis, Krokowski has developed a theory that disease is frustrated love. In a lecture on epilepsy, he proclaims:

> [This a]ffliction, which in pre-analytic times...[was] by turns interpreted as holy, even a prophetic, vision and as devilish possession...is the equivalent of love and an orgasm of the brain.[27]

To Krokowski, tuberculosis has a similar dynamic: it, too, is inhibited sexuality, and as such, it manifests itself in erotic symptoms. In addition to his weekly lectures at the sanatorium, Krokowski conducts seances where he and the patients experiment with the occult. Hans learns to mistrust Krokowski just as he has learned to mistrust Behrens as a reliable authority on the meaning of disease.

As he achieves the insights connected with what it means to be a person ill with tuberculosis, Hans Castorp becomes, from the institutional viewpoint, a model patient. He readily conforms to the regulations proscribed and prescribed for those with serious lung disorders. Presumably, this conformity with medical advice and procedure would fit any illness. Within the confinements to the rules, Hans seeks to acquire and to retain a sense of worth and importance. As his innocence is replaced by sophistication, he becomes knowledgeable of himself as a tubercular. He accepts his own condition and establishes a fraternity with those who share his fate:

> It was a gay company in which the three...sat and looked about them. There were white teeth Englishmen in Scotch caps talking in French to highly scented ladies dressed from head to foot in bright colored woolens–some of them even wore knickerbockers; an

American with small, neat heads on which the hair was plastered down, pipe in mouth, wearing shaggy furs, the skin side out; bearded, elegant Russians looking barbarically rich, and Malayan Dutchmen all sitting among the German and Swiss population as well as a sprinkling of indeterminate types, perhaps from the Balkans or the Levant. Hans Castorp showed a certain weakness for the motley, semi-barbarous world.[28]

In the beginning of the novel, Castorp thinks of himself as in perfect health. His thoughts under these circumstances are preoccupied with projections of a contributing participant in family, society, and nation. As he comes to think of himself as ill, Hans is content to occupy a marginal role. After dwelling for a time on the mountain, Hans becomes an invalid, the meaning of whose life no longer requires what was formerly defined as right, good, and proper. Facing disease and death, Hans becomes in his own eyes a full person. He successfully rebels against the temptation to become a mere social or political functionary. Moreover, he also refuses to be reduced to an anatomical specimen. Hans Castorp's attainment of human status entails a growth from the abstract to the concrete, from appearance to reality, and from spectator to participant. The philosophical Castorp must re-think concepts such as "honesty," "courage," and "rationality." Definitions no longer threaten Castorp's humanity. Honesty, courage, and rationality are re-constituted within his experience. Mann, the author, appraises his character, Castorp. In *A Sketch of My Life* he writes, "Yes certainly the German reader recognized himself in the simple minded yet shrewd young hero of the novel. He could and would be guided by him."[29]

The explorations of disease and death in *The Magic Mountain* provide evidence contrary to Engelhardt's assertion that "little work has been done to develop a phenomenology of illness states."[30] The philosopher of medicine might agree with Mann's own immodest assessment: "I was early aware that the Davos story had something to it."[31] In the final paragraph, Mann reaffirms this *something*:

Farewell honest Hans Castorp. Farewell life's delicate child. Your tale is told. We told it to the end...We have told it for its own sake, not for yours. For you were simple. But after all, it was your story, it befell you. You must have more in you than we thought...We shall see you no more...Moments there were when out of death and the rebellion of the flesh there came to thee, as thou tookest stock of thyself, a dream of love. Out of this universal feast of death, out of this extremity of fever, kindling the rain-washed evening sky to a fiery glow, may it be that Love one day shall mount?[32]

CONCLUSION

Engelhardt's essay, "Illnesses, Diseases, and Sicknesses," anticipates a phenomenology of illness. Mann's novel, *The Magic Mountain*, provides both content and structure for such a phenomenology. To Mann the six definitive characteristics which distinguish the tubercular experience are:

1. Tuberculosis has its source from without. Its cause is an invasion of the human organism by a specific bacteria. These bacteria may have been invited or welcomed by the victim, but they are always *other*. Hans recognizes this *otherness* which produces panic: "He had repeatedly to rest by the way, feeling the color recede from his face and cold sweat break out on his brow; the wild beating of his heart took away his breath."[33] Hans learns to measure the extent and power of his infection in terms of both psychological and physiological-anatomical processes. A high temperature, fatigue, depression, and erotic excitement are each indicators of bacterial invasion.

2. Hans' first-hand experience is corroborated by the accounts of others. One who feels ill is isolated from the physical environment, from other people, and from past experiences. Those who remain healthy appear strange to the ill and *vice versa*. Gradually or suddenly the victim becomes aware that he/she has become special, different, and alienated from what is ordinarily accepted as "normal." Disorientation occurs. The ill become inexplicably indifferent to ordinary stimuli and to conventional rules of conduct. They may become acutely susceptible to physical, social, or metaphysical stimuli which the healthy ignore. Hans concludes:

> It was that a certain fundamental fact of life which is conceded the world over to be of great importance, and is a fertile theme of constant illusion, both in jest and in earnest, that the fundamental fact of life bore up here an entirely altered emphasis...It had an accent, a value, and a significance which were utterly novel and which set the fact itself in the light to make it look much more alarming than it had been before.[34]

3. The categories of time, space, relation, quality, and quantity are radically altered by the tubercular disease. Description and analysis of the categorical changes becomes difficult. Mann's novel explores the life world of the sick and contrasts it with a healthy world. Time and temporality are radically effected. Hans notes:

I shall never cease to find it strange that the time seems to go so slowly...When I look back in retrospect, that is, you understand, it seems to me I've been up here goodness knows only how long. It seems an eternity back to the time I arrived.[35]

Mann, as omniscient author, comments further: "Hans Castorp did not keep inward count of the time as does the man who husbands it notes its passing, divides and labels its units."[36]

4. The inward life of the reflectively ill produces images, narratives, arguments, and models. The educated clientele which constitute the sanatorium population in *The Magic Mountain* explore introspectively their mental life. In so doing, they strive to give significance to their symptoms and to the lives of which they are a part. Settembrini asks, "Did you know that the great Plotinus is said to have made the remark that he was ashamed to have a body?"[37] To which Hans replies, "What have you against the body?... I'm getting out of my depth, but I won't give way... What can you have to say against the body?"[38]

5. Illness eventually becomes to those who have accepted their destiny as diagnosed tuberculars their sole reason for *being*. As incapacity and death appear, the individual freely releases his/her life to alien forces which overwhelm the body and the soul. The patient ceases to rebel, to fight, or to struggle. Hans anticipates his own death:

Whoever hears about it afterward imagines it as horrible, but he forgets that disease... so adjusts its man that it and he can come to terms. There are sensory appeasements, short circuits, a merciful narcosis–Yes, oh yes, yes.[39]

The disease the accompanying experience of which Engelhardt utilizes for a phenomenology of illness is gonorrhea. It is difficult to compare venereal disorders with the more serious tuberculosis of the lungs. Gonorrhea, when promptly treated, is not life threatening. It is inconvenient, uncomfortable, and embarrassing; but its symptoms do not terminate or seriously alter one's train of experience. Lifestyle may be altered and some ordinary functions made painful, but gonorrhea's symptoms seldom approach the range and depth of a tubercular disorder. Except facetiously, few consider the contraction of gonorrhea to be ennobling. Ethical considerations are superficial and even amusing. Present and former lovers must be notified, and medical authorities must be informed. The attitude of the victim toward him/herself may change toward self-loathing, unworthiness, or moral taint. But even the vivid imagination of H. Tristram Engelhardt, Jr. cannot make gonorrhea equal tuberculosis. Dr. Engelhardt would probably concede that the drastic cases fictionally represented in *The Magic Mountain* are a more significant source of insight for the phenomenology of illness which he recommends than the specific pathology explored in "Illnesses, Diseases, Sicknesses." Nonetheless, either malady and its repercussions can be used to develop a phenomenology of illness.

NOTES

1. H. Tristram Engelhardt, Jr., "Illnesses, Diseases, Sicknesses" in *The Humanity of the Ill: Phenomenological Perspectives*, ed., Victor Kastenbaum (Knoxville, TN: University of Tennessee Press, 1982).

2. Engelhardt, "Illnesses, Diseases, Sicknesses," 144.

3. J. H. Van den Berg, *The Psychology of the Sickbed* (Pittsburgh: Duquesne University Press, 1966), American edition of *Psychologie van het Ziekbed* (Nijberk: G. F. Callenbach N. V., 1966).

4. Van den Berg, *The Psychology of the Sickbed*, 28.

5. Erwin Straus, *Event and Experience*, Translated by Donald Moss and re-published as the first part of *Man, Time, and World* (Pittsburgh: Duquesne University Press, 1982), 3-142. Originally published as *Geschehnis und Erlebnis* (Berlin: Springer-Verlag, 1930).

6. Medard Boss, *Grundriss der Medizin und der Psychologie* (Bern: Verlag Hans Huber, 1975). Translation is available in English.

7. Karl Jaspers, *Strindberg and Van Gogh*, trans. O. Grunow and D Woloshin, (Tucson: University of Arizona Press, 1977). Originally published as *Strindberg und van Gogh: Versuch einer pathographischen Analyse unter vergleichender Heranziehung von Swedenborg und Holderlin* (Bern: Bincher, 1922. 3rd ed, Munich: R. Piper & Co, 1951).

8. Ludwig Binswanger, *Being-in-the-World*, trans. Jacob Needleman, (New York: Basic Books, Inc., 1963).

9. A more exhaustive list of narratives built on this theme is enumerated in Jeffrey Myers' *Disease and the Novel: 1880–1960* (New York: St. Martin's Press, 1985). A similar list is supplied in Susan Sontag's *Illness as Metaphor* (New York: Vintage Books, 1979).

10. Fritz Kaufmann, "The Philosophy of Thomas Mann," *Philosophy and Phenomenological Research* 4, no. 2, (December, 1943).

11. Kaufmann, "Thomas Mann," 304.

12. Kaufmann, "Thomas Mann," 304.

13. Thomas Mann, *A Sketch of My Life*, trans. by H. T. Lowe-Porter, (New York: Alfred A. Knopf, 1960). Originally published in German as "*Lebensabriss*" in *Die Neue Rundschau* (Berlin: S. Fischer, 1930). Subsequently published in English in a limited edition by Harrison of Paris in October, 1930.

14. Mann, *A Sketch of My Life*, 62.

15. Mann, *A Sketch of My Life*, 47.

16. Engelhardt, "Illnesses, Diseases, Sicknesses," 142.

17. Mann, *A Sketch of My Life*, 289ff.

18. Engelhardt, "Illnesses, Diseases, Sicknesses," 142.

19. Engelhardt, "Illnesses, Diseases, Sicknesses," 143.

20. Thomas Mann, *The Magic Mountain*, trans. H. T. Lowe-Porter (New York: Alfred A. Knopf, 1934), 128. Originally published as *Der Zauberberg* (Berlin: S. Fischer Verlag, 1924).

21. Mann, *The Magic Mountain*, 129ff.

22. Thomas Mann, "The German Republic," 5, quoted in *The Order of the Day*, 44.

23. Mann, *A Sketch of My Life*, 47.

24. Mann, *The Magic Mountain*, 256.

25. Mann, *The Magic Mountain*, 587.

26. Mann, *The Magic Mountain*, 338.

27. Mann, *The Magic Mountain*, 380.

28. Mann, *The Magic Mountain*, 399.

29. Mann, *A Sketch of My Life*, 62.

30. Engelhardt, "Illnesses, Diseases, Sicknesses," 154.

31. Mann, *A Sketch of My Life*, 67.

32. Mann, *The Magic Mountain*, 899.

33. Mann, *The Magic Mountain*, 159.

34. Mann, *The Magic Mountain*, 301.

35. Mann, *The Magic Mountain*, 136.

36. Mann, *The Magic Mountain*, 289.

37. Mann, *The Magic Mountain*, 317.

38. Mann, *The Magic Mountain*, 316.

39. Mann, *The Magic Mountain*, 301.

9

PERSONS, PROPERTY OR BOTH?
ENGELHARDT ON THE MORAL STATUS OF YOUNG CHILDREN

JOHN C. MOSKOP

In his many contributions to the bioethics literature over the past quarter century, H. Tristram Engelhardt, Jr. has addressed the question of the moral status of children a number of times, sometimes in passing and occasionally at greater length.[1] Engelhardt typically distinguishes the moral status of younger children, including infants, from that of older children and adults; in this paper I will focus on his discussions of younger children.

Engelhardt draws one conclusion clearly and consistently in all of his writings on this subject–he embraces a Kantian conception of persons as self-conscious, rational beings able to make and act on moral judgments.[2] Only such beings, Engelhardt argues, have attained the status of autonomous moral agents; their existence is a necessary condition for the possibility of a moral community. Engelhardt points out that *young children clearly do not qualify* for the moral status of persons in this full-blown Kantian sense. They lack the attributes of self-consciousness, rationality and possession of a moral sense necessary for making moral judgments. Older children, once they acquire these attributes, do become persons in this strict sense of the term.

Since younger children are not persons in the strict sense, what is their moral status? On this question, Engelhardt's writings convey a sense of ambivalence on two different levels, one explicit and the other largely implicit. In his most recent writings on the subject, Engelhardt explicitly laments "the painful contrast between general secular morality and content-full canonical morality."[3] He notes that many specific moral communities, as, for example, those organized around a particular religious faith, may ascribe to infants and fetuses a moral status equivalent to that of persons in the strict sense. Because such beliefs are dependent on the particular moral insights of a faith community, however, they are not features of a general secular ethics and thus cannot form the basis for public policy in a secular pluralistic society. Engelhardt emphasizes this unbridgeable gulf between the moral systems of specific communities and the more limited secular morality governing the interactions of "moral strangers" within a pluralistic society, that is, persons who do not share a concrete moral vision.

B. P. Minogue et al. (eds.), Reading Engelhardt, 163–174.
© 1997 *Kluwer Academic Publishers. Printed in the Netherlands.*

Engelhardt's account of the general secular morality binding moral strangers also contains an implicit ambivalence about the moral status of young children. This ambivalence is suggested by the existence of two separate and unreconciled accounts of children's moral status. On the one hand, Engelhardt proposes an account of the moral status of young children as persons in an extended, "social" sense of that term. This account contends that although young children are not persons in the strict sense, "nearly the full rights of persons strictly are accorded" to them, for several reasons.[4] On the other hand, in both the first and the second editions of *The Foundations of Bioethics* Engelhardt also proposes an account of property rights which suggests quite a different understanding of the moral status of young children. Based on the principle that one owns what one produces, Engelhardt concludes that parents have limited ownership rights over their young children.[5]

At first blush, these different accounts of the moral status of young children appear to dictate very different consequences regarding their treatment. Consider, for example, the much discussed case of Jehovah's Witness parents who refuse a life-saving blood transfusion for their infant.[6] If the infant has a right to life equivalent to that of competent adults, then we should intervene to rescue him or her, but such a right is, according to Engelhardt, based on a particular moral vision which cannot be independently established and which the parents presumably do not share. If the infant is a person only in an extended, social sense of that term, it is not immediately clear whether such a social sense of personhood is powerful enough to justify intervention against the will of the parents. If the infant is owned by his or her parents, they would presumably be free to control how he or she is treated without outside interference. As this example suggests, much is at stake in establishing the proper moral status of young children.

In his discussions of the moral status of children, as in so many of his other recent writings, Engelhardt stresses the limits of secular ethical argumentation. In fact, he finds it disquieting that secular moral reasoning can establish only very limited claims regarding the moral status of children.[7] In this paper, I will re-examine Engelhardt's two "secular" accounts of the moral status of young children, arguing that despite the limitations of general secular morality, Engelhardt's and others' arguments can be deployed to protect children from harmful treatment.

YOUNG CHILDREN AS PERSONS IN THE SOCIAL SENSE

Engelhardt first discusses the moral status of children in a series of articles published between 1973 and 1976,[8] most notably in his 1974 article in *Ethics*, "The Ontology of Abortion." He returns to the subject and offers his fullest treatment of it in Chapter 4 of *The Foundations of Bioethics*, "The Context of Health Care: Persons, Possessions, and States."[9] In these writings, Engelhardt is pursuing two broad objectives: (1) to defend the morality of abortion prior to fetal viability while maintaining a general moral prohibition on infanticide and (2) to defend treatment limitation and euthanasia for severely disabled infants.

Engelhardt rejects potentiality-based arguments against abortion; he contends that it is not the potentiality to acquire the morally significant attributes of rationality, self-consciousness, etc., but rather the actual possession of those attributes that constitutes personhood with its attendant rights and protections.[10] This poses an obvious problem, however, since infants, young children, and the profoundly developmentally disabled or senile also lack the attributes of rationality, self-consciousness, autonomy, and moral personality. It is in response to this problem that Engelhardt proposes his social conception of personhood.

Even though infants, young children, and some other human beings are not persons in the strict sense, Engelhardt claims that societies confer personhood upon them in more limited senses, with corresponding sets of rights and protections.[11] Engelhardt refers to these as social senses of personhood, since they are based on the social roles and relationships held by these individuals within human communities. We confer the status of social personhood, Engelhardt argues, because this practice has a number of good consequences. He lists several of these consequentialistic reasons in the following passage from *The Foundations of Bioethics*:

> A social role of person can be justified for infants and others in terms of (1) the role's supporting important virtues such as sympathy and care for human life, especially when that life is fragile and defenseless, and (2) the role's offering a protection against the uncertainties as to when exactly humans become persons strictly, as well as protecting persons during various vicissitudes of competence and incompetence, while (3) in addition securing the important practice of child-rearing through which humans develop as persons in the strict sense.[12]

If it is morally appropriate to confer the status of personhood on infants and young children, why not confer it on fetuses as well? The first of the above reasons, protection of defenseless human life, would seem to apply to fetuses as well as infants. In response, Engelhardt stresses the discontinuities between pre- and postnatal human life.[13] Though we may not be able to pinpoint exactly when individual humans become persons in the strict sense, we do know that this occurs after, not before birth; birth is thus a conservative, but surely safe boundary for protecting the moral status of persons strictly. Engelhardt also argues that the sentient experience of pre-viable fetuses is much more limited than that of infants, or adult mammals of other species, and thus, our concern to prevent the suffering of sentient beings applies more strongly to infants than to fetuses. Finally, Engelhardt notes that infants enter into social relationships in which they are cared for by their parents and others. We value these relationships and hence seek to protect and foster them by conferring special moral status on infants and young children. Fetuses, in contrast, are hidden within their mothers' bodies; the mother-fetus relationship is primarily bio-logical, not social.[14]

Engelhardt recognizes an additional reason for protecting infants and young children which is not consequentialistic.[15] If the moral community protects the lives of children, almost all of them will eventually become persons in the strict sense. The behavior of parents and others towards children will profoundly affect the lives of these future persons. Therefore, we owe duties not to act towards children in ways which will harm the persons they will become.

Through the concept of social personhood, then, Engelhardt seeks to grant a protected moral status to infants and young children while at the same time differentiating them from persons strictly, that is, rational moral agents. We recognize social personhood primarily for the benefits such a practice brings about. Important as these benefits may be, the recognition of social personhood is not as stringent a moral imperative as that of respect for persons strictly. We can, Engelhardt argues, permit limitations on the conferral of rights to infants or young children when the burdens of such a conferral greatly outweigh the benefits. Engelhardt argues, for example, that the foreseeable burdens of pro-longing the lives of severely disabled newborns may so exceed the benefits of doing so that we may not be obliged to prolong those lives. In this way Engelhardt can allow the practices of treatment limitation and euthanasia for severely disabled newborns.[16]

In summary, Engelhardt introduces the concept of social personhood to explicate the moral status and claims of infants, young children, and others. Recognizing this status, Engelhardt claims, allows us to grant "nearly the full rights of persons strictly" to young children.[17]   Nevertheless, Engelhardt recognizes, critics will find this defense of the moral status of children unacceptably weak. Engelhardt's comments on children and property rights, to which we now turn, are likely to reinforce the suspicions of such critics.

YOUNG CHILDREN AS PROPERTY

In a later section of the same chapter of *The Foundations of Bioethics* in which he discusses the social senses of personhood, Engelhardt addresses a critical issue for his libertarian approach to bioethics, namely, the justification of property rights.[18] Engelhardt begins this section by asserting ownership of one's own body, talents, and abilities; then he defends one's ownership of the services of others acquired through voluntary agreements.

The next paragraph begins as follows:

> One also owns what one produces. One might think here of both animals and young children. Insofar as they are the products of the ingenuity or energies of persons, they can be possessions. There are, however, special obligations to animals by virtue of the morality of beneficence that do not exist with regard to things. Such considerations, as well as the fact that young children will become persons, limit the extent to which parents have ownership rights over their young children.[19]

Later in the paragraph Engelhardt adds, "At the point that an entity becomes self-conscious, the morality of mutual respect would alienate the property rights of the parents over the children or other animals."

In his summary of "the principle of ownership," Engelhardt restates these claims as follows:

> Young children and mere human biological organisms are owned by the people who produce them. Ownership rights may be limited not only by the principle of beneficence, but by the circumstance that the young child (or fetus) will become a person.[20]

These brief, tantalizing claims are essentially all that Engelhardt has to say about parental ownership of young children in either edition of *The Foundations of Bioethics* or, to my knowledge, anywhere else. Although his further discussion of ownership rights suggests that such rights include the right to possess, control and transform one's property without interference from others, Engelhardt does not indicate how these rights apply to young children or how they are limited by the sentience and the future personhood of children. Neither does Engelhardt even mention in this section the status of young children as persons in his social sense or the implications of that status for the ownership rights of parents in their children.

I will now take up this unfinished business, examining in greater detail these two accounts of the moral status of young children and the relationship between them.

CONSENSUS ON CHILDREN'S RIGHTS

Engelhardt first addresses the issue of the moral status of young children as part of the broader problem of justifying moral distinctions among different groups of human beings–fetuses, infants, children, adults and individuals with profound disabilities. This problem is a central and difficult one for bioethics and for ethical theory generally. Lacking a compelling argument for the moral significance of all who are biologically human, Engelhardt focuses instead on the moral agency of adults and older children and on the social significance of infants and young children. As we have noted, he claims that the social person-hood we confer on young children includes nearly the full rights of persons strictly. Engelhardt does not, however, attempt to enumerate those rights, and hence we may ask what they are.

Though Engelhardt does not say so explicitly, presumably such rights would include a right to life, at least in the sense of a right not to be killed, since that is a fundamental right of persons in the strict sense. He does point out that young children do not possess a right to respect for their autonomous choices, since they lack the ability to make such choices. As Engelhardt reminds us, because young children cannot recognize and express their own needs and interests, we who are persons strictly must do so on their behalf. It is also left to us to weigh the interests of young children against those of other morally significant beings.[21] This poses a problem for specifying the rights of children, since moral agents disagree about the nature and importance of children's interests; there is no single authoritative ranking of the benefits and burdens to be allocated to different groups.

Since we lack a demonstrably infallible moral guru or a single compelling moral theory which can identify all of the legitimate rights of children, must we give up the attempt to specify them? Despite these limitations on moral inquiry, we need not abandon our efforts. Instead, we can seek to identify or create a consensus within society regarding the rights of children. John Rawls argues that persons and groups with different ideological, philosophical, or religious commitments may nevertheless agree on a significant set of reasonable doctrines for their society.[22] Though Rawls does not apply this idea to the moral status of children or to specific societies, I believe that there exists at least a limited consensus about a variety of basic rights of children in the United States today, including rights to life, to protection from injury, to material and emotional support, and to education. This consensus is reflected in a variety of state and federal laws governing homicide, child abuse and neglect, and public education.

This consensus about children's rights is not purely *ad hoc*; instead, it can be guided by the considerations Engelhardt offers, the social value of caring for young children and the duty to prevent harms to the future persons those children will become. To act on this latter duty, persons must reflect on how their behavior toward children will affect the children's future selves. Thus, Tibor Machan suggests that parental authority and obligations can be dis-covered by answering the question, "What would one's child have wanted one to do for (and maybe to) him or her when she turns out to be a grown person?"[23] Engelhardt's appeals to beneficence, social personhood, and future personhood offer an ethical framework which can guide the formation of a social consensus. Such a consensus can, in turn, define and implement specific rights of children.

Consensus about the enforceable rights of children may vary somewhat from society to society. I recognize that the United States and Bangladesh, for example, will likely define medical neglect of children in different ways. Such consensus will also change over time–children in the United States today are protected against exploitation as wage laborers more fully than they were one hundred years ago. I am, nevertheless, uncomfortable with Engelhardt's dis-cussion in *The Foundations of Bioethics* of Jehovah's Witness parents' refusal of blood transfusions for their infants.[24] Engelhardt comes very close to concluding that such refusals should be honored, hesitating only on the grounds that we can require treatment as a condition of access to community supported health care. I believe a stronger prohibition is in order here on the grounds that denial of clearly effective life-saving treatment to infants would violate establi-shed consensus regarding children's rights to life. Jehovah's Witnesses cannot exempt themselves from this consensus, at least as long as they remain members of the larger society.

Engelhardt's arguments regarding children are quite general, that is, they apply to all moral agents in their dealings with children. An additional argument, which Engelhardt does not invoke, focuses on the specific duties of parents regarding their own children. Becoming a parent obviously involves several choices. Except in the case of rape, persons choose to engage in sexual activity, perhaps for the purpose of procreation, or perhaps with conception and pregnancy as undesired consequences. Should pregnancy occur, the couple, or at least the woman, faces another choice about whether to bear the child or terminate the pregnancy. After birth, the woman (or couple) can choose to keep the child or give it up for adoption. In other contexts, Engelhardt emphasizes that voluntary choices create responsibilities. He argues, for example, that the choice made by older children to remain dependent on their parents imposes duties of obedience on those children.[25] If this is the case, then parents' choices to conceive, bear, and keep a child should also impose duties on the parents to care for their child, in view of his or her special moral status and state of vulnerability and dependency. Engelhardt acknowledges elsewhere that guardians have special fiduciary responsibilities to their wards.[26] Parents' voluntary actions in bearing and keeping their children provide a good reason for imposing such fiduciary responsibilities on them.

PROBLEMS WITH "PROPERTY"

As we have noted, Engelhardt focuses less on the fiduciary duties of parents than on the ownership rights that they acquire by producing children. I suspect that these claims about ownership of children evoke an immediate and strong negative response in many readers. Engelhardt's use of property language reminds us that children did have the legal status of property in ancient Roman and medieval societies and did suffer greatly from cruelty, neglect and exploitation in those societies.[27] In his defense, Engelhardt clearly would not permit such abuses of children; he asserts that parental ownership rights over children are limited. Given the negative connotations of ownership and property language applied to children, and the special moral status and rights Engelhardt believes should be conferred on children, are there still good reasons for describing children as the property of their parents, even in a limited sense?

Engelhardt might claim that his description of children as property is an essential part of a consistent and comprehensive account of property rights, a basic element in his theory. "Making babies" does bear some resemblance to producing other goods over which one can claim ownership, but there are also significant disanalogies. For example, we have noted Engelhardt's claim that one's body is primordially one's own. What are the grounds for this claim?

If one must consciously assert one's ownership over one's body to possess it, then this kind of ownership applies only to persons strictly. If, however, this ownership is based simply on inhabiting and using one's body, for example, to eat or to move, then it should extend to young children as well as to adults. Engelhardt argues that one comes to own things by forming or transforming them as one wills; one's ability to form or transform children according to one's will is limited, however, as parents are often painfully aware, and the paradoxical result of raising one's children is that they do not become more completely one's own property, but rather persons in their own right who cannot be anyone's property (at least, without their own consent). Thus, Engelhardt's claim that children are a kind of property has, at best, an imperfect fit with other types of property rights he recognizes. These disanalogies between children and other objects raise questions about the appropriateness of describing children as property.

We should also note that in his discussion of property rights in *The Foundations of Bioethics*, Engelhardt often uses the term 'property' in a non-standard sense, extending its meaning beyond current usage. Describing parents as having limited ownership of their children is but one example of this extended usage. Engelhardt also describes a person who has contracted to receive services from another as owning a part of that other person.[28] What is meant here seems to be that one person has a claim on or right to control some of the actions of another. If this is all that is meant by saying that parents are limited owners of their children, however, it hardly seems an outrageous proposition. Parents are, after all, expected to assume substantial control over the lives of infants and young children. We recognize such control as appropriate for several reasons. First, control is often necessary for the care and well-being of young children, since they are unable to care for themselves or protect themselves from harm. Second, we recognize parenthood as a valuable kind of human activity and hence seek to honor parents' interests in having a major influence on the lives and values of their children.[29] We grant this control to parents because they are the ones who have chosen to produce a child, thereby taking on the role of parent with its attendant rights and responsibilities. Parental control of children is thus a far cry from the slave-owner's control of his slaves. Slaves object to their bondage, but young children lack the capacity to consent or object to being controlled by others. Unlike slavery, parental control is not absolute, but limited by the rights of children; parents are thus bound not to kill, maim, sell, exploit, abuse or neglect their children.

Interpreted thus broadly, there seems little to object to in Engelhardt's claims that parents have limited ownership rights over their children. In fact, this usage seems analogous to the use of 'property' in the law to refer to one's legal interests in an object, rather the object itself. In order to prevent misunderstanding, however, it might be wiser simply to abandon the terms 'property' and 'ownership' in non-legal descriptions of the parent-child relationship, due to their misleading connotations in this context.

CONCLUSION

What, then, should we conclude about the moral status of young children? Are they best understood as persons, or property, or both? Young children are not, Engelhardt emphasizes, persons in the sense of morally responsible agents who can claim our respect for their free choices and actions. There is, nevertheless, a strong social consensus in support of protecting and enriching the lives of young children; Engelhardt's arguments for ascribing a different sense of personhood to children can explain and support that existing consensus. It can also account for commonly recognized differences in the moral status of young children and responsible adults.

If young children are persons, can they also be someone's property? Yes, Engelhardt would respond, and so can older children or adults, in the sense that others can make legitimate demands on their behavior. Engelhardt acknowledges that persons are owned by other persons only in limited ways. Nevertheless, because we do not generally use the terms 'property' and 'ownership' in these contexts, I suspect that such usage is more likely to mislead and alarm readers than to enlighten them. There is an important point to be made here, however–we do grant substantial control over infants and young children to their parents because those parents have chosen to produce offspring and to take on this role, with its legitimate rights and responsibilities.

Properly qualified and interpreted, young children can be understood as both persons and property, but the necessary qualifications and interpretations are, in this instance, at least as important as the terms 'person' and 'property.'

NOTES

1. H. Tristram Engelhardt, Jr., "Viability, Abortion and the Difference Between a Fetus and an Infant," *American Journal of Obstetrics and Gynecology* 116 (1973): 429-434, also "The Ontology of Abortion," *Ethics* 84 (1974): 217-234, "Ethical Issues in Aiding the Death of Young Children," in M. Kohl ed., *Beneficent Euthanasia* (Buffalo, New York: Prometheus Books, 1975), 180-192, also "On the Bounds of Freedom: From the Treatment of Fetuses to Euthanasia," *Connecticut Medicine* 40 (1976): 51-55, also *The Foundations of Bioethics* (New York: Oxford University Press, 1986), lastly *The Foundations of Bioethics*, Second Edition (New York: Oxford University Press, 1996).

2. Engelhardt, *Foundations* (1986), 104-109; *Foundations* (1996), 135-140.

3. Engelhardt, *Foundations* (1996), 146-147.

4. Engelhardt, *Foundations* (1986), 119; *Foundations* (1996), 149.

5. Engelhardt, *Foundations* (1986), 129; *Foundations* (1996), 156.

6. Engelhardt himself uses this example in *The Foundations of Bioethics* to illustrate the tension between parental rights to choose treatment for their children and societal intervention to protect children from harm. See *Foundations* (1996), 329-330.

7. Engelhardt, *Foundations* (1986), 120-121; *Foundations* (1996), 150.

8. Engelhardt, "Viability, Abortion and the Difference" (1973), "The Ontology of Abortion" (1974), "Ethical Issues" (1975), also "On the Bounds of Freedom" (1976).

9. Engelhardt, *Foundations* (1986), 104-156, and *Foundations* (1996), 135-188.

10. Engelhardt, "The Ontology of Abortion," 223-225, and *Foundations* (1986), 110-113.

11. Engelhardt, *Foundations* (1986), 115-121.

12. Engelhardt, *Foundations* (1986), 117.

13. In his most recent writing on this subject in the second edition of *The Foundations of Bioethics*, Engelhardt appears to have abandoned the sharp distinction he had previously drawn between the moral status of fetuses and that of infants. In the following passage, for example, Engelhardt seems willing to allow a social sense of personhood to be applied to fetuses as well as infants: "Still, in general secular terms a protected social role might be justified, or at least established within particular formal or informal agreements, for *embryos*, infants and others...." *Foundations* (1996), 147; emphasis added.

14. Engelhardt, "The Ontology of Abortion," 231.

15. Engelhardt, *Foundations* (1986), 115.

16. Engelhardt, "Ethical Issues," 183-185; *Foundations* (1986), 117-119; *Foundations* (1996), 148-149.

17. Engelhardt, *Foundations* (1986), 119.

18. Engelhardt, *Foundations* (1986), 127-135; *Foundations* (1996), 154-166.

19. Engelhardt, *Foundations* (1986), 129; *Foundations* (1996), 156.

20. Engelhardt, *Foundations* (1986), 134; *Foundations* (1996), 165.

21. Engelhardt, *Foundations* (1986), 109-110.

22. John Rawls, *Political Liberalism* (New York: Columbia University Press, 1993), 133-172.

23. Tibor R. Machan, "Between Parents and Children," *Journal of Social Philosophy* 23 (1992): 17.

24. Engelhardt, *Foundations* (1986), 289-90; *Foundations* (1996), 329-330.

25. Engelhardt, *Foundations* (1986), 129.

26. Engelhardt, *Foundations* (1986), 287-288; *Foundations* (1996), 327-328.

27. D. Archard, *Children: Rights and Childhood* (London: Routledge, 1993).

28. Engelhardt, *Foundations* (1986), 128-129; *Foundations*, (1996), 155-156.

29. E. Page, "Parental Rights," in B. Almond and D. Hill, eds., *Applied Philosophy* (London: Routledge, 1991), 73-89.

10

TRIS ENGELHARDT AND THE QUEEN OF HEARTS:
SENTENCE FIRST, VERDICT AFTERWARDS

MARGARET MONAHAN HOGAN

The bioethics of H. Tristram Engelhardt, Jr. presents a challenge. On the one hand, his grasp of this moment in the history of philosophy, the post-modern period, and its impact on the intersection of morality, medical practice, and public policy is incredibly precise. On the other hand, his direction for the remedy–a philosophical position anchored in the choices of mutually consenting, rationally developed adults–and, as a consequence, some of his particular conclusions are seriously flawed. In both his direction for the remedy and in the particular conclusions his work resembles the rule of the irascible Queen of Hearts in the Wonderland Kingdom encountered by Alice in her journey through the looking glass. In his general position, Engelhardt constructs a community in which only fully developed, self-conscious human beings count as persons, while in her domain the Queen permits only red roses. Engelhardt allows the conferral of personhood on lesser humans by fully developed, self-conscious human beings and the Queen allows the non-red roses to be painted red. In his conclusions, Engelhardt, like the Queen, wants to deliver the sentence–death–before he allows for the sufficient examination of the evidence and the determination of the verdict.

In his response to the contemporary moment, Engelhardt takes up the task of fashioning an ethic for biomedical problems that can speak with rational authority across a plurality of moral viewpoints present in this historical period which, in his view, is post-Christian, post-scientific, and post-humanist. In the absence of faith and the failure of reason to discover a content-full moral framework, Engelhardt articulates his theory, "The Will to Morality" which, he claims, provides "a moral framework that can be shared by moral strangers in an age of both moral fragmentation and apathy."[1] The central notions that constitute the matrix of "The Will to Morality" are the following:

(1) a content-full secular morality cannot be discovered;
(2) we are moral strangers;
(3) peaceful negotiation is the only possible way to secure a general moral framework;

175

B. P. Minogue et al. (eds.), Reading Engelhardt, 175–188.
© 1997 *Kluwer Academic Publishers. Printed in the Netherlands.*

(4) only human beings who are autonomous, i.e., fully developed, rational, and self-conscious are persons:
(a) personhood is a matter of accomplishment;
(b) only persons are bearers of rights in the strict sense; and
(c) human non-persons are vulnerable.

While Engelhardt is partially correct in regard to (1), (2), and (3), his philosophy of person (4) is inaccurately framed and inadequately developed. This paper will briefly respond to the incompleteness of (1) and (2) and, then, will develop a more complete response to (4), the inadequate philosophy of person. From within the context of these responses, a more structured matrix will be fashioned to facilitate and to direct (3), the negotiation of the possible peaceful community. The response suggests that human beings live their lives in various relationships and in varying degrees of dependency. And it further suggests that if there is to be peace, the vulnerable are in need of protection. In summary, Engelhardt has an inadequate epistemology which results in an incomplete metaphysics which yields an improper ethics.

Engelhardt moves too quickly from his assessment that a content-full secular morality cannot be discovered to the conclusion that there is not some content available to be discovered. Two notions need to be developed here. One has to do with the activity of reason; the other has to do with the objects of reason. Between an understanding of the role of reason as limited to discovering "the already out there now reality" and an understanding of the role of reason as empowered to construct reality there is a middle position. The middle position holds that sometimes reason discovers and sometimes reason creates. Reason is directed, and sometimes constrained, in constructing by that which reason discovers, that is, reason is fettered to truth. Reason is guided in discovering and creating by its own method–the ongoing, recurrent, related, cumulative, corrective set of operations employed in every cognitional enterprise yielding results that are cumulative and progressive.[2] This method moves from experience, to inquiry, to understanding, to judgment. It moves from the *quid sit* question that initiates inquiry to the *an sit* question which demands verification and does not rest until that verification is accomplished.[3] It is this method which guides human inquiry within a horizon that has expanded beyond the classical worldview of the past to the contemporary cultural moment with its historicist context. This method does not guarantee the possession of truth but lays out a path toward truth not as certain knowledge of the necessary, the essential, the universal, but as the probable affirmation of the particular and concrete.

In regard to possible concrete objects of reason, there are, between the emptiness of abstract heuristic guidelines such as "do good; avoid evil" or "be a peaceable member of a willed moral community" and the richness of content laden particular moral traditions such as that which can be found in the narrative schools of thought, specific markers to be discovered which place limits on and give direction to moral theory. Engelhardt has developed one–the will of the autonomous rights-bearing isolated individual. There is at least one other. This marker lies in our nature as related beings. It is the source of the principle of beneficence and the activity of intersubjectivity. Furthermore, it lies latent in Engelhardt's treatment of mutual respect, of beneficence, and of intersubjectivity. This being-in-relation counters Engelhardt's categorical claim that we are moral strangers and attenuates his elitist philosophy of person. While we are moral strangers in one sense–in the sense that we are holders of different moral traditions whose possible points of convergence we have chosen to ignore–there is another sense in which we, as related beings, are not moral strangers. We exist in real relationships to one another. And from these specific relationships to each other, concrete duties to each other arise and are defined. In addition, the human beings who anchor these relations possess individual identity, that is, their lives do not receive definition only in terms of the relations. They have significance in themselves quite apart from the relationships. An adequate moral theory attends both the beings who constitute the relationships and the link which defines the relationships. Engelhardt misses the linkage entirely and errs in his segregation of some human beings who anchor specific relations into classes of person and non-person.

Human relations vary. Some are quite close–even intimate. Some are distant–so distant that it takes a concerted effort to experience them. Some are problematic; some are so effortless as to appear natural. Some of these relationships are physical; some are moral. Some are freely chosen; others occur without choice. Some are symmetrical; others are asymmetrical. Some of the more obvious relationships are those of husband and wife, mother and fetus, parent(s) and family, family and community, physician and patient, attorney and client, experimenter and subject, teacher and student, the community of scholars...membership in the world community. These relationships suggest definition and give content to our responsibilities and duties. These relationships limit and structure the activity of "the willing" in peaceful negotiation.

It is our existence as related beings that is the source of our traditions of community and hospitality, of mutual respect, and of liberty as ordered. These relationships constitute the links in the web of sociality. Insufficient attention to these links provides only a partial sense of reality. And we are guilty of insufficient attention to these links.

An examination of human lives as embedded in relationships suggests the following: (a) autonomy is always a limited accomplishment achieved over time after a long period of dependency and often followed by another period of dependency; (b) living the rich human life often places human beings in asymmetrical relationships of varying degrees of dependency throughout life; (c) autonomy is constrained by the relationships which define one's life; and (d) relationships to others sometimes require the acceptance of disadvantages for the sake of the other.

This understanding of human life as woven in relationships gives direction, even substance, to the negotiation of the guidelines for the peaceable community. In the absence of a common moral authority, in the absence of the discovery of a final, rational, canonical perspective, and in the presence of individuals whose limited autonomy is temporary and defined by specific relationships, we, who live together, must both create and discover solutions to the moral problems we encounter. Whether or not we choose to solve our moral problems is dependent on our choice–hence the "will to morality" is crucial. However, the deliberation that guides the will must be informed by the reality discovered. The goals of peace and the emergence of the community require great protection for those who are dependent. Those who have achieved relative autonomy or those who exercise specific autonomy are required to protect those in conditions of dependency. Here the values of care, nurture, and relation, espoused by some feminists have a powerful role to play. This same observation has also been made by communitarians such as Mary Ann Glendon who wrote in *Rights Talk*:

> As mothers and teachers [women] have nourished a sense of connectedness between individuals, and an awareness of the linkage among present, past, and future generations. Hence the important role accorded by many feminists to the values of care, relationship, nurture, and contextuality, along with the insistence on the rights that the women's movement in general have embraced. Women are still predominately among the country's caretakers and educators and many are carrying insights gained from these experiences into public life in ways that are potentially transformative. Their vocabularies of caretaking are important sources of correctives to the disdain for dependency and the indifference to social bonds that characterize much of our political speech.[4]

Knowledge of human relations and the beings who are the terms of the relationship does not depend on belief in a creator God as the source of nature as normative. Furthermore, knowledge of these relationships does not depend on a privileged intuitive power to recognize a nature as morally normative. Knowledge of these relationships and their terms arises from the concerted and ongoing work of experience, inquiry, understanding and judgment, followed by more experience, inquiry, understanding, and judgment. Knowledge of the relations and terms provides a foundation to derive prescriptions from descriptions in the same way that knowledge of the role of a quarterback offers direction to the aspiring athlete or the knowledge of the role of the Snow Queen offers guidelines to the fledgling ballerina or knowledge of the nature of the heart offers direction to the surgeon.

Pregnancy provides an example of human lives embedded in relationship. The relationship is constituted by two human beings variously described as woman and fetus or mother and child. They exist as really related to each other. An adequate morality requires that attention be directed both to the relationship and to the beings who constitute the relationship. Directing attention to the relationship reveals the union to be asymmetrical. Directing attention to the beings in the relationship reveals an isomorphic symmetry, that is, each related being is a human being at a particular point on the human development trajectory.

Examination of the pregnancy relationship reveals several things. There is a physical union–a union of being. There may be a moral union–a union of purpose. That there is a physical union there is no doubt. However, this relation is more complex than most physical unions. If it were a kind of relationship that characterizes most physical unions, that is, a relationship of whole to part where the part is not necessary for the continuation of the whole and where it may be the case that the part threatens the life of the whole, there would be very little to discuss. However, since pregnancy is a temporary relationship between two physically whole human beings, one immature and the other more mature, a more complicated set of questions arises.

This temporary physical union is also a moral union–a union of purpose. Neither of the human beings who constitute the relationship is determined to accomplish the totality of existence within this relationship. Since each of the two entities has meaning outside the relationship, then the discussion of problems within the relationship cannot be resolved only in the limited examination of the relationship. The woman is a relatively autonomous being. Her life is characterized by a set of ends that extend beyond the pregnancy. For the duration of the pregnancy the fetus is a radically dependent being. While the growth and development of the fetus is intrinsically directed, the continued existence of the fetus is possible only within the nurturing environment supplied by the woman. The accomplishment of the ends of the fetus which lie outside the pregnancy require the cooperation of the woman. When the union is chosen either explicitly or implicitly, its status and the obligations of the more powerful member are less problematic from an ethical perspective. The more powerful accepts the disadvantages which occur for the sake of the more dependent. When the union occurs without implicit or explicit consent a more problematic relationship is constituted. The obligations that arise from a non-voluntary relationship are a function of the need fulfilled by the relationship and the status of the beings who constitute the relationship. In attending to that relationship as a physical union the appropriate question may be: what obligations might be claimed to arise where the life of one human being is so radically dependent on the other for such a limited period of time? In attending that relation as a moral union the appropriate question may be: what limitations may be placed on the activities of the more powerful when they find them-selves in relationships that are not of their own choosing? Attending those questions might defuse the prevailing rights-claiming and rights-trumping that marks the contemporary abortion debate and might facilitate peaceful negotiation. However, the approach to these questions requires more know-ledge of the beings who constitute the relationship. And it is here that Engelhardt's philosophy of person enters into the discussion.

When Engelhardt turns his attention to the beings who form the bases of the relationship, he applies his philosophy of person to them. In that philosophy, he segregates human beings by degrees of autonomy into categories of personal human life and non-personal human life. His core claim is that only human beings who are fully developed, rational, and self-conscious are persons. The elements that shape his view are (a) personhood is a matter of accomplishment; (b) only persons are bearers of rights in the strict sense; (c) human non-persons may have rights conferred upon them by human persons; and (d) human non-persons are vulnerable. When applied to the beings involved in the pregnancy relationship this means that the woman is a person and the fetus is a non-person. The woman may be a bearer of rights and the fetus has rights only if the woman so chooses.

This philosophy of person with its division of human beings into two classes–"[p]ersons, not humans, are special"[5]–and with its claim of significant moral difference–"[a]dult competent humans have much higher intrinsic standing than human fetuses or adult frogs"[6]–receives a multifaceted defense. The defense is tied to the principle of autonomy and it derives from Engelhardt's assessment of the fetus in terms of potentiality and probability. An exposition of Engelhardt's defense will be followed by a response to its inadequacies.

To be a person, Engelhardt claims, one must be autonomous. Only autonomous beings are capable of mutual respect. The constitution of a moral community requires personal beings. The required characteristics for the status of person are "self-conscious, rational, free to choose, and in possession of a sense of moral concern."[7] Those who do not have these characteristics are non-persons. Engelhardt says: "[f]etuses, infants, the profoundly mentally retarded and the hopelessly comatose provide examples of human non-persons. Such entities are members of the human species. They do not in and of themselves have standing in the moral community."[8] And, even more forcefully, he says:

> [I]t is nonsensical to speak of respecting the autonomy of fetuses, infants, or profoundly retarded adults, who have never been rational. There is no autonomy to affront. Treating such entities without regard for that which they do not possess, and never have possessed, despoils them of nothing. They fall outside the inner sanctum of morality.[9]

In developing his position, Engelhardt chooses the language of potentiality and probability to frame his dismissal of the fetus from the category of personhood. He presents an undifferentiated understanding of potentiality with a distinction between abstract and concrete potentiality, between material continuity and substantial discontinuity, and a deficient discussion of probability.

Engelhardt presents potentiality as a rather simple affair. If one is potentially something, then one is not yet that something. It is an all or nothing affair. He says: "[i]f fetuses are potential persons, it follows clearly that fetuses are not persons ... If fetuses are potential persons they do not have the rights of persons."[10] By way of analogy he argues that "if X is a potential president, it follows from that fact alone that X does not have the rights and prerogatives of actual presidents."[11]

In describing the fetus as possessing abstract potentiality, he contrasts the potentiality of the fetus with the concrete potentiality of the sleeping person.

In this limited discussion of concrete potentiality versus abstract potentiality, framed in terms of states of consciousness, he says:

> [T]he potentiality of the sleeping person is concrete and real in the sense of being based upon the past development of a full blown person. Unlike the fetus, the sleeping person has secured the capability of being fully human and has exercised it in the world. Far from a promissory note, the potentiality of the sleeping person to awaken is presented in concrete actuality in the physical substratum of that person, in his intact and functioning cortex. In this case the concept of person and personal presence depends heavily upon an intact normally developed brain; it presupposes some doctrine of the concomitance of mental personal life with an appropriate physical substratum. Further it requires recognizing the singular role of this intact substratum in weaving together the otherwise discontinuous life of the mind....The discontinuity of sleep...is bridged and woven together in mental life.[12]

Further, he maintains that the human person emerges from the human animal in a process best described in terms of material continuity and substantial discontinuity. This discontinuity, Engelhardt claims, is based on the development of new properties. He says: "it is easier to construe the situation as a development from biological properties to personal properties with a consequent and substantial change in the significance of the bearer of properties."[13]

Finally, in his application of the notion of probability to preborn beings, he claims that because research reveals that forty to fifty percent of human zygotes do not survive to become fully developed self-conscious rational human beings, it is more appropriate to consider the human zygote a 0.4 probable person.[14]

When one becomes a fully developed self-conscious being one gains significance and becomes a bearer of rights which may not be transgressed. Before one accomplishes such significance, one is not a person in the strict sense. However, rights for non-personal humans may be socially derived, that is, rights may be bestowed on human animals by the activity of already existing human persons on the basis of a utilitarian or consequentialist calculus. In setting value to non-personal human life, Engelhardt says:

> The value of animal life which is not the life of a person, must be determined by other persons...The value of an animal's quality of life is thus set by persons in two senses. First, if the animal has no developed conscious life, persons may find no intrinsic value in such life and the predominant value may be the value that the life has as an object for persons. Second, even if the animal has an inward life that in a prereflective sense has a value for that organism, persons must still compare the value with other competing values.[15]

Until the personal properties emerge or once the personal properties are lost, one is vulnerable. When this philosophy of person is applied to the beings involved in the pregnancy relationship the woman is a person and the fetus is a non-person. The woman is a bearer of rights and the fetus has rights only if the woman so chooses. Thus, in Engelhardt's peaceable community, the white roses have to be painted red.

Engelhardt's demarcation of biological human life from personal human life as determined by the relative accomplishment of autonomy and other characteristics of personhood is artificial, arbitrary and, even more, it is elitist. Its central error lies in his construal of the notion of potentiality. Potentiality does not simply describe a "have" or "have not" state of affairs. Potentiality is a rich notion with an ancient pedigree. Its legacy continues to the present.

The fetus is a human being in act. Within that being resides the potentiality–active natural remote potentiality–to become a more fully developed human being who may achieve a degree of autonomy or may accomplish whatever characteristics are used to define personhood. A nuanced explication of potentiality requires attendance to the distinctions of potentialities as active/passive, as natural/specific potentiality, and as remote/proximate. In active potency the being goes from not acting to acting and is also the agent of the action; for example, the human being may develop or go, by its own agency, from being not conscious to being conscious. In passive potency, a human being has the capacity to receive a modification but the agency of the modification is an external agent. The present reality of the fetus in relation to the adult human being is not that of passive potentiality which requires extrinsic agency for actualization. In the act that is the fetus there resides the active natural potentiality to become a more fully developed human being. Engelhardt's example of the potential presidential candidate who becomes president and enjoys presidential privileges is an example of a passive potentiality, that is, the extrinsic agency of the voters is required.

There are two distinct factors that make up the notion of active potentiality. One is constitution or nature and the other is tendency.[16] The fetus is, by its constitution, determined as a human being and is, by tendency, determined to become–in a fashion prefixed by its constitution–rather than not. Since the tendency of the fetus in regard to fuller human development proceeds in a completely determined manner and since it cannot become something other than what the constitution determines it to be and since it cannot of itself not become, it may be said that the potentiality of the fetus for more fully developed human life is an active potency.

Active potentialities are designated either natural or specific. In the accomplishment of an active specific potency, the agent has a degree of freedom in the actualization of the potency. The agent may specify the manner in which to actualize the potency. Active natural potencies are accomplished in a completely determined manner. The agent is not free to choose whether or not to actualize the potency. In addition the agent is not free to specify the manner in which to actualize the potency. Factors external to the agent, such as the destruction of the normal environment or dismemberment, can inhibit the actualization but the agent cannot inhibit the actualization.

A further distinction is made between those potentialities which may be designated remote and those which may be designated proximate. This distinction is a function of time and development. The presence of the proximate potentiality allows the possibility of immediate realization. The presence of the remote potentiality allows the possibility of future activity and future realization. However, the remote precedes the proximate and is the necessary condition for the existence of the proximate in terms of both constitution and tendency. The proximate is the further developmental specification of the remote. In regard to specific functions characteristic of more developed stages of human life there exist in the fetus the remote potentialities which specify the proximate potentialities necessary for action. In the chromosomal material, there is all that is necessary–in a relatively unachieved state of affairs–for the becoming of the neocortex which serves as the proximate potency for higher mental processes.

These distinctions suggest the inadequacy of Engelhardt's position. Engelhardt's distinction between the concrete potentiality of the sleeping person for human activities and the abstract potentiality of the conceptus for human activities is a strange distinction. On one hand, it seems to embody the distinction used in medical practice in problems which arise in the allocation of scarce resources when the decision is to be made between the patient that the physician knows and has treated and the similarly situated patient whom the physician does not know and has not treated. The former is perceived as concrete, while the latter patient is perceived by the physician as abstract. On the other hand, the concrete/abstract distinction seems rooted in the person/personal consciousness distinction, that is, one is a person so long as one is conscious of oneself. From the perspective of the first distinction, the reality of each patient is the same; the difference lies in the relation of the physician to each of the patients. From the perspective of the second distinction, Engelhardt appears to be reducing the person to personal consciousness. He mistakes an attribute for the whole. He makes consciousness the determinant of the person, rather than viewing human beings as persons who have the capacity to be conscious. That is, human persons are beings who are (1) sometimes conscious, that is, accompanied by the awareness of the self as a subject, (2) sometimes conscious with the awareness of the self as an object, and (3) sometimes (a) in act—as the fetus or as the sleeping person or as the person under anaesthesia—or (b) in action—so immersed in a problem or an activity or an encounter—that awareness or consciousness of self is lost. These different states are states of one being who continues throughout the states. This condition has been described as:

> The conscious life of the person is not the whole person; it is that in which the being of the person is actualized and this implies that a person is more than consciousness and that his or her body is to be distinguished from consciousness.[17]

From both perspectives, Engelhardt's analysis suffers from an inadequate notion of potentiality and from a lack of appreciation of the reality of the fetus. The fetus, or even earlier, the embryo or zygote, does exist and in its act resides the potentialities that may be actualized in the life of the individual. The potentialities are not in action but are present nonetheless. They may be abstract on the side of the observer but they are real and therefore concrete on the side of the fetus. In order for the activities of the higher central nervous system to be possible in the adult human being the cerebral cortex must be present (proximate potentiality). In order for the cerebral cortex to be present in the adult it must be present (remote potentiality) in the conceptus.

The description of the fetus as "an animal with great promise of becoming more than just an animal"[18] suffers from the same inadequacies as the distinction between abstract and concrete potentialities, namely, an inadequate perception of the reality of the fetus and an inadequate notion of potentiality. The possibility of the fetus's becoming a human being, i.e., Engelhardt's fully developed self-conscious person, is more than just a promise. By virtue of its active natural potency, "which is a guarantee of the future insofar as the agent is concerned,"[19] the fetus will develop itself (tendency) into an adult human (constitution).

Engelhardt's questioning of the appropriateness of identifying the "what or the who that the fetus is" with the "adult 'who' which develops out of the fetus" is framed in terms of material continuity and substantial discontinuity. If there is discontinuity it seems appropriate to inquire as to the source of the properties of personal life and the subsequent change in the significance of the bearer of the properties. If discontinuity is maintained, the source cannot be the fetus. Engelhardt does not designate a somewhere or a someone else. His difficulty seems once again to stem from his impoverished notion of potentiality. For example, he maintains, "The genetic basis for the development of the physiological substratum of consciousness is not yet that substratum."[20] The genetic basis for the physiological substratum of consciousness may not yet be that substratum, but it is not nothing. It is not a simple case of have or have not. It, the genetic basis, is that from which will develop the physiological substratum of consciousness. In the genotype there is the remote potentiality–an active natural potency–that is the necessary condition for the emergence of the proximate potentiality–the physiological substratum–of consciousness. Personal properties are present in the reality of the conceptus, a being who is in the process of building a body of a particular kind, but whose organs are not yet in operation. This reality has been described in this fashion, "it would be proper to say that it is an actual human person with a body whose full development is already in dynamic process."[21]

Finally, in Engelhardt's discussion of probability as it relates to the possibility of the human zygote's being born, he confuses predictions of the future with descriptions of present states of existence. He fails to distinguish between classical laws and statistical laws. Classical laws describe regularities–a one to one causal relationship..."other things being equal."[22] An example of a classical law in operation is syngamy–the union of the human sperm and the human ovum with the restoration of the diploid number of chromosomes along the mitotic spindle which marks the beginning of a new human life. Here there is an anticipation of invariance, the mark of a classical law. Another is the law of gravity–the anticipation of constant velocity. Statistical laws relate to probabilities, that is, assessments based on relative actual frequencies. The statement that only forty percent of fertilized ova survive to be born may be used to formulate a probability statement, that is a statistical assessment of the likelihood that a fertilized ovum will survive to be born. It says nothing of the nature of the surviving being. What one might conclude from this probability statement is that existence is precarious at this period in one's life. At the other end of the life continuum, it may be the case that only forty percent of those who reach the age of seventy-five live to be eighty. That does not make those who are now seventy-five only 40% persons. It simply means that those who have reached the age of seventy-five are rather vulnerable in a statistical sense.

Engelhardt's distinction between human biological life and human personal life is an artificial distinction without adequate philosophical foundation and cannot serve to segregate human beings into categories of non-vulnerable rights bearers and vulnerable non-rights bearers for the purpose of killing the vulnerable. The status of personhood as a matter of conferring value should include all members of the human community regardless of their degree of development. A more adequate philosophy of person holds that (a) all human beings have value, that is are rights bearers; (b) the human community is constituted by some humans who are dependent and some humans who are relatively autonomous; (c) autonomy, which is preceded and followed by states of dependency, is a matter of relative accomplishment; (d) the accomplishment of the peaceable community requires that dependent vulnerable beings, including the conceived but not yet born, be protected. The application of this philosophy of person to the physical union and the moral union of the non-voluntary pregnancy would require the recognition that the relationship is constituted by two human beings possessing value. Each human being endures a degree of dependency. The woman is dependent on the larger community; the fetus is dependent on the woman. Care of both seems the appropriate response of the peaceable community.

And so, finally, sufficient attention to evidence changes the verdict and stays the death sentence for dependent vulnerable human beings.

NOTES

1. H. Tristram Engelhardt, Jr., *Bioethics and Secular Humanism* (Philadelphia: Trinity Press International, 1991), xi.

2. Frederick E. Crowe and Robert M. Doran, ed., Bernard Lonergan, S. J., *Insight: A Study of Human Understanding* (Toronto: University of Toronto Press, 1992).

3. Lonergan, *Insight: A Study of Human Understanding*.

4. Mary Ann Glendon, *Rights Talk* (New York: Free Press, 1991), 174.

5. H. Tristram Engelhardt, Jr., *The Foundations of Bioethics* (New York: Oxford University Press, 1986), 104.

6. Engelhardt, *Foundations*, 104.

7. Engelhardt, *Foundations*, 105.

8. Engelhardt, *Foundations*, 107.

9. Engelhardt, *Foundations*, 108.

10. Engelhardt, *Foundations*, 111.

11. Engelhardt, *Foundations*, 111.

12. H. Tristram Engelhardt, Jr., "The Ontology of Abortion," *Ethics* 84, 3 (1974): 217-34.

13. Engelhardt, "The Ontology of Abortion," 225.

14. Engelhardt, *Foundations*, 111.

15. Engelhardt, *Foundations*, 111.

16. Gerard Smith and Lottie Kendzierski, *The Philosophy of Being* (New York: The Macmillan Company, 1961), 105.

17. John F. Crosby, "The Personhood of the Human Embryo," *The Journal of Medicine and Philosophy* 18 (1993): 407.

18. Engelhardt, "The Ontology of Abortion," 225.

19. Francis Wade, "Potentiality in the Abortion Discussion," *Review of Metaphysics* 29 (1975): 245.

20. Engelhardt, "The Ontology of Abortion," 226.

21. Joseph T. Mangan, "The Wonder of Myself: Ethical–Theological Aspects of Direct Abortion," *Theological Studies* 31 (1970): 130.

22. Lonergan, *Insight: A Study of Human Understanding*, 88.

11

THE FOUNDATIONS OF *THE FOUNDATIONS OF BIOETHICS*: ENGELHARDT'S KANTIAN UNDERPINNINGS

CYNTHIA A. BRINCAT

In these days of post-modernism and anti-essentialism actualized within the context of the relatively recent appreciation of the supposed failure of the Enlightenment Project, it is rare to hear terms like "rights," "guarantees" and "freedom." Surprisingly, these very terms are used by Tristram Engelhardt, a most contemporary thinker. Not so surprisingly, these very same terms are used by Immanuel Kant. In what follows, I show how it is that Engelhardt employs the above terms as the criterion for what he advocates as the foundation of bioethics. In doing so, I demonstrate that Engelhardt's foundation for bioethics, as a morality of mutual respect, is strikingly similar not only in its consequences, but in its basis, to Kant's civil commonwealth–a society based on right. Finally, after assessing the similarities between Kant and Engelhardt, I address their crucial difference. This difference consists primarily of Kant's recognition that for there to be peace instead of merely the cessation of war, the move to a content-rich ethic must be made. Whether or not this move can be made successfully brings us to face the role of hope, or its glaring absence, in the foundations of bioethics and ethics alike.[1]

MORAL DISSONANCE, OR THE PROBLEM OF NORMATIVE RELATIVITY: WHATEVER HAPPENED TO THE GOOD OL' DAYS?

Clearly, the current world, moral or otherwise, is far from peaceful. Even in communities that are ostensibly without conflict, it is sometimes the case that particular moral world views are violently contentious. This is demonstrated as we witness the way in which it has become increasingly dangerous to those who hold the opposite views of a select and violent few. In conflicts over abortion, logging rights, or access to semi-automatic weapons, those who hold certain viewpoints have made their views known, especially to their foes, by means of threats, violence and destruction. It seems that we shall always have this violent fanatical fringe to fear. Yet, what about the majority of us who engage in moral discourse? We disagree, yet are not quite ready to take up arms, bombs, or various other violent means against those with whom we disagree. Our times are rife with dissent and its resulting frustration.

189

B. P. Minogue et al. (eds.), Reading Engelhardt, 189–203.

Engelhardt maintains that this dissent comes about as a result of our conflicts over the normative terms that give our moral lives meaning. Not only do we disagree as to what is good or bad and right or wrong, but we also disagree as to what these terms mean. Good and right are no longer held unanimously by means of substantiation by government, church or society. Furthermore, if good and right ever were held unanimously, universal allegiance to such norms was, in most instances, certainly a product of coercion. Consequently, moral discourse, according to Engelhardt, has become something of a semantic melting pot bubbling over with multiple articulations of the normative terms which have typically served as the foundation of moral theories.[2]

The semantic relativity of terms like good and bad has become recognized as the predominant moral *modus operandi*.[3] From this keystone, Engelhardt argues that in their varied and various employments, these multifarious normative terms serve as the foundations for our myriad moral viewpoints. It is these viewpoints, with their primary conflict at a semantic, foundational (or meta) level, which lead to the differences and conflicts over ethics in our current world. In sum, not only do we disagree as to what is good or bad and right or wrong in ethics and bioethics—we also disagree as to what these terms mean. From this discord of dissent, how are we to come to any sort of moral meeting ground other than the graveyard?[4]

FACING OUR DEMONS: A RESPONSE TO NORMATIVE PLURALITY

In response to the lack of a shared singular moral world view, Engelhardt proposes that we first face, then accept, the current situation of ethical and bioethical discourse. There is a plurality of moral opinion, specifically as evidenced in bioethics. This plurality is not some sort of ethical dysfunction, it will not go away. Engelhardt rightly points out that the current situation within bioethics "calls out for a recognition that bioethics is a plural noun. There is not one bioethics."[5] Bioethics and its consequences, responsibilities and policies differ widely relative to the parties which are wielding the term.

Furthermore, Engelhardt argues that once we come to this realization of the semantic plurality of ethics and bioethics, we are also forced to conclude that the discussion of ethical issues "[n]ow transpires within the compass of secular pluralist societies."[6] This is a large leap, yet one that is not unreasonable. In asserting that we have "lost" a unified unanimous moral viewpoint, Engelhardt not so tacitly points to the Reformation as that which stole away our certitude.

Without the certainty of "the Church," for the most part, our ethical discourse transpires within a secular and pluralistic context.

In short, Engelhardt advocates that we give up the pursuit of a unified moral perspective from which to address bioethical concerns. We must recognize that relative to moral and bioethical issues society holds a multitude of views. It no longer makes sense, he claims, to speak of a unified societal or communal moral perspective, and perhaps it never did. Engelhardt rejects the possibility of there ever again being a *universally justifiable* way to go about moral or bioethical discourse. This is an important point and bears repeating. There will never again be an universally accepted notion of good/bad and right/wrong. Insofar as these terms are semantically relative there is no non-question begging justification for their status. In defending one particular notion of good over any other, one will eventually be reduced to (or rewarded by) asserting that this is just what we *mean* by *good*.[7]

Consequently, Engelhardt does not defend the view that there is one notion of bioethics and everyone else has previously gotten it wrong, will never get it right and thus we must settle for a notion of a bioethics based on mutual agreement. He is not concerned with coming up with the best, the most moral, or any other type of bioethics. Rather, it is his view that it was a mistake ever to have thought that there was one correct notion of bioethics to the exclusion of any other. As he says, "bioethics is a plural noun."[8]

ENGELHARDT'S MORALITY OF MUTUAL RESPECT: THE BEST THAT WE CAN DO IS PEACE AS THE CESSATION OF WAR

As a result of his surrendering to the plurality of bioethics, Engelhardt has but one self stated concern relative to the atmosphere of expressive multiplicity. He articulates this concern as "how to fashion an ethic for biomedical problems that can speak with rational authority across the great diversity of moral viewpoints."[9] Thus Engelhardt's program seeks the most expedient and efficacious of ethical systems in which health care can be delivered. In doing so, moral agents would be given recourse to appeal to rational authority in order to come up with biomedical policies to which they could as a society agree. That is, after diagnosing the current ills of modern moral discourse, Engelhardt realizes that the diseased state of a secular pluralist ethic creates a situation where it is very difficult for health care to be delivered. Hence, Engelhardt proposes a procedural ethic as a therapy for this diseased body of moral discourse. The result is an ethic that will be able to speak with rational authority across the difficulties of delivering health care, while at the same time taking into account the plurality of opinions that are in operation in the arena of health care deliverance. In this ethic, Engelhardt is not trying to educate people on how things should be, or so he says. Instead he is attempting to create an environment in which everyone can be not only true to themselves, but true to each other insofar as moral agents are treated with mutual respect.

Such an ethic of mutual respect can only be brought about through the specific conditions of a particular environment in which rational authority would be allowed (or required) to reach across the boundaries of various and differing moral perspectives. The conditions providing adherence to such rational authority could only be those to which all would agree. As such, these conditions would not be justified (nor justifiable), but rather they would be "disclosable in the very nature of ethics itself."[10] The situation which allows for the appearance of this seemingly self-evident, minimum criterion of what ethics is, Engelhardt characterizes as follows:

> If one is interested in resolving moral controversies without recourse to force as the fundamental basis of agreement, then one will have to accept peaceable negotiation among members of the controversy as the process for attaining the resolution of concrete moral controversies.[11]

In the din of moral discourse, Engelhardt thus articulates the calming comfort of peaceful negotiation as the way to proceed. In this procedural ethic, various moral perspectives shall be able to be pursued in an environment that guarantees the possibility of their pursuit insofar as this pursuit does not hinder the very same of another. This environment becomes actualized as the parties to moral controversy implicitly (or explicitly) agree that their conflicts will be resolved not by force, but by peaceable negotiation.[12]

Engelhardt's procedural ethic of peaceful conflict resolution is based on respect for autonomy, recognition of equality among persons, and the implicit freedom one has as a member of a moral community. [13] Under such an ethic, one is unable to "establish *a* particular moral viewpoint as *the* proper moral viewpoint."[14] If a moral perspective is to be agreed upon and a policy to have been fashioned, "one must have reasons that all have endorsed."[15] These reasons must be able to be maintained regardless of the individual moral perspectives of those party to the dispute. The authority of the general, unified moral perspective comes from mutual consent, a mutual consent mitigated by respect for freedom and autonomy. Furthermore, Engelhardt explains that this consent "must be actual or plausibly integral to resolving issues by agreement without the presumption of a common moral vision."[16] Through consenting to this very general, consent-governed moral perspective, we are, according to Engelhardt, thereby provided with the only remaining framework for moral discourse as well as for the deliverance of health care. In order to be efficacious, ethics is robbed of its vision. But is it?

Engelhardt is not misled. A morality of mutual respect is not an exhaustive nor limiting depiction of moral discourse. It is necessarily vague in order to remain uncommitted to a particular subscription to a particular notion of the morally good life. Just because a certain set of conditions is introduced to allow people to come to some sort of general agreements and solutions to the specific problems of the distributions of health care (Engelhardt's procedural ethic), it is not the case that all moral agents will share the views that are thereby being proscribed. Instead, it is very possible that an individual will personally object to the specific consequences of the deliverance of health care, while at the same time agreeing with the conditions that have allowed for this specific consequence. Engelhardt leaves us with the advocation of an environment that will provide the conditions under which various moral views as to what constitutes the good life are able to be expressed in their multiplicity.

So, there are two tiers to Engelhardt's peaceable community of mutual respect. On the first level, there is agreement as to what minimally an ethic is, as peaceful conflict resolution. This level creates an environment in which access to the second tier, where particular moral viewpoints can be expressed, is guaranteed. It is through this second tier that one learns what good and bad, right and wrong mean through their expression in particular moral communities. The inclusion of content is not an integral part of the first general level of moral discourse. As Engelhardt describes: "It is only within the embrace of a particular community that one learns whether it is right or wrong, worthwhile or not, to do the things one has a secular moral right to do."[17] Thus the first tier of moral discourse is devoid of content in order to avoid conflict, and guarantees one's "secular moral right" to the pursuit of moral content in Engelhardt's second tier. Through Engelhardt's two-tiered approach to moral discourse we have seemingly safeguarded not only our own views, but those of others as well.

KANT'S CIVIL COMMONWEALTH: ENTER THE POSSIBILITY OF A TRUE AND LASTING PEACE

Engelhardt constantly asserts that this two-tiered approach will leave us with the peaceable resolution of ethical conflicts. My response to this is two-fold. First, there is no peace where there is moral dissent. Although ideally there is only dissent in Engelhardt's second content rich moral tier, the conflict is there nonetheless. Engelhardt's plan is terribly effective for ending the wars of moral discourse on the first tier, but is this where our ethical conflicts stop? No, ethical conflicts do not center around a minimum criterion for ethics, but begin and end in the richness of a moral life. Engelhardt's procedural ethic does not leave us with peace, but merely the cessation of war. It is a postpone-ment of war, and in its advancement, as the means of proceeding in our moral discourse, it limits our possibilities for a true peace or at the very least our hopes for the possibilities of a true peace.

Second, and in response to the first point, I suggest by means of Kant a possibility for a true and lasting peace. In doing so, I defend Kant from Engelhardt's criticisms. Like Engelhardt, Kant articulates two realms of moral interaction. In the first realm, he presents a morality of mutual respect as the minimum criterion for his peaceable society, the civil commonwealth. Through the civil commonwealth, Kant articulates political right as that principle which serves as the basis of society, through the way in which poli-tical right grounds the formation of the state, just as a procedural ethic grounds the formation of our discourse. This realm allows for the simultaneous pre-sence of diverse moral viewpoints insofar as their pursuit is protected by right.[18] In his second realm, Kant like Engelhardt recognizes that there is more to moral discourse. Yet, unlike Engelhardt, Kant advocates a content rich specific moral understanding in this second realm, that of the ethical common-wealth. In this second realm, the two discrete tiers of discourse are now collapsed into one, and a third comprehensive tier of moral discourse is introduced. In articulating Kant's two realms, where three different tiers appear, I defend Kant from Engelhardt's accusation that Kant "smuggled concreteness into moral principles."[19] In truth, Kant smuggles no concreteness into his principles of right. Rather, Kant unabashedly celebrates the concrete-ness of his moral principles as they become manifest in his conception of a moral community, the ethical commonwealth. It is in the preparation to this celebration that my exposition of Kant begins.

KANT'S FIRST REALM: THE TWO-TIERED STATE OF RIGHT

In what follows, I outline the two realms that Kant proscribes for moral discourse. In the first realm, that of the civil commonwealth, Kant maintains the separation of the two tiers of moral discourse that Engelhardt articulates. It is with this realm that my exposition begins, after which I outline Kant's second realm, that of the ethical commonwealth, which introduces a third tier to the discussion. I maintain that this third tier is an inevitable move insofar as it includes the collapse of the separations between the two original tiers that both Engelhardt and Kant describe. Thus the primary difference between Engelhardt and Kant is that Kant recognizes the inevitability of a move to this third tier, while Engelhardt only makes such a move by means of his criticism of Kant, without recognizing he has done so.

In his corpus, Kant articulates a program for the civil commonwealth. The realm of the civil commonwealth, a discrete move in Kant's overarching plan to make morality real in the world, provides the opportunity for humanity to escape from its state of nature.[20] For the sake of this discussion, the nature and task of the civil commonwealth will not be my focus. Instead, this discussion focuses on the way in which Kant includes both of the tiers that Engelhardt describes. The first and primary tier present in this realm, that which forms the foundation of Kant's peaceable society, is based on the principle of right. In the civil commonwealth, right is the rule of that system which has as its basis autonomy. As Kant describes:

> The concept of an external right in general derives entirely from the concept of freedom in the external relations among men...Right is the limitation of each person's freedom so that it is compatible with the freedom of everyone, insofar as this is possible in accord with a universal law...[21]

Hence right supplies us with systematized moral principles in the form of laws that allow the guarantee of an environment in which we can pursue our particular moral goals. These particular moral goals are the constituents which provide content for both Kant's and Engelhardt's content-rich second moral tier. The pursuit of this second tier, for Kant like Engelhardt, has its very basis in freedom. If there is to be an expression of any particular morality, Kantian or otherwise, this freedom, which makes the expression of particular moralities possible, must be in place. To translate this Kantianese into an Engelhardtian turn of phrase, Kant has created an environment by means of the civil commonwealth in which freedom must be present as a condition of the existence of the commonwealth (Engelhardt's environment of a minimum criterion of morality). In being present, this freedom guarantees the individual's pursuit of his or her own moral interests. Through right, Kant provides a system that allows for the protection of the minimum rights of individuals within the context of his civil system.

As both Kant and Engelhardt stress, in being moral agents we are free, and this freedom and its pursuit must be protected. Otherwise, we are left with nothing like a morality of mutual respect. We are left instead with a morality of might makes right, a morality of all out war without postponement or cessation. Freedom must be able to be expressed if morality is to have any veracity, and the expression of freedom is guaranteed by right. Thus it is through right as "the sum of the conditions under which the choice of one can be united with the choice of another in accordance with a universal law of freedom"[22] that the social commonwealth is formed. If right is to be respected, Kant, like Engelhardt, advocates that moral individuals come together under conditions of mutual agreement in order to safeguard a minimum criterion of procedural morality. Kant specifically advocates that we come together to form a nation since

> ...before a public lawful condition is established, individual men, peoples and states can never be secure against violence from one another, since each has its own right to do what seems right and good to it...[23]

Like Engelhardt's first tier, Kant, through the civil commonwealth, addresses the plurality of our normative terms in order to demonstrate the need to establish a means through which we can peacefully manage our diversity. There is no content snuck into this realm. Truly, Kant does have in mind a picture for what should seem "right and good," but the manifestation of this picture does not yet appear.

The individual's pursuit of her own personal moral vision and happiness is protected in the civil commonwealth. Kant stresses that a civil state is the only form that a commonwealth may take if it is to be grounded in right, thereby protecting the freedom and autonomy of the individuals that make up that state in order that "each person remains at liberty to seek his happiness in any way he thinks best so long as he does not violate that universal freedom under law and, consequently, the rights of other fellow subjects."[24] As each person's pursuit of happiness and hence what each determines as good or bad and right or wrong is protected, Kant demonstrates his recognition of the two realms of moral discourse at work in Engelhardt. At this point in the Kantian project, there is no attempt at filling in the content of this second individually determined tier of moral discourse. Instead, in articulating the civil commonwealth, Kant is merely presenting the way in which our individual moral interests are preserved.

KANT'S SECOND REALM: THE ETHICAL COMMONWEALTH; OR WHERE MORAL CONTENT IS NO LONGER A CRIME AND THE TWO TIERS ARE ONE

After the formation of the civil commonwealth, Kant is not satisfied that he has completely accounted for the human moral condition. It is not enough for him to have safeguarded moral diversity. Instead, Kant here advocates a specific moral vision that is to be made manifest through the ethical commonwealth, a commonwealth based on the peaceful preconditions begun in the civil commonwealth. The individual members of this consummate articulation of the Kantian project are those who accurately fall prey to Engelhardt's accusation of collapsing into one realm the two discrete tiers of moral discourse previously described. In collapsing the two tiers, individuals in this realm enter a third tier through which the prior two are integrated. This is a problematic development, if moral development is to stop with Engelhardt's limited (and limiting) postulation of the two separate tiers of discourse. But, discourse is not naturally separate, as we shall see, and an integration of the two prior tiers is the purpose of the ethical commonwealth. This realm is not set up to preserve the plurality of moral discourse. Instead, Kant here introduces his notion of a content-rich moral community and the way it should be made manifest. For the sake of this discussion, the nature and task of the ethical commonwealth will not be my focus. Instead, my discussion focuses on the way in which it is here that Kant introduces the amalgam of the two prior tiers that Engelhardt describes. The ethical commonwealth is thus not based on right (the principle of the first tier) nor virtue (the normatively plural principle of the second tier). Rather it is based on the laws of virtue or moral right (*tugend gesetzen*).[25]

The distinction between this second realm and the prior one is made very clear insofar as Kant describes the following command: "Man ought to leave his Ethical State of Nature in order to become a Member of an Ethical Commonwealth."[26] That place from where humanity is retreating is the civil commonwealth, which removes us from our brute state of nature, but is unable to overcome our ethical state of nature. In calling for the establishment of the ethical commonwealth, Kant differentiates it from the civil commonwealth as he states that it is to be based in its structure on the civil commonwealth, but it is to go beyond the civil commonwealth insofar as it is required "to impress these laws (of virtue) in all their scope upon the entire human race."[27] Hence the ethical commonwealth gives vision and content to the schema that allowed for multiple understandings of a content-rich ethic as expressed in the civil commonwealth, and in doing so, we are freed from our ethical state of nature.

Once again, to put Kant in an Engelhardtian context, a third tier is present in the ethical commonwealth. This tier is an amalgam of the prior two. As such, in this third realm, all moral pursuits are not equal, and consequently the general procedural ethic, which in the former realm sought to protect a plurality of perspectives, now seeks to bring about the specific content-rich ethic that is advocated. At this point in the Kantian corpus it is no longer appropriate to speak of right or of virtue. Instead, moral discourse is governed by moral right as the manifestation of a move beyond the two distinct realms.

The recognition that these two realms are separate in Kant's work is crucial only insofar as the recognition allows Kant to escape from Engelhardt's criticism. Engelhardt accuses Kant of not allowing for the expression of various moralities, and this is completely accurate when considering this second realm of the Kantian ethic as here presented, the ethical commonwealth. Yet the ethical commonwealth, through the above, has been differentiated from that of the civil. In the civil commonwealth, there are two tiers present in Kant's realm and they are kept separate. Hence various moralities are able to be expressed, as long as their expression does not impinge upon the freedom of another. For here, the human race is in an *ethical* state of nature and not completely morally integrated. In short, Kant does allow that our two tiers can be separate, and he provides a mechanism to serve that purpose. Yet he does not see that separation as the highest purpose for humanity as it leaves us in two tiers and hence in discord.

ENGELHARDT'S POSTPONEMENT OF WAR

I hope it is clear at this point clear that within the Kantian corpus there is an eye for teleology. This is the case insofar as the *telos* of Kant's moral person includes the integration of the two Engelhardtian tiers of moral discourse. This consummate articulation of a moral life in Kant leads us to move beyond first and second tiers into a third, integrated tier. However, the general inevitability of the collapsing of two moral tiers for not only the Kantian moral person, but moral persons generally, becomes evident when we analyze Engelhardt's discussion of Kant. In treating Kant's depiction of a moral person, as portrayed in *The Groundwork*, Engelhardt accuses Kant of smuggling concreteness into the moral life. In truth, concreteness is not smuggled into a moral life, it is present. Engelhardt himself recognizes that each of us, in being human, operates in two moral tiers, one of which is very content rich. Hence it is trivially true to accuse Kant's moral individual of operating on two tiers. This is true of all moral persons, even those described by Engelhardt. This aside, the bite of Engelhardt's criticisms consist in his accusations that Kant "does not provide a justification for a principle of beneficence."[28] Engelhardt accuses Kant of borrowing from his specific content-rich moral tier where freedom is affirmed "as a cardinal value" by sleight of hand to bolster his first tier.[29] This supposedly benign first tier Engelhardt describes as "an ethic of respect for persons," something in and of itself unobjectionable.[30] However, when freedom is used as a justification for beneficence, as is done by Kant, Engelhardt points out that Kant's tiers collapse and Kant thereby has smuggled moral content into a place where it should not have gone.

The Kantian moral person, according to Engelhardt, is stumbling through the moral life in, dare we say, an integrated manner, residing in both tiers. This dual residence, according to Engelhardt, eliminates the possibility of a first tier for Kant. Hence, Engelhardt asserts that Kant's moral person, in operating autonomously and holding that autonomy as a moral ideal, "thus steps beyond the support of Kant's actual argument" which would "require an appeal to a particular moral sense." One consequence of this appeal consists in the fact that "Kant does not allow suicide, although in the case of a competent person there is surely consent."[31] Truly, Kant does not allow suicide. The integrated Kantian moral agent, operating in a third tier, would not will suicide either. However, in the civil commonwealth, suicide would have to be permitted, perhaps not sanctioned, but nevertheless permitted. Thus Kant does not allow suicide, since Kant's integrated moral agent operates in a third moral tier. However, any moral agent who has not made such a development, and is a member of the civil commonwealth, which still keeps the first and second tier separate, would allow suicide since not allowing it would infringe upon the interests of another, thereby violating Kant's principle of right.

What is missing in Engelhardt's depiction of Kant is the journey through which we arrive at this integrated life where something becomes "not allowable." It is as if Engelhardt is describing the end product of a long labor without acknowledging that a labor had, in fact, taken place. As Engelhardt adds in the footnote to the prior passage, "for Kant choices regarding one's self are not different from choices regarding others."[32] Instead, I would like to assert that for Engelhardt choices regarding one's self are not different from choices regarding others. Engelhardt's accusation that Kant collapsed his two tiers is really a realization that in taking a stand for or against anything we typically move into a third tier that integrates the two and calls us towards a realm of such agents. In failing to distinguish that Kant has two moral realms, set up in such a way as to lead to the complete person who integrates both tiers into a third tier (where granted, suicide is not allowable), Engelhardt points us to the way in which we too shall eventually have a third tier. This dialectical, although Kantian, third is our end insofar as we are human. It is not a borrowing from one tier to bolster another, it is our commitment to a content-rich realm while at the same time attempting to make our world a moral one, even if that entails merely what we *mean* by *moral*. Yet, in doing so, we are constrained by a minimum notion of respect that requires we pursue our own interests, moral or otherwise, only insofar as they do not infringe upon those of another.

KANT AND ENGELHARDT: PEACE VS. ITS POSTPONEMENT

Although nearly identical, the foundations of the peaceable communities of Engelhardt and Kant differ in a crucial teleological respect. Engelhardt sees the peaceable community for which we should aim as the best that we can do in these days of secular pluralism. But Kant sees the civil commonwealth as peaceable only insofar as it entails the cessation of war, and thus the civil commonwealth is a minimum expression of morality, and a mere stage in the development of Kant's consummate articulation of a moral society. This teleological differentiation is subtle, but crucial. In failing to recognize it, Engelhardt falsely accuses Kant of "smuggling moral content" into his ethical project as he accuses Kant of collapsing the principal categories of autonomy and beneficence. So, Engelhardt fails to credit Kant for realizing that there is a difference between what we should do and what we should be compelled to do.

For Kant, the full expression of his moral view goes beyond (or falls short of) Engelhardt's demand of a peaceable community as the mere cessation of warring factions. This is the case because Kant articulates the civil common-wealth as a mere moment in the moral life. For it is only after the moral development of the society progresses beyond the civil commonwealth and develops into the ethical commonwealth that humanity achieves Kant's consummation of a moral life. In this way, the ethical commonwealth includes the addition of a particular moral viewpoint as to what is the good life, where that good life is a notion of society not merely ruled by right, but by moral right. Moral right comes about through moral conversion as the only condition for an actual peaceable community as truly peaceful and not merely calmed.[33] The peace of this community consists in the absence of conflict in the second moral tier since everyone at this level holds the same view.

Alas, as Engelhardt aptly points out, the inclusion of a particular moral viewpoint cannot be justified by non question-begging reasons. Hence the ethical commonwealth includes not *the* notion of the good life, but merely the Kantian notion of the good life. Consequently, it is only Kant's foundations for a moral society that Engelhardt advocates, and not Kant's hopes for a truly peaceful community.

So, where does this leave us? Do we opt for a content poor ethic and its guarantee of conflict resolution, tacking on content only insofar as it avoids conflict (a sort of conditional moral commitment)? Or, do we opt preliminarily for a content-poor ethic that evolves into a content-rich ethic with promises, perhaps vainglorious of true and lasting peace. Neither view of ethics can be defended without question begging. Even a procedural ethic based on mutual agreement has its roots in a non-justifiable commitment to a minimal notion of ethics as peaceable resolution to conflict. Perhaps the decision is based on efficacy. If so, then Engelhardt's procedural ethic, with or without hope for true and lasting peace, is by far our best alternative. Perhaps instead is the inevitability of a hope for a true and lasting peace, demonstrably inevitable as we often collapse the two tiers for others (witness Engelhardt's discussion of Kant) and for ourselves, regardless of the organization of tiers, since our lives at their best, moral or otherwise, are integrated and cohesive. And in having moral content, hope seems to arise sooner or later, as Pindar explains, "Hope cherishes the soul of him who lives in justice and holiness."[34] With Engelhardt we have the cessation of war. But the price we shall have to pay is the loss of hope, justice and holiness.[35]

NOTES

1. All references to Kant will be made in English. Bibliographic reference will cite *Kants gesammelte Schriften*; Königliche Preussische Akademie der Wissenschaften (Berlin and Leipzig: Walter de Gruyter & Co., 1904-), abbreviated as KgS. This will be followed by reference to the English translation.

2. See H. Tristram Engelhardt, Jr., "Health Care Reform: A Study in Moral Malfeasance," *The Journal of Medicine and Philosophy*, (October, 1994): 501-516.

3. The position asserting the relativity of moral terms, semantic or otherwise, is not new. The position has roots in as various of sources as Nietzsche (see especially *Beyond Good and Evil*) and Wittgenstein (see especially *On Certainty*). For an excellent discussion of the specifically semantic relativity of moral and other crucial philosophical issues see Paul Moser, *Philosophy After Objectivity*, especially Chapter Four, (Oxford: Oxford University Press, 1993).

4. See Kant, "Towards Perpetual Peace, a Philosophical Sketch" contained in the collection *Perpetual Peace and Other Essays*, translated by Ted Humphrey (Indianapolis: Hackett Publishing, 1983). (KgS Band 8, 341; Humphrey, 107ff).

5. H. Tristram Engelhardt, Jr., *The Foundations of Bioethics* (New York, Oxford: Oxford University Press, 1986), 4.

6. Engelhardt, *Foundations* (1986), 4.

7. Engelhardt makes this point specifically on page three of *The Foundations of Bioethics*. By no means do I wish to present this view as outlandish by the use of scare quotes. This view is held by others, not the least of which is Alasdair MacIntyre, see *After Virtue* (Indiana: University of Notre Dame Press, 1981) especially Chapter Four. My use of scare quotes is only a means to highlight that these terms are semantically relative and were never meaningful to those who were not included in the language game in which they took effect.

8. Engelhardt, "A Study," 510.

9. Engelhardt, *Foundations*, 3.

10. Engelhardt, *Foundations*, 41. Furthermore, through this assertion Engelhardt demonstrates how he too falls prey to the way in which moral assertions are unable to be defended except by means of question begging (i.e. the conditions for a procedural ethic would be "disclosable in the very nature of ethics itself." The *very nature* of ethics has yet to be satisfactorily determined (italics mine).

11. Engelhardt, *Foundations*, 41.

12. Engelhardt, *Foundations*, 41.

13. Engelhardt, *Foundations*, 41-42. Although the parallels between Engelhardt's and Kant's system will be treated later in the paper, it is of interest to note the similarities between the above passage and the following passages in Kant: see "Perpetual Peace," 350 (112) and "On the Proverb that may be True in Theory, but is of No Practical Use," contained in the collection *Perpetual Peace and Other Essays*, translated by Ted Humphrey (Indianapolis: Hackett Publishing) 1983. (KgS, Band 8, 290; Humphrey, 72).

14. Engelhardt, *Foundations*, 42.

15. Engelhardt, *Foundations*, 43.

16. Engelhardt, "Health Care Reform," 508, in which he cites *The Foundations of Bioethics*, 2nd ed. (New York: Oxford University Press, 1996).

17. Engelhardt, *Foundations*, 49.

18. All translators cite the difficulty of translating the term *Recht* into English. With that stated, I will follow standard procedure, using the term right for the German *Recht*.

19. Engelhardt, *Foundations*, 69.

20. That Kant has a plan for making morality real in the world is not completely without controversy, especially to Hegelians. The following authors are excellent representatives of this type of Kantian exposition and interpretation: Sharon Anderson-Gold, Thomas Auxter, Georg Cavallar, Mary Gregor, Harry Van der Linden, Allen Wood, and Yirmiahu Yovel, just to name a few.

21. Kant, "On the Proverb that may be True in Theory," 290 (72).

22. Kant, *The Doctrine of Virtue*, translated by Mary Gregor (Cambridge: Cambridge University Press) 1991. (KgS, Band 6, 230; Gregor 56).

23. Kant, *Doctrine of Virtue*, 312 (Gregor, 124).

24. Kant, "On the Proverb that may be True in Theory," 298 (78).

25. Here Kant explains: "Hence an ethical commonwealth can be thought of only as a people... *under laws of virtue.*" See *Religion Within the Limits of Reason Alone*, translated by Greene and Hudson (New York: Harper Torchbooks, 1960). B(KgS, Band 8, 99; Greene and Hudson, 91).

26. Kant, *Religion Within the Limits of Reason Alone*, 96 (8).

27. Kant, *Religion Within the Limits of Reason Alone*, 94 (86).

28. Kant, *Religion Within the Limits of Reason Alone*, 105.

29. Kant, *Religion within the Limits of Reason Alone*, 106.

30. Kant, *Religion Within the Limits of Reason Alone*, 105.

31. Kant, *Religion Within the Limits of Reason Alone*, 106.

32. Kant, *Religion Within the Limits of Reason Alone*, 132.

33. With regard to Kant's presentation of moral conversion, see Book Three of *Religion Within the Limits of Reason Alone*.

34. Pindar, Fragment 214.

35. This paper has benefitted greatly from conversations with and the editorial assistance of Dr. Gabriel Palmer-Fernández. Needless to say, all remaining weaknesses are those of the author.

12

ENGELHARDT, HISTORICISM AND THE MINIMALIST PARADOX

BRENDAN P. MINOGUE

At the core of H. Tristram Engelhardt's bioethical vision is a paradox, which I will call the minimalist paradox. The individual elements of this paradox serve to justify and explain many of the positions most closely associated with his *Foundations of Bioethics.*[1] However, Engelhardt does not acknowledge the significance of paradox or antinomy within his ethics. Engelhardt has no references to either topic in the first or the second edition and therefore it is fair to say that the paradoxical character of our moral lives is left untreated within his most important work. This absence is especially curious given the influence that Kant's ethical theory has had on Engelhardt. For Kant not only admits the importance of paradoxes within our intellectual architecture but also conceives of the antinomies as *sine qua non* for appreciating the meaning of the moral life. For example, according to Kant, if we fail to understand the conflict between being free and at the same time being subject to a moral law, then the nature of our moral life will remain largely unintelligible.[2] In this paper I will first identify the elements of this minimalist paradox within *The Foundations* and describe how these elements play a vital role within Engelhardt's minimalist approach to secular or public bioethics. Secondly, while I am sympathetic to minimalism as an ethical methodology within a pluralistic society, my primary concern is to display how this minimalist methodology has evolved within Engelhardt's work from a conceptually based method to a historically conditioned method. This evolution, I believe, is more understandable if we assume that Hegel's influence is gaining ascendancy within Engelhardt's vision of bioethics.

THE PARADOX

The minimalist paradox involves two claims. First, according to Engelhardt, because the secular or minimal state cannot give a secular justification for a host of restrictions on individual autonomy, including laws forbidding commercial surrogacy, active voluntary euthanasia and abortion, the secular state must be skeptical about prohibiting such behaviors. For Engelhardt, skepticism is at the root of the stranger motif that he explicitly employs to subvert substantive, secular ethics. Strangers cannot justify values across their cognitive boundaries and this inability is the basis for the secular imperative to

B. P. Minogue et al. (eds.), Reading Engelhardt, 205–219.

remain neutral on a host of controversial bioethical topics. The conceptual rule which explains this neutrality is simple: knowledge that X is immoral requires justification that X is immoral, and since the secular state cannot justify opposition to the above behaviors across religious and ideological boundaries, it follows that the secular state must be skeptical of commercial surrogacy, active voluntary euthanasia, abortion, etc. For Engelhardt, justifying that such behaviors are immoral from a neutral standpoint requires appealing to what is outside the minimal, secular or formal restriction against using persons against their will. This secular skepticism or neutrality gives us the first element of the paradox: *the secular state is ignorant of the moral quality of active euthanasia, commercial surrogacy, abortion, etc.* (**A**).

The second element of the paradox is closely connected to the first. Skepticism about the above behaviors flows from the failure to justify the immorality of these behaviors. For Engelhardt, since the secular state has failed to justify the immorality of these behaviors to its diverse members, the secular state *must permit* these behaviors. A permissive attitude, according to Engelhardt, is the only morally legitimate attitude that the secular state can take, as soon as it is clear that it cannot justify prohibition. For Engelhardt there seems to be no middle ground between permission and prohibition. Thus, while secular moral knowledge regarding these behaviors is minimal, *it is not zero.* There is sufficient moral knowledge to justify permitting these behaviors since secular skepticism necessarily entails secular permission. This, however, constitutes the second element within the paradox: *the secular state is not ignorant of the moral quality of active euthanasia, commercial surrogacy, abortion, etc.* (**B**).[3]

We can thus summarize the paradox with this question: How can Engelhardt's secular state be both morally ignorant of these behaviors and at the same time knowledgeable enough about them to morally permit them? Another interrogative formulation of this paradox is "How can secular moral knowledge come from secular moral ignorance?"

The sense of paradox is only increased if we examine Engelhardt's view of the relation between secular skepticism and secular permission. Must the secular state permit what it cannot justify? This somewhat simple Engelhardtian rule ignores two important considerations. First, while it may be *conceptually obvious* to Engelhardt that the secular state must permit what it is skeptical about, it is not *factually obvious* that presently existing secular states follow this demand nor is it obvious that historical secular states have followed his conceptual requirement. Minimalism, the view that secular states must permit anything which is not an instance of using persons against their will, is surely at the heart of Engelhardt's bioethics, but it rests on the philosophical assumption that we may disregard the behavior of actual, secular states within our philosophical speculations regarding the scope of the permissible within a legitimate secular state. Disregarding the behavior of actual states is crucial to this strategy since examples of non-minimalist secular states proliferate throughout history. The requirement that we disregard actual secular ethics in order to find a minimal secular ethic is at the heart of the minimalist paradox, and it is unfortunate that Engelhardt has not turned his extensive analytical skills toward this critical issue. The second question that Engelhardt ignores is to whom must we justify a behavior before it is determined to be unjustified? At one extreme the committed skeptic may never accept that even the most obnoxious behavior violates the requirement to avoid using persons.[4] On the other extreme, the naive citizen often accepts the slightest evidence as sufficient to prohibit behavior.

SKEPTICISM AND PERMISSION

Let us now turn to a closer examination of Engelhardt's conviction that there is a necessary connection between skepticism and permission. *There is some reason to think that he is right.* The *Roe v. Wade* decision, for example, appeals to widespread ethical disagreement over abortion to justify its permissive approach. This decision is thus consistent with Engelhardt's principle that skepticism requires permission.[5] However, while there is some evidence connecting skepticism and permission, there is also significant evidence against the idea that there is a necessary connection. Furthermore, there is good evidence to warrant the belief that there is plenty of middle ground between skepticism and permission. Indeed, *Roe v. Wade* itself is a good example of jurisprudence which is both permissive restrictive. Third-trimester or post-viability abortions are not protected by *Roe v. Wade.* Indeed one can easily interpret the decision as generally prohibiting late stage abortions. This decision does not entail that doubts about the morality of abortion imply that we are duty bound to permit unconditionally all instances of abortion. Despite the presence of skepticism on the part of many people about third-trimester, nontherapeutic abortions, the *Roe* decision takes a substantive liberal position on abortion by admitting some ignorance but not complete ignorance. In short, doubt, skepticism and social uncertainty only infrequently yield unrestricted permission.[6] In similar fashion, many secular states forbid the commercial marketing of human organs for purposes of transplantation despite significant argument that such restriction violates the autonomy of individuals. Such prohibitions frequently rest on evidence that creating a market in such organs is exploitative.[7] Prohibitions against the sale and use of recreational drugs and active euthanasia are additional examples of actual, secular governments prohibiting or variously restricting behaviors even in the face of vast skepticism. These examples suggest that for actual secular communities, as opposed to philosophically abstract secular communities, *the relations between our knowledge and permission is underdetermined rather than necessary.* In summary, there may be something like a *prima facie* or contingent linkage between restricted permission and skepticism but there is no necessary connection or logical implication between them.

Because of this tendency to conceptually represent the relations between skepticism and permission, Engelhardt's minimalist method in ethics proceeds as if justification within the secular domain is determinate and qualitative rather than underdetermined and quantitative. Secular states seem to accept the latter rather than the former view account. Such states often manage conflict by establishing ignorance about abortion or commercial surrogacy or active euthanasia but they also appeal to voting procedures following extensive compromises. The extent and form of the permissible is not simply determined by the presence or absence of knowledge. Examples such as these suggests that what a secular state chooses to be skeptical about is not something which is conceptually fixed and independent of historical influence. Secular governments simply change what they accept as the minimal duties of a secular state and, just as there is no canonical account of the good, there is no historically immune, canonical account of the minimal duties of the secular state.[8] Secular moral strangers may not be able to determine which God is the real God but they can often achieve sufficient agreement, albeit compromised agreement, to proscribe or regulate behaviors even in the presence of significant and deep moral disagreement. One could choose to protect this supposed necessary connection between skepticism and permission by claiming that if any apparently secular state did not follow this requirement, then it was only an apparent secular state and not a legitimate or genuine secular state. This strategy surely immunizes Engelhardt's position from historical and actual verification, and transforms his minimal liberal ideal into an empty tautology.

THE MEANING OF SKEPTICISM

One way of understanding Engelhardt's conceptual account of the relation between secular skepticism and permission involves the suggestion that he misunderstands skepticism. For Engelhardt, skepticism involves both the suspension of propositional judgement about a behavior and the permission of that behavior. Surely skepticism requires suspending judgment, for by definition, skepticism involves neither affirming nor denying the truth of propositions. Being morally skeptical is no different. If we are skeptical about commercial surrogacy, active voluntary euthanasia, abortion, etc. this means that we must withhold judgement. However, the implications of withholding judgment are another matter. Some people may think that psychological depression is an appropriate reaction to ignorance. Others are psychologically exalted and liberated by it. Some are motivated to inquiry or experimentation while others are paralyzed by admitting ignorance. How we should psychologically respond to skepticism is thus a matter of widespread disagreement. Social responses are also matters of widespread conflict. Some societies deny that they are ignorant of anything. Some turn to social experimentation while others return to the "tried and true" traditions of the past. Some societies appeal to slippery slope considerations to justify past practice while others see nothing but rational fallacy when the slippery slope is used to conserve the status quo. How society should respond politically to the presence of ignorance is not determined solely by philosophical linkage between the concepts of ignorance and permission.

It may well be that the state cannot offer a secular justification prohibiting abortion that is convincing to either all or a majority of its citizens, but even if this were true, all that follows is that the state must now decide *what to do about this fact*. The state must still decide to forbid or permit or restrict abortion. Moral skepticism, i.e., the inability to universally justify one's moral convictions, is silent on issues concerning permission or prohibition or regulation.

The problem of what to do about ignorance remains a practical one, which Aristotle managed by appealing to phronesis. We may choose to permit some things of which we are morally uncertain but we may also choose to forbid or restrict some things of which we are morally uncertain. Our secular, public beliefs, in addition to our communal, private beliefs, are not separable from this practical dimension and therefore they need not be treated as resting exclusively on a pure or universally recognized principle like the categorical imperative. Thankfully our practical lives and beliefs need not be treated as a set of propositions which can and should be derived from philosophically pure concepts such as the categorical imperative. Consent, as well as history and tradition, are relevant to the secular ethic just as they are relevant to our private, communal moralities.

Throughout history, secular states have taken a variety of approaches to ignorance. Engelhardt is surely correct when he claims that they often take a permissive approach in the presence of widespread ignorance. However, the practical demands of governing a secular state often involve compromising among competing and vastly different ideological views. The upshot of this claim is that if the secular state is to justify permissions, prohibitions or regulations of ethically controversial practices then *it must supplement its secular moral ignorance* about these behaviors with substantive values relevant to ethics, practice and politics. These values may go beyond the singular restriction to avoid using individuals against their will.[9] Such normative considerations often include estimates regarding the relative harms which may flow from competing permissive or prohibitive or regulative laws.

THE ROOTS OF MINIMALISM

Engelhardt's indebtedness to Kant is obvious. He explicitly identifies the rights and duties of the secular citizen and the secular state with those that are consonant with Kant's principle that we ought to avoid using individuals as if they were objects rather than subjects. While Kant himself does not openly adopt a minimalist method, it is easy to see why Engelhardt (and other classical liberals) represent the categorical imperative as a minimal moral rule that transcends the cultural and religious differences that divide communities within the secular state. The startling novelty of Kant's system of morals was his construction of a moral system in which respect for the moral autonomy and the moral equality of individuals were not only treated as primary and foundational within ethics but also treated as sufficient for preserving what is universal within our moral consciousness. Furthermore, the categorical imperative requires that individuals, not classes or groups, be treated as the basic unit of morality. This makes personhood alone and not national origin or religion or skin color or culture the sole determinant of moral right. Kant's doctrine of personhood enables him to determine what is relevant within formal ethics. It allows him to separate the cultural, psychological, biological and religious domains from the domain of formal ethics. For Kant considerations involving the treatment of persons define what is morally relevant.

Liberals such as Engelhardt interpret Kant as attempting to identify a *rational ground* that can function as "common rational ground" or conflict resolution across cultural barriers precisely because it is minimal or formal. Kant's attempt to avoid presupposing anything that is not given to rational consciousness, abstracted from the empirical, contingent factors makes his system of morality open to both a formalist (non-empirical) and minimalist interpretation. We can illustrate what this formalism means by appealing to skin color. Many cultures have treated skin color as a basis for justifying slavery or other harms to persons. However, if skin color is irrelevant to personhood, then it must be viewed as irrelevant to secular ethics. Kant's formalism is thus open to be reinterpreted within the liberal tradition as a search for a minimal ethic acceptable to all irrespective of culture or religion or other non-universal traits.

MINIMALISM AND HEGEL[10]

This Kantian formalism was troubled by substantive criticism. What exactly was implied by the injunction to avoid using a person? Kant thinks of the categorical imperative as having very specific implications or what Engelhardt calls moral content. For Kant, the categorical imperative not only undermines slavery but implies that lying and promise breaking are always wrong, even in Plato's case of the madman who wants someone to return to him a borrowed sword.[11] Most of us agree about the slavery case but the rules against lying and promise breaking are far more controversial. Other uncertain implications are also present. Does respecting the minimal rights of persons require respect for their consent to voluntary active euthanasia? Kant said no at the end of the eighteenth century. Is the one month old fetus a person? Does respect for the individual person justify commercial surrogacy? These last questions themselves are historically conditioned by the growth of technology and the last was itself unthinkable for the historical Kant.

These questions about the implications of the categorical imperative illustrate Hegel's conviction that Kant's formalism opened the door to rampant skepticism within the moral life. If individuals isolate themselves from the traditions of the society, as the skeptic does, then even if they should accept the abstract duty to avoid using individuals, they are still left with the difficulty of determining the concrete implications of this abstract duty. Hegel thinks of the

Kantian will as primarily negative in that the Kantian will is always attempting
to overthrow what is restricting it. But this negative sense of freedom, according to Hegel, cannot address the need to generate a positive view of freedom
as well as a positive morality. Hegel is convinced that a purely negative
account of freedom leads only to the excesses and terrors of the French
Revolution.[12] In short, Hegel's rejection of the Kantian system was tied to its
susceptibility to rampant skepticism since accepting only a purely formal,
minimal and non-historical account of the autonomous will offers us no
substantive account about how our freedom should be exercised. If we are to
avoid this problem, we must admit content or substance into the construction
of the secular ethic.

Hegel's critique of Kant can be read as an assault not so much on formalist
minimalism *per se* but as an attack on any purely conceptual attempt to articulate the meaning and implications of the minimal, secular ethic. Hegel pictured
the categorical imperative as an ethical principle that was valuable. It represented the formal dimension of ethics. The error of the Kantian system was the
assumption that this formal dimension is all there is to ethics.

For Hegel, the Kantian autonomous will is purely abstract or purely formal
in that it attempts to derive all our moral duties from the individual's reason
and will isolated from cosmic issues regarding the development of absolute
spirit and historical issues concerning the culture in which the individual is
situated. The dependence of ethics on these matters explains why the Kantian
system fails to resolve the conflict among autonomy, skepticism and the ethical
life (*Sittlichkeit*).[13] Kant attributes to reason and will the ability to justify
particular moral convictions which Engelhardt himself sees as impossible to
defend within a pluralistic culture. But such particular moral beliefs, according
to Hegel, are conditioned by history and culture and therefore not derivable
from any purely abstract principle such as the categorical imperative. For
Hegel the dependence of morality on history and culture is not something to
bemoan. Rather, history and culture are pictured as items within our moral life
that interact with and provide concrete content to the purely abstract will of the
Kantian individual. One would be unable to do ethics without assuming both
abstract and concrete values. Just as one would be unable to practice science
without admitting both an abstract, theoretical dimension and a concrete
experimental dimension. Overreliance on abstract, formal and empty moral
principles leads only to skepticism about a culture's concrete values which are
the starting points for ethics itself. The autonomous will is capable of skeptical

responses to any of the laws that historical men and women feel subject to. In short the skeptical will is capable of suspending judgment not only about such conventional values as that gentleman ought to shine their shoes but also about the rule that killing female newborns is wrong. Pure reason like pure will, if isolated from historically conditioned values, concrete wills and historically conditioned interpretations of reason will yield skepticism on both private and public moral values.

To meet this critique within his own account of the ethical life, Hegel developed the parallel distinctions between abstract and concrete reason and abstract and concrete will. The emptiness of pure will and pure reason seems to give unlimited power to skepticism, and this violates our intuition that skepticism in the moral order is something to be avoided. For Hegel our ethical life is something that cannot be reduced to or derived from either abstract principle or the mores of a given culture. Rather our moral lives exist dialectically. They emerge within the conflict between abstract reason, which he thinks is well characterized by the categorical imperative, and the content-rich principles dictated by particular cultural and historically conditioned values. The ethical life itself is something that is always in transition and it is therefore impossible to determine the fixed nature of our ethical lives. Furthermore, as our ethical lives are in transit, so too are institutions such as the secular or minimal state in transit. We create these institutions to manage this conflict between our abstract ideals and our concrete rich culture and, for Hegel, it is not at all surprising that the rules which govern the secular or minimal state are in constant change. The meaning and extent of abstract reason and pure freedom, which we may call the secular or public component of our moral lives, will always be determined by the concrete culture which gives content to our abstract ideals.

> An immanent and consistent doctrine of duties can be nothing except the serial exposition of the relationships which are necessitated by the idea of freedom and are therefore realized across their whole extent that is in the state[14]

For Hegel the individual is not pure will or pure reason isolated from concrete will and concrete reason embedded within historically conditioned culture. Similarly, the meaning and extent of concrete will and concrete reason will be restricted by abstract principle. Neither culture nor abstract reason dominates. A concrete, particular will is determined by abstract principle and similarly abstract reason is determined by history and culture. The determinants of the concrete will and concrete reason are such things as desire or emotion or religion and history. Hegel maintains that these concrete determinants, along with the abstract categorical imperative, are necessary elements within the moral or ethical life (*Sittlichkeit*).

We can illustrate the thesis that our ethical lives exist within a tension between concrete and abstract reason and will by attending to the issue of the right to national health care. One can portray the right to health care as coercive of the individual person. Some national health care systems force people to access only the system's brands of health care. They practically close off other treatment possibilities. But national health care also can be represented as a means for realizing equality of opportunity, as are public education or police protection. How we should represent the issue cannot be abstractly derived from the categorical imperative itself. The imperative by itself is too abstract, too thin to justify one manner of representation.

MINIMALISM: THE ETHICS OF AGREEMENT IN ENGELHARDT

While the impact of Kant's formalism on Engelhardt's bioethical program is extensive, he is not uninfluenced by Hegel. One can portray Engelhardt's minimalism as something that flows from his vision that the secular ethic must be determined by the categorical imperative. Given the formal, abstract and empty character of this principle, it is not surprising that Engelhardt's image of secular moral content is so thin as to leave many of our most fundamental values unprotected against the onslaughts of the stranger. For Engelhardt our secular ethical life is characterized by the "stranger" motif.[15] Strangers do not share a vision of the good birth, the good life or the good death. They do not share a vision of a good human future. Strangers do not share commensurable definitions of pleasure and pain and happiness. Furthermore they do not share religious faith and so religious discourse cannot be the basis of cultural and ethical unity.

However, in a very insightful essay entitled "*Sittlichkeit* and Post Modernity: An Hegelian Reconsideration of the State"[16] Engelhardt gives a very sympathetic interpretation of Hegel which leaves the reader with the distinct feeling that Hegel was an insightful precursor of the Engelhardtian program. He pictures Hegel's philosophy of the secular state as emphasizing diversity among competing societies which do not share moral content. Furthermore, Engelhardt argues that this "plurality of moral communities demands the moral space that civil society affords."[17] This moral space is remarkably similar to

Engelhardt's substance-free secular government. However, it is my contention that the early Engelhardt either missed an essential point within the Hegelian program or simply rejected it. For Engelhardt interprets Hegel as merely claiming that while moral content is missing from the Kantian dictum to avoid using persons, this content can be provided *only within particular moral communities.* Engelhardt fails to see the primary Hegelian idea that the secular, minimal state *is itself a practical rather than a purely abstract invention.* It emerges within particular historical settings and is carved and designed with particular goals in mind. Engelhardt is right that the secular state is not on the same logical level as the communities which it mediates. The secular state is not just another religious or ideological community. If it were, it would not be able to serve its mediating function. However, this logical distance separating secular, minimal states from their communities implies only that the secular state is less morally substantive than its component communities. The logical or categorical distance that separates communities from the state does not entail that the secular state is without moral content completely. The secular state is not a community, such as the Amish. Rather, it is a practical, concrete invention inaugurated in the west largely as a tool for diminishing bloodshed among religious communities. Its practicality introduces a greater degree of moral thinness. But Engelhardt fails to see that the secular state is itself in a dialectical relationship with the concrete communities which compose it. The secular state is not and cannot be completely isolated from the concrete communities from which it emerges. Indeed the major paradox within the Hegelian account of the state is that the secular state is neither purely formal and minimal nor purely concrete and particular. *It is a "concrete universal."*

This Hegelian view of the secular state does not forbid secular strangers from sharing a substantive as well as a formal ethic. The search for *what is both substantive and minimal* is not in principle a search for the holy grail. Reasonable strangers are surely alienated from one another. They are surely at odds over the meaning of pleasure, happiness, wisdom, and the purpose of life. Modern secular strangers do not share a common religious outlook, and therefore arguments that rest on these religious convictions lack the universality so admired by Engelhardt and Kant. But modern persons are not total strangers. A total stranger would be someone with whom we have nothing in common. Furthermore, the history of liberal states suggests that the process of developing minimal, content-rich, substantive values is not something that is ruled out *a priori.*

THE HEGELIAN INFLUENCE ON ENGELHARDT'S MINIMALISM

Ostensibly substantive secularity is what Engelhardt rules out by appeal to his Kantian formalism. For Engelhardt, respect for social agreement and individual permission are rules that are formal and minimal in nature rather than content-rich. The minimal secular ethic is an ethic of agreement and therefore substance-free. "If one cannot establish by sound rational argument a particular concrete moral viewpoint as canonically decisive (and one cannot because the establishment of such a viewpoint is exactly what is at stake), then the only source of general secular authority for moral content and moral direction is agreement."[18] Because of this formal or procedural nature, Engelhardt thinks of agreement and permission as ethical rules that are outside the realm of normative ethics. They are metaethical and because of their meta-ethical character they transcend the typical restraints imposed by normative ethics. For example, we often think of something as bad if it effects bad results. But this typical response is inappropriate when it is free choice or permitted behavior or agreed upon behavior that results in more harm than good. However, this idea that because secular liberal morality is based on agreement that it must be substance- or content-free, is what I have been at pains to question and I believe that it is also something of which Engelhardt himself has seen the limits.

Though Engelhardt is resistant to Hegel's notion that the secular ethic is paradoxically both concrete and universal, and though he persists in treating the categorical imperative isolated from communal influence, the influence of this Hegelian notion of the secular state as substantive has silently crept into Engelhardt's second edition of *The Foundations*. Formal minimalist methodology is at the heart of Engelhardt's first edition of *The Foundations*. But he begins to waver in the second edition and there are two reasons for this abandonment. While minimalism is at the heart of Engelhardt's early program, he, like Kant, had troubles clarifying the practical implications of the duty to minimally respect individual persons. Furthermore, we can see, in Engelhardt's commitment to the legitimacy of a multi-tier national health care system, the influence of the Hegelian demand to supplement the purely formal demands associated with the categorical imperative with the content-rich elements of *Sittlichkeit* in order to find a concrete interpretation of what it means to respect individual persons.

Much of Engelhardt's early work is easy to interpret as espousing a commitment to a deeply libertarian public ethic governed only by respect for

individual autonomy. The content of this libertarian ethic is min
does not allow taxing for the purpose of a national health care sy
hardt's early conceptual minimalism suggests that taxing for this v
mixing private and public spheres and transforming ones private ..u_s about
the moral excellence of health care into a universal, secular ethic. To tax for
public health would presuppose a substantive understanding and agreement
regarding the common good and this fails to meet the requirements of universality. Furthermore, taxing for national health care would involve the use of
state coercion to secure private goods to pay for national health care.

The Second Edition version of minimalism is far more willing to accept
national health care. While Engelhardt is still very suspicious of purely egalitarian national health care systems which forbid any appeal to the market, he
does not reject health care systems that provide for decent minimums.
Nowhere does he denounce the idea that a legitimate minimal state may tax for
the purposes of establishing a national health care system. Nowhere does he
denounce such systems for imposing substantive and private definitions of the
good on unwilling individuals. Second Edition minimalism surely opposes
single-tier, Canadian-styled, health care systems which restrict the rights of
citizens to secure medical services outside the national system, but Engelhardt
does not denounce two-tier systems of the sort that are common in Europe.
Indeed, he is quite supportive of these systems.

> A two-tier system with inequality in health care distribution is both morally and
> materially inevitable. In the face of unavoidable tragedies and contrary moral intuitions,
> a multi tiered system of health care is in many respects a compromise. On the one hand
> it provides some amount of health care for all while on the other hand allowing those
> with resources to purchase additional or better services. It can endorse the use of
> communal resources for the provision of a decent minimal or basic amount of health care
> for all while acknowledging the existence of private resources at the disposal of some
> individuals to purchase better basic as will as luxury care . . . The serious task is to
> decide how to define and provide a decent minimum or basic level of care as a floor of
> support for all members of a society while allowing money and free choice to fashion
> special services for the affluent.[19]

Engelhardt's Second Edition may be read as approaching the problem of
national health care in Hegelian fashion rather than in a purely formal, Kantian
fashion. The thin, public ethic driven only by respect for individual autonomy
is so thin that it is silent on the legitimacy of secular strangers to agree to form
a national health care system. In order to make the thin ethic useful, it must be

supplemented with historical and cultural values involved in public health care. Join these values with the consent of the governed, and for Engelhardt we have a justification for a substantive intrusion into the private, economic and personal lives of secular citizens.[20] The hallmark of the Hegelian system is the necessity to make compromises among conflicting libertarian and egalitarian values and this is precisely what is present within Engelhardt's support of two-tier health care systems. These systems *surely restrict* the autonomy of individuals for the sake of the common good but *they are not as restrictive* as the one-tier systems which severely restrict the patient's right to access health care opportunities outside the single system. States violate the rights of patients and providers when all forms of *private* health service are outlawed by single-payer systems, but two-tier systems which allow for alternative choices do not necessarily violate the formal requirements of the injunction to avoid using people.

The later Engelhardt seems to accept the idea that the thin secular ethic admits of at least two interpretations within the realm of health care. One could interpret the thin ethic, as the strict libertarians do, as requiring that all health care transactions be governed exclusively by free market, *laissez-faire* rules. This assumes that all health care associations must be completely private. A second Hegelian interpretation treats health care as something that can be the subject of public as well as private agreement. This second Engelhardtian interpretation represents secular ethics as having a thin, rather than substance-free content.

NOTES

1. H. Tristram Engelhardt, Jr., *The Foundations of Bioethics*, 2nd. Ed.(New York: Oxford University Press, 1996).

2. For a thorough discussion of Kant's "two worlds" (the sensible and intelligible worlds) and resolution of the antinomy between freedom and necessity, see Immanuel Kant, *The Critique of Pure Reason*, translated by F. Max Muller (Anchor Books Doubleday: Garden City New York, 1966), 369.

3. **A** and **B** are formal contradictions and appear to be paradoxical.

4. This question is at the root of Hegel's critique of Kant's formalism. Kant's approach to ethics failed to appreciate that in the hands of the committed skeptic, the requirement to respect autonomy could justify immoral behavior.

5. *Roe v. Wade*, 410 U. S. 113 (1973), 93 S.Ct. 705.

6. The recent legislative actions prohibiting brain suction abortion are an illustrations of how secular states continue to attempt to restrict abortion rights.

7. The concept of exploitation is extremely elusive. For a good review of the matter see, Alan Wertheimer, *Coercion* (Princeton: Princeton University Press, 1987), 222-239.

8. This transformation is itself evident within Engelhardt's evolving views on national health care.

9. For example, recent legislative attempts to prohibit brain suction abortion to end late term pregnancies surely involve secular government affirming that it cannot remain silent on this abortion method.

10. The main text that I draw on is G. W. Hegel, *The Philosophy of Right*, translated by T. M. Knox (Oxford: Oxford University Press, 1942).

11. This case is discussed in *The Republic* Book One, translated by Robin Waterfield (Oxford: Oxford University Press, 1993). Kant discusses this case in "On A Supposed Right to Lie From Altruistic Motives" in *The Philosophy of Immanuel Kant*, translated by L. W. Beck (Chicago: University of Chicago Press, 1949), 346.

12. Hegel, *The Philosophy of Right,* section 258.

13. For an excellent discussion, see Charles Taylor, *Hegel* (Cambridge: Cambridge University Press, 1975), 365ff.

14. Hegel, *The Philosophy of Right*, section 148.

15. Engelhardt, *Foundations*, 74-83.

16. H. Tristram Engelhardt, Jr., "*Sittlichkeit* and Post-Modernity: An Hegelian Reconsideration of the State" in *Hegel Reconsidered*, eds. H. T. Engelhardt, Jr. and T. Pinkard (Dordrecht, The Netherlands: Kluwer Academic Publishers, 1994).

17. Engelhardt, "*Sittlichkeit* and Post Modernity:" 220.

18. Engelhardt, *Foundations*, 68.

19. Engelhardt, *Foundations*, 399.

20. Engelhardt's appeal to Locke's theory of property to defend his national health care hypothesis involves appealing to an historically conditioned theory to justify this hypothesis.

13

The Unjustifiability of Substantive Liberalisms and the Inevitability of Engelhardtian Procedural Liberalism

Ruiping Fan

Through his account of the cardinal role of the principle of permission in a secular pluralist society, H. Tristram Engelhardt, Jr. has established an ethic of non-substantive liberalism, which he usually terms "a content-less secular morality." Unlike versions of substantive liberalism, what he offers is a pure procedural principle concerning moral and political authority. In this essay I will argue that versions of substantive liberalism cannot be justified through sound rational argument. Consequently, an Engelhardtian non-substantive secular morality is morally unavoidable in the contemporary world.

It is generally considered that the contemporary world is entering into a period of post-Marxism. The history of this century has witnessed how enthusiastically pursuing so-called collective interests at the price of individual liberty under a centrally-planned economic system has caused human disasters, one after another, in all Marxist-Socialist countries. Marxism, as a political and ideological authority, has collapsed in Eastern Europe and has significantly lost its cultural force in the rest of the world. Many people have recognized anew the moral strength and practical importance of Western classical liberal doctrines. A significant opportunity is available to return to the call of the classical liberal principles, especially the principles of individual liberty and an unhampered market mechanism. These two principles state roughly that competent adult individuals are entitled to do anything with consenting others as long as their actions do not harm unconsenting innocents, and outline the extent to which governments should not artificially interfere with free market mechanisms.

However, society today is also marked by a post-Enlightenment character. On the one hand, a number of Western people are no longer committed to their traditional Christian faith. On the other hand, no human intellectual inquiries have successfully disclosed a canonical, universal, and content-full view of the good life through sound rational argument. As a result, a variety of moral communities holding different and incommensurable moral assumptions and principles coexist in contemporary society. This prominent diversity of morality poses severe challenges to the intellectual foundations of classical

B. P. Minogue et al. (eds.), Reading Engelhardt, 221–235.

liberal doctrines which are rooted in Christian understandings as well as an Enlightenment faith in human reason. New versions of liberalism have been put forward. Consequently, those who claim themselves to be liberals do not all believe in the same substantive liberal doctrines. As a matter of fact, there is not a single, coherent, and universally accepted liberal theory that prevails in contemporary Western society. There is instead a plurality of substantive liberalisms.

In the following sections, I will briefly explore three sorts of substantive liberalisms (i.e., theological, utilitarian, and political liberalisms) to show why they cannot be justified through rational philosophical argument. I certainly do not imply that these three sorts exhaust all versions of important substantive liberalisms. Rather I use them as examples to illustrate why it is unlikely rationally to confirm a version of substantive liberalism in the contemporary pluralist world. Specifically, in the second section, I will discuss the theological liberalisms advocated by John Locke and Adam Smith and demonstrate the major difficulties that they must confront. In the third section I will address the utilitarian liberalism defended by John Stuart Mill and show its internal defects. In the fourth section I will assess the political liberalism advanced by John Rawls and argue why it too cannot be justified. The fifth section will then outline Engelhardtian procedural liberalism and argue that it is morally inevitable. Finally, I will briefly state my conclusions in the sixth section.

THEOLOGICAL LIBERALISM

The versions of liberalism afforded by Locke and Smith are theological. For Locke, the principle of fundamental individual liberty is derived ultimately from the supposed intentions of the Creator. As he argues, since men are "the workmanship of one omnipotent, and infinitely wise maker," they naturally have "perfect freedom to order their actions, and dispose of their possessions and persons, as they think fit, within the bounds of the law of nature," which require that "no one ought to harm another in his life, health, liberty, or possessions."[1]

Similarly, Smith developed his doctrine of liberty within a broadly theological context. According to Smith, there is a natural order of human society which is conducive to the wealth and happiness of mankind. This order is, Smith believed, derived from the beneficent arrangement of the Creator. The major condition for it is the liberty of each man to follow his natural instincts insofar as he does not violate "fair play" or hurt his neighbor. For

Smith, as long as these instincts do not bring men into collision with each other, the artificial interference of government is unjust, because it disregards the natural liberty of human individuals. Such interference is also foolish, because it hinders the orderly development of a market economy through which individuals' desires are best satisfied. Thus, Smith advocated the classical liberal principles of fundamental individual liberty and unhindered market mechanism.[2]

At first glance, it seems amazing that Smith could believe that the pursuit of individual selfish interests coincides with the greatest happiness of the whole race. But in his religious beliefs we can find an explanation for his confidence in this consistency. He continually refers to the need, through some sort of faith, to direct our private behavior toward God's wishes, "to cooperate with the Deity, and to advance as far as in our power the plan of Providence."[3] According to Smith, human individuals have been equipped with, among other things, the perspective of an "impartial spectator": "the demigod within the breast–the great judge and arbiter of conduct."[4] This "great judge" is a particular gift offered by God so that we may achieve an equilibrium among the different virtues of prudence, justice, and beneficence that we possess as humans. Thus, we are able to follow God's plan through the perspective of an impartial spectator. Unlike the utilitarian, Smith does not argue that the impartial spectator should bring us to the position of universal benevolence. His understanding is that:

> [t]he administration of the great system of the universe...the care of the universal happiness of all rational and sensible beings, is the business of God and not of man. To man is allotted a much more humble department, but one much more suitable to the weakness of his powers, and to the narrowness of his comprehension; the care of his own happiness, of that of his family, his friends, his country...[5]

In short, it is the pre-established harmony of Providence or the invisible hand of God that ensures the consistency between seeking our own benefits as individuals and achieving the happiness of the human race as a whole. For Smith, freely pursuing wealth through an unhampered market mechanism is not only the necessary expression of our natural liberty but also in harmony with God's beneficent arrangement.

Such theological defense of liberalism as provided by Locke and Smith, however, faces intractable difficulties of justification in contemporary society. First of all, the arguments were worked out within the context of a particular theology and religious faith. In today's pluralist context in which there are multiple Christian and other religious denominations, as well as many people not committed to any particular theistic faith, the basic assumptions from which Locke and Smith derived the classical liberal principles of individual liberty and the importance of a free market will not be universally accepted. Such theological liberalism has lost its original foundation through which it was justified.

Moreover, outside of their theological contexts certain particular conceptions of liberty that theological liberalism has absorbed may not make sense. For instance, Locke argues that man should be prohibited from taking his own life or enslaving himself as he pleases. This is because, for Locke, men in principle do not belong to themselves. They are God's property, whose workmanship they are, "made to last during his, not one another's pleasure."[6] Therefore:

> a man, not having the power of his own life, *cannot*, by compact, or his own consent, *enslave himself* to any one, nor put himself under the absolute, arbitrary power of another, to take away his life, when he pleases.[7]

Obviously, people who do not share Locke's theological assumptions will not accept these conclusions. For instance, Robert Nozick's conception of individual rights (or liberties) as side constraints does not provide such Lockean constraints upon individual liberties.[8]

Finally, outside of the context of the particular theology on which Smith depended, a belief in a pre-established harmony between the pursuit of individual interests and the realization of a whole nation's happiness through a free market mechanism will not hold. Those who do not share Smith's theology regarding such a perfect consistency and who yet nonetheless advocate a free market system to be maintained in contemporary society will need to produce an independent argument to explain why such a system is morally required. Those who do not accept Smith's theology but who still believe that a harmony exists between individual and general interests will need at least to recast the account that Smith provided.

UTILITARIAN LIBERALISM

Similar to theological liberals, utilitarian liberals propose and defend a classical doctrine of liberty. The most famous representative of utilitarian liberalism, Mill, advocates a classical principle of individual liberty, terming it "a very simple principle."[9] He expresses the principle this way:

> [t]hat the sole end for which mankind are warranted, individually or collectively in interfering with the liberty of action of any of their number, is self-protection. That the only purpose for which power can be rightfully exercised over any member of a civilized community, against his will, is to prevent harm to others. His own good, either physical or moral, is not a sufficient warrant.[10]

Unlike Locke or Smith, however, Mill did not intend to provide a theological justification for his principle of individual liberty. He claims that he forgoes any advantage which could be derived to his argument from the idea of abstract right or liberty as a thing independent of utility. Instead, he regards "utility as the ultimate appeal on all ethical questions."[11] This is to say that, as a utilitarian, Mill asserts the principle of liberty ultimately not because he thinks it is right, or that it is what God has commanded, but because he believes that following this principle will produce the greatest amount of total utility or general happiness in human society.[12] As he argues:

> [e]ach is the proper guardian of his own health, whether bodily, or mental or spiritual. Mankind are greater gainers by suffering each other to live as seems good to themselves, than by compelling each to live as seems good to the rest.[13]

Such utilitarian arguments for the principle of individual liberty eschew the theological elements contained in Locke's and Smith's accounts. They constitute a turn in moral language. Emphases have shifted from the nature, dignity, and the right of individual liberty to the utility, effect, and nature of the good. Needless to say, this type of approach has been significantly influential in economic, political, and legal decision-making in modern society.

However, Mill's utilitarian liberalism contains fatal defects. It may even be logically self-defeating. If maintaining the principle of individual liberty is justified on the basis of the interests of individuals, then limiting individual liberties will be morally allowable and may even be morally required whenever the constraints are expected to bring about better results for the individuals. Is it possible for utilitarian liberals, Mill included, to argue that endorsing individual liberties will, on the whole, always lead to the greatest general happiness? Mill's basic assumption is that individuals are the best judges of what is best for them. But this claim is ambiguous and in some cases dubious. It may be the case that individuals know best what their goals are. But they may not be the best judges about the best means to achieve their goals. Even if individuals are the best judges about the best means to achieve their goals, they may not be the best judges about what are the best goals that they should set for themselves. Consequently, utilitarian arguments for individual liberties logically leave immense room for interfering with individual liberties. Mill must either drop his utilitarian foundations for the principle of individual liberty, or abandon the principle itself in order to preserve his utilitarian commitment.

In addition, a utilitarian approach will naturally lead to the approval of significant governmental interventions in the market. Since the ultimate moral concern is the greatest general happiness for society, it is morally praiseworthy for governments to control the market to the extent that such interference is expected to increase general happiness. As a result, the principle of allowing a free market mechanism (which many liberals take to be a crucial element of classical liberalism) may no longer necessarily hold in this utilitarian context. Not surprisingly, Mill attempts to lay down general guidelines for state intervention in his *Principles of Political Economy*. He gives much emphasis to certain non-market values and as a result offers a significant positive account of state-enforced re-distribution. He supports a broad scope for taxes: taxes on the increase in income from land due to "natural causes"; taxes on legacies and inheritances; house-taxes or rates; and finally, preferably only in times of national emergency, proportionate taxes on incomes.[14] Contemporary readers may be shocked by the extent to which Mill was prepared to go in requiring state interference in individual private property and personal liberties. This is particularly ironic, for Mill is in other respects an enthusiastic advocate of individual liberties.

POLITICAL LIBERALISM

Rawls has elaborated the conception of political liberalism to cope with the question, how it is possible that "there may exist over time a stable and just society of free and equal citizens profoundly divided by reasonable though incompatible religious, philosophical, and moral doctrines?"[15] This version of liberalism, Rawls emphasizes, differs from other traditional types (such as theological and utilitarian liberalisms) in that it is neither general with respect to the subjects to which it applies nor comprehensive in the content it includes. It is not general because it tries only to elaborate a reasonable conception for the basic structure of modern democratic regimes. It is not comprehensive because it does not cover a full conception of the good informing what is of value in human life.[16] Rawls believes that since our contemporary social and historical conditions "have their origins in the Wars of Religion following the Reformation and the subsequent development of the principle of toleration, and in the growth of constitutional government and the institutions of large industrial market economies," only this version of political liberalism can provide a publicly recognized basis for a conception of justice. It allows for "a diversity of doctrines and the plurality of conflicting, and indeed incommensurable, conceptions of the good affirmed by the members of existing democratic societies."[17]

Unlike theological liberals such as Locke and Smith, Rawls does not intend to defend his principle of liberty and its priority from the perspective of God's providence. Neither does he attempt to ground it in a comprehensive conception of the good such as the principle of utility forwarded by utilitarian liberals like Mill. Instead, he begins with certain fundamental ideas that he believes reflect an overlapping consensus of all reasonable persons though opposing general and comprehensive conceptions that exist in contemporary democratic society. Indeed, a crucial factor in Rawlsian political liberalism "is not the fact of pluralism as such, but of *reasonable* pluralism."[18] Specifically, Rawls believes all conflicting but reasonable religious, philosophical, and moral doctrines in modern constitutional democracies share an overlapping consensus which boils down to three fundamental ideas: of society as a fair system of cooperation over time, of citizens as free and equal persons, and of a well-ordered society as one effectively regulated by a political conception of justice.[19] Through the assistance of a device of representation which he terms "the original position,"[20] Rawls believes these ideas can be elaborated into two political liberal principles:

a. Each person has an equal right to a fully adequate scheme of equal basic liberties which is compatible with a similar scheme of liberties for all.
b. Social and economic inequalities are to satisfy two conditions. First, they must be attached to offices and positions open to all under conditions of fair equality of opportunity; and second, they must be to the greatest benefit of the least advantaged members of society.[21]

To these two principles Rawls attaches certain priority rules of which the most important is that liberties are given a priority over all other primary goods, so that "liberty can be restricted only for the sake of liberty"[22] and cannot be restricted for any other form of social or economic advantage or any perfectionist values.[23] Thus Rawls establishes his political principle of liberty and its priority.

This principle of liberty and its priority, unfortunately, are difficult to defend. First, even if we accept Rawls' identifications of "the reasonable"[24] and grant his crucial assumption that all reasonable but conflicting religious, philosophical, and moral doctrines in modern democratic society share an overlapping consensus concerning the three fundamental ideas, these ideas do not necessarily elaborate into a priority of the principle of liberty. For one thing, Rawls concedes that this priority is not required under all conditions. It is required only under "reasonable favorable conditions" into which Rawls thinks at least contemporary United States has entered.[25] Rawls elaborates his conception of person as having two moral powers (i.e., the capacity for a sense of right and justice and the capacity for a conception of the good) so as to argue for the priority of liberty as necessary for persons to exercise these powers.[26] But it is far from clear why there should not be any trade-offs between a particular liberty and other goods. Is this because any particular liberty possesses a super value so that it is not worthwhile to limit it for the sake of any other values, no matter how much amount of other values we may gain, even when limiting the liberty does not significantly interfere with persons' exercising their two moral powers? Or, is this because any restriction of a liberty, no matter how trivial, will necessarily significantly harm persons in the practice of their moral powers? Rawls does not explicitly address these issues.

In any case, the literature poses a very instructive question for Rawls, which he never clearly addresses: suppose that situation A is that of a person anxious to exercise a lost liberty and who cares nothing for the extra wealth brought him by surrender of the liberty, and that situation B is that of a person living at the bottom economic level of society and who would gladly surrender a liberty for a greater advance in material prosperity, then which of the situations, A or B, will be judged worse?[27] In the Rawlsian original position, it might be that persons are not able to make a judgment about these two situations because they, being behind a veil of ignorance, cannot know which situation is in their better interests. But if they are able to choose in the original position, it is very hard to imagine that they will all make the same choice, let alone the choice that Rawls prefers. As a matter of fact, in the real world people do make quite different choices. For instance, Singaporeans generally advocate a compulsory saving system under which they are required to save 40 percent of their personal income in the Central Provident Fund to be used particularly for paying medical care, purchasing a home, paying college education expenses, etc., but which may not be used for other purposes.[28] The restriction that this system imposes on the liberty to "hold and to have the exclusive use of personal property," which Rawls emphasizes is "among the basic liberties of the person,"[29] obviously is not for the sake of any other liberties. It is placed mainly for a good that Rawls does not even consider as one of primary social goods: security–the security of healthcare, the prosperity of home-owning, etc. Singaporeans are in general willing to trade liberty for greater security and prosperity. Are they mistaken in giving security and prosperity a priority over liberty? Or is it that Singapore as a state has not reached Rawls' "reasonable favorable conditions" as the United States has, so that it may be right for Singapore but cannot be right for the United States to give priority to security and prosperity over liberty? However, because a large-scale country such as the United States includes so many different geographical and moral communities, it is hard to conceive that Rawls can convincingly argue that they all should endorse a priority of liberty no matter what their social and economic situations and their conceptions of the good life are. Rather, Rawls himself "is best understood as having engaged in a limited, but still important, goal of providing a rational reconstruction of the moral world of a liberal member of the Cambridge, Massachusetts, community."[30]

In addition, since the whole structure of Rawls' theory appears to suggest a pessimism regarding the prospects for a universalistic ethical theory, Rawlsian political liberalism is bound to be incomplete in a profound moral sense. Rawls states that since his theory of justice "is intended as a political conception of justice for a democratic society, it tries to draw solely upon basic intuitive ideas that are embedded in the political institutions of a constitutional democratic regime and the public traditions of their interpretation."[31] One cannot help asking whether Rawls' choice of liberal democratic society conveys any normative force. Does Rawls' focus on a democratic society reveal a belief that such a polity is the telos of history or of the development of human society? It seems that Rawls cannot accommodate such a belief into his theory, because with such a belief his liberalism would not be only political, but also metaphysical. What reasons then can Rawls advance for his choice? If one were to select the basic intuitive ideas which govern a contemporary non-Western society and to construct for that society principles of justice that substantially conflict with those of Rawls, would Rawls be satisfied with acquiescing in the equally arbitrary nature of both theories? Rawls has not considered grounds for accepting his view of reasonable pluralism so much as the consequences he draws from it.

The failure to justify a Rawlsian political liberalism is particularly heuristic. Rawls attempted to avoid the hard task of moral justification through entertaining a political (rather than metaphysical or fundamentally moral) conception of justice overlappingly supported by distinct comprehensive doctrines of the good life which are at home in a democratic state. As he believes, "[a] crucial assumption of liberalism is that equal citizens have different and indeed incommensurable and irreconcilable conceptions of the good."[32] However, since he presupposes a thin theory of the good which establishes a particular ranking of primary goods that is to block, for example, trading liberty for greater prosperity, the content of his theory necessarily goes beyond pure procedural requirements. No matter how thin his theory of the good is, it remains reconcilable with only some but not all comprehensive conceptions of the good that equal citizens may have. In addition, one might even question whether all democratic polities presuppose the same conceptions of equality (e.g., compare equality to act on one's own view of the good life with one's own resources and with consenting others, with fair equality of opportunity, with equality of outcome). In any event, Rawls has not only sacrificed any profound moral sense that his theory might have possessed but also failed to keep his promise regarding the "crucial assumption of liberalism." This illustrates how difficult it is to attempt to establish a substantive liberalism.

PROCEDURAL LIBERALISM

Engelhardt's account of his principle of permission can be recognized as a new defense of the classical liberal principles of fundamental individual liberty and unhindered market mechanism. Unlike those who have appealed to theological or utilitarian arguments, Engelhardt takes explicit account of our post-modern predicament. He persuasively shows that a canonical, universal, and content-full morality cannot be justified through sound rational argument because any such argument has to presuppose exactly what it needs for the justification: a particular content-full account of the good and of obligations.[33] "The recognition of this failure [to establish a canonical content-full account of the good life] marks the post-modern philosophical predicament."[34] Distinct and incommensurable moral assumptions and convictions are held by a variety of moral communities in which people lead their respectively particular moral lives. Consequently, in the post-modern society, individuals cannot avoid encountering each other as moral strangers–persons who do not share a common content-full understanding of the good or of moral obligations.[35] Neither do people share jointly recognized moral authority to resolve moral controversies between them.[36]   Given this situation, Engelhardt argues, a peaceable secular moral world can only be fashioned through a transcendental principle which lays out a necessary condition for the possibility of the moral authority of joint actions involving moral strangers.[37] Since moral authority in large-scale secular societies cannot be derived from God (because moral strangers do not listen to God in the same way) or from sound rational argument (because moral strangers do not hold morality with the same content), such authority can only be derived from the permission of individuals. As a consequence, the burden of proof will always be on the shoulders of those who would interfere with the actions and agreements of individuals and at the same time claim general secular moral authority for their interference. This circumstance conveys a moral priority to the free market and limited democracy because the "[a]uthority for actions involving others in a secular pluralist society is derived from their permission."[38] Thus, what Engelhardt offers is a pure procedural and content-less principle regarding moral and political authority, though the principle has substantive moral consequences.

This principle sustains the spirit of the classical liberal principles of individual liberty and the centrality of the market without an appeal to consequentialist considerations.[39] In a minimal necessary condition of morality (i.e., the principle of permission), Engelhardt grounds the fundamental liberty of individuals to pursue their own view of the good life with their own private resources in collaboration with other consenting individuals through a free market mechanism. In other words, given the failure to establish a binding account of justice, fairness or the good life through rational argument, governments have no secular moral authority to interfere with the peaceable actions performed by individuals on themselves, their possessions, or with other consenting individuals. For Engelhardt, the business of the state is only to honor the principle of permission rather than to impose a particular content-full doctrine of justice or beneficence. Because the state spans diverse moral communities through a political structure, it should become "a neutral limited democracy" which protects an open civil society, not a moral community with a particular content-full moral vision. The state "affords a political unity and an identity, not a social unity and identity," much less a communal unity and identity.[40]

Engelhardt restates the classical liberal principles without presupposing their original theological commitments or utilitarian assumptions. His account does not need any particular theological commitments, because the principle of permission is a transcendental premise established as a necessary condition for the possibility of the peaceable morally authoritative collaboration of moral strangers. Nor does his account invoke any utilitarian assumptions. The fundamental liberties of individuals to be left alone are embraced by default, because of the failure of reason to disclose any one canonical, universal, and content-full view of the good life as morally authoritative. Therefore, his account avoids the difficulties and defects that faced previous classical arguments.

Finally, Engelhardtian procedural liberalism does not appeal to a conception of overlapping consensus of incompatible but reasonable doctrines in a particular form of society as does Rawlsian political liberalism. Engelhardt would agree that there may be certain overlapping consensus in modern Western constitutional democracies. But he would contend that evidence has clearly shown that there is not universal agreement on the principle of liberty and its priority as a value, nor for that matter regarding the moral significance of equality. Although Rawls asserts that it is unreasonable to use state power to suppress a plurality of incommensurable yet reasonable comprehensive doctrines, he stands ready to use the coercive force of the state to prohibit communities from making trade-offs between basic liberties and other goods. Rawls thinks he has set out a political idea of the good which is so "thin" that it can be employed by the holders of any reasonable "thick" conceptions of the good life.[41] The truth of matter is, however, that he fails to distinguish the concept of liberty as a value from the concept of liberty as a side constraint, and he thereby begs the question by giving to basic liberties an absolute value. This particular ranking of goods is by no means in agreement with all reasonable comprehensive doctrines or accounts of democracy in contemporary societies. Even if Rawls' theory is not as comprehensive as traditional substantive liberalisms, it remains substantive and particular in the sense that it presupposes its own concrete order of goods. It is this particularity that remains unjustified. In contrast, Engelhardtian procedural liberalism does not assume any conception of the good. It relies solely upon the conception of freedom as a side constraint to build up the minimum necessary condition for secular peaceable moral cooperation of individuals and communities that hold distinct and often conflicting doctrines of the good life.

CONCLUSION

Every substantive liberalism is bound to begin with certain particular and content-full ideas. For instance, as we have demonstrated, theological liberalism starts with the intentions of the Creator, utilitarian liberalism with benefits to general happiness, and political liberalism with an overlapping consensus of reasonable doctrines in a modern democratic regime. Without substantive premises, there cannot be substantive conclusions. Crucially, since a set of substantive premises can always be challenged by other equally substantive assumptions, no version of substantive liberalism can be justified without begging the question, and no controversy between competing accounts can be resolved through sound rational argument. Consequently, in a pluralist secular world, moral and political authority of joint actions can only be derived from the permission of individuals. It is for this reason that an Engelhardtian non-substantive (or procedural) liberalism is morally unavoidable.

NOTES

I am grateful to H. Tristram Engelhardt, Jr. for his critiques, clarifications, and suggestions regarding the first draft of this essay.

1. J. Locke, *Second Treatise of Government*, ed. C. B. Macpherson (Indianapolis: Hackett Publishing Company, Inc., 1980), 4-6.

2. It seems that these ideas do not often come to the surface in Smith's discussions on economics, A. Smith, *The Wealth of Nations* (New York: The Modern Library, 1937). This might be because he aims at dealing more with detailed ideas rather than these primary principles. In any case these principles are a part of his writings. For a similar point, see L. Stephen, *History of English Thought in the Eighteenth Century*, Vol. II (New York: Harcourt, Brace & world, Inc.,1962), 274.

3. E. G. West, "Introduction to the Theory of Moral Sentiments," *The Theory of Moral Sentiments* (New York: Arlington House, 1969), x.

4. A. Smith, *The Theory of Moral Sentiments* (New York: Arlington House, 1969), 385-388.

5. Smith, *Moral Sentiments*, 348.

6. Locke, *Second Treatise*, 6.

7. Locke, *Second Treatise*, 23.

8. R. Nozick, *Anarchy, State and Utopia* (Basic Books, Inc., 1974), 30-35. Unfortunately, Nozick does not offer any arguments for his conception of rights (or liberties) in his libertarian theory. His theory simply starts with the assumption that '[i]ndividuals have rights, and there are

things no person or group may do to them (without violating their rights)' (ix). But he does not explain why individuals have rights or ought to have rights. We don't know in what ground he would provide his critiques with regard to ethical theories (especially those traditional theories) in which rights-based consideration is no part of their moral languages. Thus, as Engelhardt points out, Nozick's presentation of right as a side constraint "is offered in his account somewhat as a surd given." H. T. Engelhardt Jr., *The Foundations of Bioethics* (New York, Oxford: Oxford University Press,1996), 97n.86.

Fortunately, as I show in Section V, Engelhardt's transcendental account of secular morality provides a forcible argument for Nozickian individual rights as side constraints. According to Engelhardt, given the failure to establish a canonical, universal, and content-full vision of the good and of moral obligations through sound rational argument, and given the sociological fact that distinct and incommensurable moral visions coexist in contemporary secular pluralist societies, only a transcendental principle which lays down the possibility of moral authority of joint actions can make a secular morality possible. This principle is the principle of permission, which states that "[a]uthority for actions involving others in a secular pluralist society is derived from their permission" (*The Foundations*, 122). Without the consent of an individual, others do not have moral authority to do things on him/her. Thus, individual rights (or liberties) as side constraints get established.

9. J. S. Mill, *On Liberty* (New York: Prometheus Books, 1986), 16.

10. Mill, *On Liberty*, 16.

11. Mill, *On Liberty,* 17.

12. Gerald Dworkin argues that in addition to the utilitarian argument for the principle of liberty, Mill also offers a non-utilitarian one. I simply ignore this alternative account of Mill in the text since the utilitarian argument is in any case Mill's major concern. See G. Dworkin, "Paternalism," in *Philosophy of Law*, eds., J. Feinberg and H. Gross (Belmont: Wadsworth Publishing Company, 1995) 214-215.

13. Mill, *On Liberty,* 19.

14. J. S. Mill, *Principles of Political Economy*, ed. Augustus M. Kelley (New York: Bookseller, 1969), Book V.

15. J. Rawls, *Political Liberalism* (New York: Columbia University Press, 1993), xviii. My interpretation of Rawls' theory mainly depends upon his most recent volume *Political Liberalism* rather than the earlier book *A Theory of Justice* (Cambridge: Harvard University Press, 1971). I simply ignore the issue of what differences in thought there are between the two books.

16. Rawls, *Political Liberalism*, 13.

17. J. Rawls, "Justice as Fairness: Political not Metaphysical," *Philosophy and Public Affairs* 14 (Summer 1985): 225.

18. Rawls, *Political Liberalism*, 144, emphasis added.

19. Rawls, *Political Liberalism*, 149.

20. Rawls, *A Theory of Justice*, 3-4; Rawls, *Political Liberalism*, 13.

21. Rawls, *Political Liberalism*, 291.

22. Rawls, *A Theory of Justice*, 302.

23. Rawls, *Political Liberalism*, 294.

24. Rawls, *Political Liberalism*, 49-50.

25. Rawls, *Political Liberalism*, 297.

26. Rawls, *Political Liberalism*, 294-324.

27. H. L. A. Hart, "Rawls on Liberty and Its Priority," *Reading Rawls*, ed., N. Daniels (Stanford: Stanford University Press, 1989), 251-252.

28. M. G. Asher, "Compulsory Savings in Singapore: An Alternative to the Welfare State," *NCPA Policy Report* No. 198.

29. Rawls, *A Theory of Justice*, 61; Rawls, *Political Liberalism*, 298.

30. Engelhardt, *The Foundations*, 51.

31. Rawls, "Justice as Fairness," 225.

32. Rawls, *Political Liberalism*, 303.

33. Engelhardt, *The Foundations*, Ch. 2.

34. Engelhardt, *The Foundations*, 8.

35. H. T. Engelhardt, Jr., *Bioethics and Secular Humanism* (Philadelphia: Trinity Press International, 1991), xiv.

36. Engelhardt, *The Foundations*, 7.

37. Engelhardt, *The Foundations*, 69.

38. Engelhardt, *The Foundations*, 122.

39. By focusing on the permission of individuals, Engelhardt affords a more accurate expression of the principles. For instance, his account avoids certain problems relating to the term "harm" used in the classical statements. People may be harmed, for instance, in normal business competitions. This makes the classical expression that "one is entitled to do anything that does not harm the other" very problematic.

40. H. Tristram Engelhardt, Jr., "*Sittlichkeit* and Post-modernity: An Hegelian Reconsideration of the State," in *Hegel Reconsidered*, eds., H. T. Engelhardt, Jr., and T. Pinkard (Dordrecht, Boston, London: Kluwer Academic Publishers, 1994), 218.

41. Rawls, *A Theory of Justice*, 396-397; Rawls, *Political Liberalism*, xix.

14

SECULAR? YES; HUMANISM? NO: A CLOSE LOOK AT ENGELHARDT'S SECULAR HUMANIST BIOETHIC

FAITH L. LAGAY

Students, teachers and practitioners of the medical humanities examine their collective professional conscience regularly, asking themselves such fundamental questions as: What does the humanist tradition have to offer the 20th- and 21st-century practice of medicine? How is that tradition brought to bear on medicine's problematic issues? How does biomedical ethics pursued without humanism's influence differ, if at all, from the medical humanities? Moreover, given the pluralism and fragmentation of today's postmodern society, how relevant is a tradition built upon the literature, history, and moral philosophy of classical Greece and Rome as augmented by two-and-a-half millennia of scholarship provided mostly by (to use Bernard Knox's term) "dead white European males"?[1] When they converge, these inquiries force those in the medical humanities to ask whether the humanities and humanist tradition make a significant contribution to the study and practice of bioethics, one without which bioethics would be morally impoverished.

Many in the medical humanities field welcomed the 1991 publication by physician, philosopher and bioethicist H. Tristram Engelhardt, Jr., *Bioethics and Secular Humanism: The Search for a Common Morality.*[2] The book appeared to pose and answer the very questions the medical humanities community pondered. In it, Engelhardt seeks a least common denominator of shared humanity to which a pluralist society's moral strangers can have recourse when they must resolve bioethical dilemmas. To locate that common human quality, he turns to the secularization of society since the Middle Ages and to the humanist tradition, drawing upon broad and careful scholarship. After examining these traditions at length, he promulgates a bioethic which most readers anticipate will partake of secular humanism.

I challenge apposition of the term humanism to Engelhardt's secular bioethic. Because I am convinced that effective approaches to solving problems in a pluralist society *ought* to be humanistic, I think the derivation of Engelhardt's procedural common morality is well worth investigating, particularly his desire to connect with the humanist tradition. Juxtaposing them, I conclude that Engelhardt's procedural bioethic differs fundamentally from

B. P. Minogue et al. (eds.), Reading Engelhardt, 237–258.
© 1997 *Kluwer Academic Publishers. Printed in the Netherlands.*

humanism's approach. Humanism is rhetorical where Engelhardt is philosophical. Humanism addresses the mess and chaos of pluralism rather than seeking to go beyond (or beneath) that chaos in search of a minimalist ethic acceptable to all. Humanism embraces positive notions of human value historically identified with the tradition. Engelhardt argues that no value-laden (or content-full, as he calls it) bioethic can be discovered that will be acceptable to all, not even a secular bioethic that is free of religious commitments. An engaged humanist's approach to solving problems would differ, in fact, so drastically from Engelhardt's proposed procedure that the humanist umbrella cannot possibly cover both. In this paper I do not take the desirable next step of outlining what a humanistic bioethic would comprise. Rather, using *Bioethics and Secular Humanism* to outline Engelhardt's model, I hope to demonstrate that too much is sacrificed when humanism is left behind.

THE NEED FOR A SECULAR BIOETHIC

To establish an acceptable starting point for negotiation among moral strangers, Engelhardt seeks a basis for moral judgments that is not "beholden to any particular faith or moral tradition but grounded in the very requirements of a rational ethic or in the nature of man or reality itself."[3] In other words, one that is secular, strictly speaking, of *this* world, separate from ecclesiastical or divine things. The pursuit of a secular foundation for bioethical negotiations leads the author to the humanist tradition. "That which distinguishes humanity" is the core meaning of the protean term humanism.

Engelhardt explains his choice of this secular humanism thus:

> [H]ow in an increasingly secular world, marked by both religious disbelief and a diversity of religious commitment, do we fashion a health care policy that can be intellectually justified in general secular terms? One of the alluring strategies has been to appeal to the character of human nature. If one can read off from human nature what the true human goods are, then perhaps one can establish a common secular morality and provide the foundations for a content-full secular bioethics.[4]

Engelhardt conveys a sense of urgency about finding a neutral framework for negotiating conflict in pluralist societies. Should such a framework not emerge, he predicts, intuition will confront intuition, tradition will confront tradition, ideology will confront ideology, religion will confront religion, and emotion will confront emotion.[5] These confrontations will be settled forcibly. The more powerful will simply impose their views unless reason can somehow reassert its former ability to limit that power. There is, then, an imperative for those who would avoid forcible imposition of policy, behavior, and regulation. The imperative to avoid force drives Engelhardt's quest on humankind's behalf and becomes the necessary condition of his secular bioethic.

The moral framework Engelhardt constructs is procedural.[6] Moral content must be sacrificed, Engelhardt maintains, because it is inseparably bound to a ranking of values no longer shared by moral strangers. Prior sources of moral knowledge in Western culture–religion, nature and reason–can no longer justify grounds for moral discourse that are satisfactory to all.

FORMER FOUNDATIONS FOR MORAL KNOWLEDGE

It is worthwhile to look briefly at the weaknesses in each of these former foundations. Traditional belief structures have been eroding steadily since the late nineteenth century when Nietzsche made the death of God a valid topic for philosophy. The effects of his outrageous (for the times) declaration have now become commonplace. Engelhardt quotes Peter Berger's recognition that, today, theology provides insufficient moral justification:

> Probably for the first time in history, the religious legitimations of the world have lost their plausibility not only for a few intellectuals and other marginal individuals, but for broad masses of entire societies.[7]

The result is a "problem of meaningfulness" that, as Berger says, infects "the ordinary routines of everyday life."[8]

Absent a shared belief in an omnipotent and all-loving creator, Nature cannot be called upon as an example of right action. Nature is, Engelhardt tells us, "merely the products of physical processes," and, as such, has "no moral significance outside a context of moral interpretation."[9] The judgments "natural" and "unnatural" have no intrinsic moral significance, no claim on our moral action.

Reason itself no longer supplies indisputable grounding for moral action. This represents the greatest loss because moral argument, when behaving its rationalist best, aspires to reliance on reason. Engelhardt acknowledges the fundamental limitation of reason early in the book: "the content of a moral vision cannot be discovered by appeal to reason alone."[10] He does not emphasize as strongly as several of his contemporaries do the fact that reason never did provide irreducible first premises for moral discourse.[11] MacIntyre points out that Enlightenment philosophers were the first to tangle with the notion of morality as a subject of study entirely separate from law, religion and aesthetics, subjects with which it had theretofore been conflated. Rational justification of the newly discrete notion of morality became a central concern for many of them. They appeared to succeed because, despite the varied forms of Christianity to which they subscribed, all accepted fundamental Christian imperatives. It was the acceptance of similar Christian beliefs that held things together in what appeared to be "a seamless fabric of morality and public authority."[12] In a recent unpublished paper, Engelhardt explains that commissions such as the National Commission for the Protection of Human Subjects of Biomedical and Behavioral Research appear to succeed in "bridging moral disagreements and in conveying the sense of a common underlying morality" for much the same reason, namely, that those selected to serve on such commissions share similar moral, ideological and political underpinnings, despite membership in superficially different moral communities.[13]

If first truths cannot be had by way of reason, what of the possibility that universal moral truth can emerge from experience? Can a common emotional response to experience be taken, as the Scottish moral philosophers argued, as evidence of an innate moral sense? This road is blocked for Engelhardt by the is/ought fallacy, the naturalistic fallacy, to which Hume first drew attention. This philosophical position asserts that "it is not possible to argue from facts to values. From what *is* the case, one cannot establish what *ought* to be done."[14] Even broad consensus in emotional response to the experienced world does not correspond to truth about "ought." For example:

> From the fact that all people on earth are likely to die if event X occurs, and that most individuals are appalled by this prospect, though a few are not, nothing logically follows as to whether it would be morally good or bad if all people died, given event X. Perhaps there are causes worth the death of all mankind. Perhaps their death is followed by a more than compensatory afterlife? To derive ought statements from mere factual statements, one must have already interpreted the facts within a particular moral or faith tradition.[15]

Considering human individuals exclusive of and prior to specific functions or roles they may have, one cannot demonstrate by force of reason what those individuals ought to do, only how they should reason about what ought to be done.

ENGELHARDT'S PROCEDURAL BIOETHIC

The inadequacies of these former and potential bases for a content-full common ethic thus established, Engelhardt formulates a procedural ethic. The procedure is abstract, "an *intellectual possibility* available to be willed by individuals whenever they meet as moral strangers and wish to resolve controversies peaceably and with common moral authority" (emphasis mine).[16] By "willing" to act morally, individuals who wish to resolve controversy with recourse to neither force nor religion transform the possibility into reality. They do so by their willing consent to establish moral authority through collaboration.[17]

Engelhardt's bioethic is a "commitment to resolving controversies between moral strangers without primary recourse to force but with common morality."[18] In traditional moralities, content is given or decreed, and the extent to which one is judged to be moral can be measured by one's commitment to acting in accord with that content. In Engelhardt's procedural ethics, the essence of morality is a commitment to the form rather than to the content. One values peaceable rather than forcible settlement and is therefore willing to be, with others, a maker of moral content. Once content-full moral principles are formulated by willing negotiators, those who wish to be moral observe the pre- and pro-scriptions because of their commitment to abide by the outcome of the agreed-upon formal procedure, not because they agree that the outcome is right or good.

The single requisite condition for participation in negotiation is mutual respect, simply the non-use of others without their consent and the acknowledgment that others as entities may agree or refuse to negotiate. Negotiators grant one another respect, not because of any value intrinsic to the concept of respect or to one's co-negotiators, but because respect is a necessary condition for negotiation; it furnishes the framework for a common moral world without arbitrary ranking and imposition of values. Used in this way, mutual respect is not, strictly speaking, a value but, rather a restraining principle, a necessary and sufficient condition for the conduct of negotiation.

Having granted themselves moral authority through agreement to negotiate, Engelhardt's agents do then legislate moral content. It is critical to the process that the agents so engaged act not as members of their particular moral communities, but as agents who have willed to be part of the moral content-establishing procedure. In the moral world thus created, individuals can maintain the proposition that "X has the moral right to do A, but it is wrong."[19]

The bureaucratic ethical decisions reached by negotiators do not express globally binding moral obligations. Rather these decisions exist as a set of general rules created for administration of common resources. If the formal procedure has been observed in decision-making, moral individuals will abide by the content regardless of whether it is right in terms of their commitments to other, content-full moral systems. Likewise, moral "outlaws" may be forcibly coerced to abide by the agreed-upon products of negotiation.[20]

MISGIVINGS

Engelhardt's secular bioethic is understandable. Its basic premises—non-use of others without their consent and the right of any individual not to negotiate—ensure that collective authority over any person must be conveyed by that person and that individuals have the right to abstain from the common moral project. Using his procedural bioethic framework, negotiators can build health care entitlements as well as multiple and unequal health care systems, and they can fashion regional joint health care endeavors.

I worry, however, that the presence of only a constraining principle (non-use of others without their consent) in the absence of any welfare consideration of beneficence fails to safeguard morality adequately. Seeking only to resolve moral dilemmas without force, value-stripped negotiators might agree on a course of action that none, individually, views as moral. Such a result is all the more possible if negotiators are able, as in Engelhardt's ideal scenario, to leave their individual moral communities behind them when entering into negotiation.[21] In his 1995 paper, Engelhardt admits that negotiators' decisions and policies

> will be beyond secular good and evil, since good and evil cannot be specified in general secular terms. They [particular choices and structures] will simply either possess or not possess the authority that moral strangers can understand that they convey to their common endeavors.[22]

The procedural bioethic thus serves as a political expedient for keeping the peace rather than serving as a common morality.

Engelhardt's bioethic also seems to sell the power of reasoning short. Because human reason is unable to provide one preeminent, rationally conclusive, content-full moral vision, Engelhardt dispenses with using reason to discover any morality. He does not consider that, while it is unable to discover first truths, reason can become a powerful tool for discovering moral knowledge when used as it is in the humanist-rhetorical tradition.

My principal objection to the procedural, secular humanist ethic that Engelhardt constructs, though, is that it isn't humanism. Content-less, his common morality stands for little that is distinctively human. Engelhardt says that individuals are salient in his procedure, but, as with Rawls' placing of agents in the "original position," these individuals must act as ideal types rather than real, historically situated people. What is more, they are not valued for their human-ness:

> Within the sparse morality of moral strangers, one cannot talk about persons as being valued or as having moral worth. They, and their consent, are simply necessary for a morality of moral strangers.[23]

Engelhardt's revised humanism focuses

> not on *humanitas*, but on what one might term *personitas*–the nature of persons as constituting a practice of peaceable negotiation that sustains a moral language for moral strangers.[24]

Dynamic as the term "humanism" is, Engelhardt's departure is so radical that his secular humanism bioethic is no longer humanism at all.[25] And he knows it. On page 11 he acknowledges that his humanistic bioethic will be a grammar for moral discourse. As such, "it will cease to be a humanism and will instead be a general morality that need not be restricted to humans."[26] Yet in the remaining 128 pages (41 comprising the chapter on humanism) he defends his bioethic in light of the humanist tradition. I take this as a bid for its admission to the tradition, but I reject the bid. In doing so, I look strictly and closely at the derivation of Engelhardt's humanism from the *humanitas* tradition.

THE HUMANIST TRADITION

One approaches the term "humanism" and its cognates–*humanitas*, humane, humanist, humanity–with due respect, observing the warnings of those who have gone ahead. Today the word "humanity" can mean "little more than being 'nice,'" as John Stephens notes in introducing his extended discussion of *humanitas* and its key role in the Italian Renaissance.[27] At the other extreme, "to call someone a secular humanist can be to use fighting words" as Engelhardt says in the first sentence of *Bioethics and Secular Humanism*.

As contemporary writers note, *humanitas* has been developing as a concept for two and one-half millennia, since before the golden age of Greek culture. But even some historians deal loosely with the term. Engelhardt quotes Paul O. Kristeller, one who does not take the term loosely:

> For many historians . . . have cheerfully applied the term "humanism" in its vague modern meaning to the Renaissance and to other periods of the past, speaking of Renaissance humanism, medieval humanism, or Christian humanism, in a fashion which defies any definition and seems to have little or nothing left of the basic classicist meaning of Renaissance humanism.[28]

Engelhardt seeks to avoid these pitfalls of interpretation in the closely re-searched chapter, "Humanism, Humaneness and the Humanities." The lengthy treatment reveals the humanities in their full complexity and richness.[29]

The cognates and definitions with which Engelhardt limns the concept of humanism are as follows: (a) *Humanitas* as human-ness refers to "that which marks humans apart from animals."[30] It includes a striving after the measures of cultivated humanity, what humans do to make the most of their distinctive-ness. (b) Humane as humanitarian connotes the qualities of mercy and philan-thropy. (c) Humanity, when used in an evaluative rather than in a species-identification sense, refers to excellence or nobility of intellect, education, sentiment, cultivation. (d) A humanist is a teacher, scholar, or student of the humanities. (e) The humanities are those studies appropriate to definition (a), the cultivation of human-ness. (f) Humanism comprises the scholarship, particularly study of the literature and moral philosophy of the ancients, engaged in by humanists. (g) Humanism, in a sense other than the scholarship referred to in definition (f), denotes prudence, poise, balance, the golden mean in the sense of proportion. This quality of humanism was the goal of the Greek education curriculum, the *paideia*. (h) Humanism can refer to a creed or set of values that draws generally on Renaissance confidence in human capacity. (i) Secular Humanism in Engelhardt's sense is "a philosophical basis for moral understanding and negotiation among moral strangers."[31] In this last entry, Engelhardt grants his version of procedural morality definitional status as humanism. I will argue that he must situate this meaning within the others that, together, form the humanist tradition if his bioethic is to be a humanist bioethic. To discover whether he succeeds in literally insinuating his definition into the tradition, I will look at the constellation of meanings more closely.

Humanitas, Humane, and Humanism. Meanings (a), (b) and (g) apply most closely to the tradition's sources: the moral/aesthetic/intellectual curriculum developed by the Greeks and refined by the Romans. Both *humanitas* and the related *humanus* referred in the Greco-Roman world to that which distinguished humans from animals and hence, to civility, nobility, dignity, refinement, culture. From at least early Roman times, a dispute of the chicken-and-egg sort appears to have waged between the "humane disposition" and "education for culture and refinement" aspects of the definition. Stephens insists, as Engelhardt does not, on the primacy of human feeling–meaning (b). "The basic meaning of the word [*humanitas*] is human feeling," Stephens says.[32] Engelhardt emphasizes that the philanthropic aspect of meaning (b), a "certain bearing towards one's fellow man," was the product of education rather than a species-natural inheritance.[33] Interestingly, both authors cite the same passage from Aulus Gellius (ca. A.D. 130-180) in defending their divergent opinions. Stephens insists that humanitas "came to mean intellectual accomplishment as well as human feeling because knowledge was necessary to an understanding of the nature and community of mankind."[34] In noting the inherent ambiguity, Engelhardt comments, "*Humanus* and *humanitas* identified that which was proper to humans: both a development of the special capacities of humans and a concern *to do good to* one's fellow man."[35] I emphasize his words to highlight the positive action this ancient definition demands of *humanitas*. It demands more than the non-use of others without their consent.

In contemporary discourse, the term dignity probably captures most closely the *humanus* notion of the inherent worth of persons as reasoning, caring beings. The concept of dignity descends in its current philosophical form from Kant but goes back to Renaissance philosopher Pico della Mirandola's *Oration on the Dignity of Man* and even beyond. In general terms, it is the faculty for self-conscious reflection that elevates humans above other species and enables them to possess a sense of self-respect.

Philosopher Charles Taylor and Political Scientist Robert Goodin profess anew that dignity is constitutive of human persons. For Taylor, dignity is inescapably part of who we are; it is our sense of ourselves as commanding respect.[36] Taylor's very positive notion of respect approximates the humanist idea of *humanus* much more closely than Engelhardt's negative basis for respect. Goodin says, very practically, that consideration for individuals' dignity must be part of the equation of public policy decisions. Values associated with dignity, he says, go beyond material preferences and cannot be measured on a utilitarian scale. For Goodin, to recognize an individual's dignity is to grant the individual formal legal rights. Further, it entails a welfare obligation to see that the individual has a minimum of those goods which are central to maintenance of that dignity.[37]

Humanity and the Humanities. Dignity as used by these contemporary thinkers relates also to the humanity of meaning (c), which notices and appreciates degrees of nobility in humans. Definition (c), however, evaluates more than the inherent component of one's humanity–one's natural deserving-ness of self-respect. It also judges the success or failure of training in the human arts that is applied to make the most of natural or intrinsic nobility.

The Greek educational system that would inspire scholars and academicians more than 1000 years later and become the seed the humanities of meaning (e) was the offspring of rhetoric. In the rhetoric/philosophy split I alluded to earlier, the rhetoricians–Sophists at first–focused even more on humanity-in-the-here-and-now than did the philosophers; "The Sophists helped to secularize Greece," Engelhardt says.[38] They also enjoyed a durable freedom from com-mitment to specific philosophic theories. Abandoning what they saw as a vain search for ultimate and universal truths, the rhetoricians sought instead the best possible judgment, given a certain set of circumstances. Isocrates strongly influenced ancient rhetoric with his belief that, properly undertaken, the practice contributed to the development of moral character. After Isocrates, who was a contemporary of Plato's, a rhetoric-based curriculum dominated educational thinking in the ancient world.[39]

Christianity altered the notion of *humanitas* inherited from the ancients to suit its own purposes. Early Christians retained the basic urging and sentiments of *humanitas*, now justified on otherworldly grounds. Humans ought to treat one another with love because God so commands. Man's God-like, though much limited, faculty of reason should be directed toward understanding the transcendent. While Greek philosophy, *mutatis mutandis,* was acceptable, much of the rhetorical tradition was not. The Church Fathers viewed rhetoric's denial of ultimate truths as relativistic sophistry. Augustine achieved an accommodation of sorts between Christian doctrine and rhetoric in the fourth century. A teacher of rhetoric before his conversion, Augustine applied rhetoric's method of inquiry to the study of scripture.[40] By so doing, he legitimated the use of formal classical methods of inquiry among the growing numbers of Christians. Augustine's accommodation helped rescue rhetoric from the rigid codification it was undergoing in late imperial Rome and insured its transmission into the Middle Ages. At the same time, it established a theological strand of rhetoric quite different from Isocratean/Aristotelian or Ciceronian deliberative rhetoric. In essence, classical rhetoric's invention of arguments (Cicero's *De inventione*) became the "discovery of what should be understood by Christians."[41] Consequently, the secular grounding and content so important to the *studia humanitatis* were lost to Western European culture until the Renaissance.

Humanist and Humanism. Lexical entries (d) and (f) in Engelhardt's list came with the Renaissance. Fourteenth-century Italy gloried in the rediscovery of ancient civilization. For one thing, Roman culture and history offered Italy a rich national heritage. Even more, however, the Italian scholars and tutors, court secretaries and other civil servants who came to be called humanists by the late 1400s responded to the pre-Christian, humanity-based focus of the Greco-Roman *studia humanitatis*. The ancients had discovered a basis for right action in their own world rather than in their gods', through reason rather than revelation, and in celebration of the human body rather than in its denigration. They had justified *sophrosyne*–the sense of prudence, balance, avoidance of extremes, and grace, in both body and mind–on humanity's account.

Renaissance humanists translated, studied and taught the grammar, rhetoric, poetry, history and moral philosophy of the ancients with the goal of perfecting their natural talent through both the discipline of the study and the imitation of virtuous lives. Their scholarly interest in classical writings was the humanism of definition (f). Other periods of revival and study of classical literature have occurred following the initial movement of the early fourteenth to late sixteenth centuries, and the studies that could be rightfully be subjects of humanism have changed.

Humanism and Secular Humanism. Sometimes such movements developed into what Engelhardt calls capital-H Humanism; that is, they came to embrace a specific creed or set of values. The secular humanist sect viewed today as a religion by the U.S. Supreme Court is an example. These definition (h) Humanists do more than study the humanities; they wish to preserve human values and attempt to change social context to do so, if necessary. Called "interventionist" humanists by Engelhardt, they generally espouse the realization of human potential and hold values that express confidence in human capacities.[42]

The Humanities. Were education the topic, the Humanities of definition (e) would be most problematic. Originally referring to the *studia humanitatis*–the grammar, rhetoric, poetry, history and moral philosophy of the ancients mentioned above–the humanities meant a classical education when the term entered the English-speaking world in the eighteenth century.[43] Volumes have been written descrying the fate of the humanities in education since the mid-nineteenth century, but that fate is beside the point here, inasmuch as Engelhardt's bioethic appears uninterested in the educational aspect of humanism.

Engelhardt's Secular Humanism. It is primarily and almost exclusively the non-religious, humanity-based aspect of the tradition with which Engelhardt connects. He is seeking moral justification in reason not revelation, in the secular realm, not the transcendent or divine realm. Engelhardt develops his idea of secular in Chapter Two of *Bioethics and Secular Humanism*, "The Secular as a Neutral Framework." The idea as developed there furnishes all the non-religious, humanity-based moral justification that Engelhardt's bioethic uses. He approaches the concept of secular, secularization and secularism in the thorough, historic manner of Chapter Three's approach to humanism, humaneness, and the humanities. Engelhardt discusses several clusters of meaning for secular. The first of these is, "the secular as a morally neutral framework through which believers and non-believers can collaborate one with another." About this meaning Engelhardt says, "It is this first sense of secular that is most important for this volume. It is this sense of secular that governs in 'secular bioethics,' a bioethics accessible to peaceable individuals independently of their special moral, ideological or faith traditions."[44]

MISSING HUMANISM IN ENGELHARDT'S BIOETHIC

My claim regarding his secular humanist bioethic is twofold. First, Engelhardt does not need the humanist tradition he so thoroughly limns to establish a purely rational foundation for morality. Second, should he nonetheless wish to situate his secular bioethic in this tradition, he will encounter many *constitutive* and *authoritative* human values, judgments, feelings, and notions of positive good that belie the rationalism of his bioethic. Engelhardt wants humanism to be, according to meaning (i), a philosophical basis for moral understanding and negotiation among moral strangers. But humanism, a *tradition*, lacks the coherence that marks philosophy.[45] It is not that clear or formal. Consider, moreover, what Engelhardt does *not* take from the humanist tradition just described.

Positive Beneficence. "The concern to do good to one's fellow man" to which Engelhardt gives equal billing in the ancient *humanus/humanitatis* controversy, he nevertheless drops in favor of "non-use of others without their consent." To do good would be to act on a given conception of the good life, which could easily be a deal-breaking obstacle to negotiations in a pluralist society.

Value Judgment. The evaluative recognition of particular excellence or nobility in a given member of the human species is missing from Engelhardt's bioethic: "we cannot talk about persons as being valued or having moral worth," he reasons. "They, and their consent, are simply necessary for a morality of moral strangers."[46] In the final paragraph of the treatise, Engelhardt writes, "We are left with a moral perspective within which not only gender, race, and culture become morally irrelevant, but species membership itself."[47]

If I am correct in calling the inherent, untutored component of *humanus,* and the respect with which we recognize it, "dignity," then I must conclude that dropping this positive value as a necessary regulator to bioethical decision-making is too great a sacrifice. Granted, there is nothing to stop Engelhardt's negotiators from arriving at agreements which respect humans simply because they are humans. But neither is there anything in his procedural ethic to assure that humans will always be accorded respect simply because they are humans. Respect for dignity is not a gatekeeper to negotiation. Mutual respect is a necessary condition for marketplace exchanges and may be a sufficient condition for them. It is not a sufficient condition for human interactions in the humanist tradition.[48]

Cultivation of Humaneness through Education. Absent from Engelhardt's bioethic is the inextricable connection between knowledge and humaneness that made it difficult if not impossible for the ancients to distinguish nature's role from nurture's in our humane behavior. This ancient connection resonates in the humanist, humanism, and humanities cognates (Meanings d-g). Renaissance humanists studied classical moral philosophy and rhetoric because, for classical philosophers and rhetoricians, *humanus* signified a native capacity for human virtue realized through knowledge. Knowledge and the getting of practical wisdom were essential prerequisites for the good life and good citizenship. Bernard Knox postulates that humanities' forerunner–the *paideia*–arose once the Greeks, having discovered democracy, realized that the populace must be educated to judge wisely and govern itself well.[49] The notion that a value-stripped cosmopolitan is best suited to formulate public policy would shock ancient proto-humanists and Renaissance humanists as well as many humanists of today.

Here I acknowledge an anticipated charge: a connection between knowledge and right action might well have been valid in the *polis* and even in the classical Roman world where greater consensus prevailed regarding right action and virtue. In a pluralist society, though, knowledge supports multiple and varied premises of virtue and right action. For example, the more law, theology, history, philosophy and embryology that opposing abortion issue partisans bring to their arguments, the more challenging the debate. This is true. Yet, the linkage of knowledge, virtue and desire for right action is intrinsic to humanism. This aspect of humanism–that its study fosters moral development which may then be put to service in friendship, citizenship and negotiation among moral strangers–does not interest Engelhardt. Though he neither wants nor can use this notion, it remains an essential component of humanism.

Humanism's Contextuality. Engelhardt neglects other essentials of humanism in his secular bioethic, for example, context. Humanism has changed over the centuries because it is contextual. The first humanists revived classical learning and applied it to the life and problems of fourteenth-century Italy, altering it in the process. They translated texts and sought to learn what those texts revealed about the (chiefly) men and events of a thousand years before. William Bennett's definition of the humanities during his tenure as chairman of the National Endowment for the Humanities recognizes this context-sensitivity:

> The humanities tell us how men and women of our own and other civilizations have grappled with life's enduring, fundamental questions: What is justice? What should be loved? What deserves to be defended? What is courage? What is noble? What is base? Why do civilizations flourish? Why do they decline?[50]

It is against the various backgrounds and textures the humanities preserve that likenesses stand out across time. Once the enduring questions Bennett asks pop into the foreground, humanists can study more readily the interplay between the answers on the one hand and the times and the cultures on the other (foreground and background). Once again, this may not be pertinent to a secular bioethic, but it is constitutive of humanism.

Humanism's Rhetorical Origin and the Role of Emotion. Engelhardt touches upon the importance of rhetoric to humanism, acknowledging that for all its chaos it "has an attractive beauty of its own."[51] Yet his preference for philosophy's single-minded commitment to reason wins the day. He does not mention emotion, for instance. Rhetoricians, both ancient and Renaissance-cra, recognized that discourse was ineffective without emotion (*pathe'*). Rhetoricians grant emotion a key place in discourse because "the essence of man is determined both by logical and emotional elements and as a result, speech can reach human beings [only] as a union of *logos* and *pathos*."[52]

Greek rhetoricians and poets–and Aristotle–recognized the role emotions play in the getting of self-knowledge and practical wisdom. Plato, on the other hand, distrusted poets and sophists because both employed *pathe'* as a tool for achieving their objectives. He denounced emotion for many reasons. It resembled instinct more than reasoning; drew its content from experience and the particulars of experience rather than from the unchanging universals and abstractions of contemplation. Emotions were changeable and ephemeral and caused discontent.[53] Greek tragedians and comedic playwrights understood that arousal of emotion offers, as Nussbaum puts it, "an occasion for an activity of knowing that could not even in principle be had by the intellect alone."[54] Receptivity to and experience of emotion advances a certain type of learning, knowledge of one's own vulnerability and limitations as well as awareness of (as Nussbaum's title declares) the fragility of goodness in the face of conflicting duties and even at the hands of fate. This kind of self-knowledge gives one practical wisdom that can "enrich future deliberative efforts."[55]

Engelhardt does not talk about emotion, so I think it is fair to assume that emotions are not critical to his framework as they are to the practice of rhetoric. When he dispenses with value ("we cannot talk about persons as being valued or having moral worth") he banishes the many emotions evoked by our almost instinctual reactions to people, things and ideas. I am willing to grant that emotional knowledge may have little to contribute to the exchanges of the marketplace, but it is bioethics, after all, that is under consideration here, matters of life, death, suffering and taking account of what is intrinsically important in our lives. The richness of human emotion in the context of value is indispensable to humanism.[56]

SECULAR? YES; HUMANIST? NO

All Engelhardt really takes from humanism is a quality readily supplied by "secular." His first definition for "secular" in Chapter Two is "a morally neutral framework through which believers and non believers can collaborate with one another." Yet the stature of his bioethic seems to depend in some way important to him upon its inclusion in the humanism tradition. His thorough examination of the tradition, however, only exposes more dramatically that his procedural bioethic does not engage what is distinctively human. Engelhardt knows that his bioethic really ceases to be humanism and admits in his final paragraph:

> Even this modest success has its price. By providing a moral standpoint for moral strangers, secular humanism sets itself free from its historical roots and deprives itself of its traditional content. The higher truth of *humanitas* is *personitas.*[57]

Summarizing his bid for inclusion in the humanist tradition, Engelhardt says of meaning (i):

> Only if this last sense of humanism can be justified will individuals who meet as moral strangers find that they share enough to frame common health care policies which they should recognize as having moral and intellectual authority.[58]

This comment confuses matters. At first it seems as though Engelhardt could be saying that his definition must be justified as a sense of humanism in order that moral strangers be able to find a basis for negotiation. But that cannot be his meaning. His procedural bioethic can form a neutral framework for the resolutions of differences among moral strangers whether or not that framework can be situated in the humanist tradition. Engelhardt must mean that only if this philosophical basis for common moral understanding and negotiation among strangers can be intellectually justified, that is, given moral authority in terms of the nature of mankind and the human condition, only *then* will individuals who meet as moral strangers find that they share enough to frame common health policies that they accept as licit. On this meaning, the statement is valid, but it accomplishes nothing by way of tying his bioethic to humanism. He declares his philosophical basis for negotiation to be meaning (i) but does not justify its presence as part of the tradition.

CONCLUSION

This paper does not attempt to sketch an outline of a truly humanist bioethic; that is another project. My sense is that such a bioethic will be in the rhetorical tradition, admitting of values and emotions and focusing on particulars. I am not alone in endorsing the so-called "extraordinarily vague but still fruitful notion" of humanism in a time characterized by competing systems of rationality, justice and morality. Stephen Toulmin and Robert

Proctor, both cited elsewhere in this paper, believe that western civilization has been at a juncture like this one before, and that a return to humanism is a better course than seeking safety in formal systems–the course taken by the rational philosophers of the 17th century when, as now, society appeared to be falling apart at the seams. Thinkers in this camp point out aspects of philosophical and scientific thinking that have come full circle: now, as before Descartes, the observer is no longer separate from the observed as an independent subject confronting a discrete object. Skepticism is again rampant, directed now toward science and reason as well as religion. Unitary systems of explanation are discredited. We have discovered the limits of both scientific rationalism and Lockean individualism. We cannot act as morally un-situated, objective subjects, try as we might.

On the positive side, many of the values we hold as humans are shared among most humans. It is their ranking, as Engelhardt acknowledges, that provokes discord. Does autonomy have primacy over beneficence? When these values conflict, is it more important to protect the entrepreneur's liberty to amass billions in personal wealth than to secure fair equality of opportunity for the least advantaged in society? A humanist/rhetorical approach opens for negotiators the possibility to reach best judgments in particular cases without declaring the absolute and universal primacy of one value over another. In the next judgment, or the next, the ordering of values may change. Humanists insist that values and preferences infiltrate negotiations, despite efforts to suppress them, and that humanity will always have individual, diverse, time-sensitive and culture-sensitive meanings. I think humanism gains dual advantage here, first in its authentic grasp of the situation at hand and, second, in its willingness to begin negotiations at that point, no matter the differences. Moreover, I believe that the 2,500-year tradition of humanism lends breadth and depth to the disparate meanings of individual humanity in ways that foster discovery of commonality and similarity. Humanism thus enhances rather than restricts our ability to resolve disagreement–in this particular case, or that particular case–among members of diverse moral communities.

NOTES

1. Bernard Knox, *The Oldest Dead White European Males* (New York: W. W. Norton & Company, 1993).

2. H. Tristram Engelhardt, Jr. *Bioethics and Secular Humanism: The Search for a Common Morality* (Philadelphia: Trinity Press International, 1991).

3. Engelhardt, *Bioethics and Secular Humanism*, 104.

4. Engelhardt, *Bioethics and Secular Humanism*, 104.

5. Engelhardt, *Bioethics and Secular Humanism*, 118.

6. The argument presented here from which Engelhardt draws the conclusion that a bioethic in contemporary pluralist society must be content-less and procedural is a recapitulation and summary of the argument he constructed in 1986 in *The Foundations of Bioethics* (New York: Oxford University Press, 1986), 17-65. The 1986 construction is more painstaking and easier to follow, especially in developing the key notion of mutual respect as the necessary condition for establishing ethics as a means of peaceably negotiating moral disputes. Ethics, for Engelhardt, is an enterprise in conflict resolution, rather than a body of value-based principles.

7. Peter L. Berger, *The Social Reality of Religion* (London: Penguin, 1969), 130, cited by Engelhardt, *Bioethics and Secular Humanism*, 4.

8. Berger, *The Social Reality*, 130.

9. Engelhardt, *Bioethics and Secular Humanism*, 108.

10. Engelhardt, *Bioethics and Secular Humanism*, 18.

11. See for instance Alasdair MacIntyre, *After Virtue: A Study in Moral Theory* (Notre Dame, Indiana: University of Notre Dame Press, 1981), Ernesto Grassi, *Rhetoric as Philosophy: The Humanist Tradition* (University Park, Pennsylvania: The Pennsylvania State University Press, 1980), and Stephen Toulmin, *Cosmopolis: The Hidden Agenda of Modernity* (Chicago: The University of Chicago Press, 1990). The awareness that first truths are not demonstrable by reason but are revealed or apprehended, grasped by "insight" as Grassi puts it, is one hallmark of the path taken by rhetoric in antiquity as it diverged from philosophy. Grassi, whose interest is also humanism, looks to the Renaissance and to Vico's working out of this matter of first truths. According to Vico by way of Grassi, humanity creates and invents the first connections between itself and its world. The primary apprehending of relationships is not deductive. There are no prior truths or identities from which to infer (Grassi, 8). In Vico's view, first truths are the products of human *ingenium,* that is, our capacity for insight and imagination, and truths thus grasped are expressed metaphorically not rationally. Starting in the here-and-now and reasoning backward toward a universally acceptable premise takes the moral investigator just so far. At reason's deductive limit stand truths that can be known only by way of revelation (e.g., that man was created by God in His image) or discovered through the *ingenium* of philosophers and scientists of various epistemological traditions (e.g., Plato's ideal forms, of which each material example is a less-than-perfect imitation or Descartes' *cogito ergo sum*). As MacIntyre says in proclaiming the literal "interminability" of present day rival moral arguments, "[f]rom our rival conclusions we can argue back to our rival premises; but when we arrive at our premises argument ceases and the invocation of one premise against another becomes a matter of pure assertion and counter assertion" (MacIntyre, 1981, 8).

12. Engelhardt, *Bioethics and Secular Humanism*, xvi. In discussing his three paths–discovery, invention, interpretation–to moral philosophy, Michael Walzer summarizes the rationalist philosophers' state of affairs using Descartes as example. While Descartes claimed in the *Discourse on Method* to be undertaking a profound philosophical journey of invention and construction, from scratch, as it were, he in fact "really launched on a journey of discovery," uncovering and offering as new and proved "facts" of either revelation or common human experience seen with new clarity. Michael Walzer, *Interpretation and Social Criticism* (Cambridge, Massachusetts: Harvard University Press, 1987), 9.

13. H. Tristram Engelhardt, Jr., "Bioethics and the Philosophy of Medicine Reconsidered." Paper delivered at the Institute for the Medical Humanities, University of Texas Medical Branch at Galveston, February 16, 1995.

14. Engelhardt, *Bioethics and Secular Humanism*, 104. This philosophical position is contested by certain contemporary philosophers. MacIntyre, for example, argues that with functional concepts, e.g., the concept of a watch or of a farmer, value judgment is part and parcel of the factual definition–a watch measures time, a farmer produces crops. Therefore, a watch which does not measure time and a farmer who does not produce crops do not meet the factual requirements of the definition. These examples demonstrate that "any argument which moves from premises which assert that the appropriate criteria are satisfied to a conclusion which asserts 'this is a good such-and-such' will be a value argument which moves from factual premises to an evaluative conclusion" (55). Charles Taylor, quoting from Bernard Williams, makes the point that there are a host of key value terms, such as courage, brutality, gratitude, which cannot be described without the benefit of normative language. Charles Taylor, *Sources of the Self*, (Cambridge: Harvard University Press, 1989), 54-5; Bernard Williams, *Ethics and the Limits of Philosophy* (London: Fontana, 1985). And a central tenet of pragmatism holds that "knowledge cannot be separated from evaluation; fact cannot be separated from value." Bruce A. Kimball, "Pragmatism," in *The Condition of American Liberal Education,* ed. Robert Orrill (New York: College Entrance Examination Board, 1995), 26.

15. Engelhardt, *Bioethics and Secular Humanism*, 104.

16. Engelhardt, *Bioethics and Secular Humanism*, 122.

17. Engelhardt does not explain his "will to morality," although, not insignificantly, he invests it with the power to "set nihilism aside" (120). His mention of nihilism brings Nietzsche into the discussion. Like Nietzsche's will to power, Engelhardt's will to morality arises from a metaphysical wasteland in which truths are shown to be nothing other than individual values and opinion. Whereas Nietzsche concludes from this that those who propound "truths" are merely demonstrating their individual will to power, Engelhardt would have us ignore truth and value altogether and agree upon a shared will to moral behavior.

18. Engelhardt, *Bioethics and Secular Humanism*, 119.

19. Engelhardt, *Bioethics and Secular Humanism*, 124.

20. Kurt Baier expresses this idea well by way of explaining Benthamite utilitarianism at the time: "The individual citizen is bound by the law only in the sense that the sanctions attached to it make it prudent but not morally obligatory for him to follow it." Kurt Baier, "Ethics: Teleological Theories" in *Encyclopedia of Bioethics*, Vol. 1, ed. Warren T. Reich (New York: The Free Press, 1978), 419-20.

21. In its second chapter, *Bioethics and Secular Humanism* employs the term "cosmopolitan" to denote post-modern, "yuppy"–like individuals who have no true ties to any specific religious or moral tradition or homeland, though they may observe fragments of any of these traditions. Their loss of faith, tradition and sense of community–and even family membership– results "in a comfortable ultimate meaninglessness, not a loss of meaning" (p. 35). Suffering has no transcendental significance for cosmopolitans. Illness is only an obstacle to achieving one's goals. To become a negotiator within Engelhardt's common moral framework is to assume this cosmopolitan frame of reference. Although Engelhardt gives "meaningless-ness" a comfortable, positive ring (it's *not* loss of meaning), the negotiators' sole commitment is "the non-use of another without that individual's permission." Embodied thus with cosmopolitans, Engelhardt's transcendent bioethic comes to earth in a familiar form. It gives us the morality of the unrestricted marketplace, in which participation is by consent, all that is solid may be liquefied,

and traders have no reason to respect the ultimate goals, values, and purposes of other traders, or even to have their own.

22. Engelhardt, *The Foundations of Bioethics*, 2nd ed. (Oxford: Oxford University Press, 1996), 19.

23. Engelhardt, *Bioethics and Secular Humanism*, 136.

24. Engelhardt, *Bioethics and Secular Humanism*, 125.

25. Engelhardt calls humanism "an extraordinarily vague but still fruitful notion," *Bioethics and Secular Humanism*, 44.

26. Passages such as this one suggest the influence of the attack on humanism which flows from Continental phenomenology and is effectively represented today by Gianni Vattimo. The thesis is that a "crisis of humanism" necessarily attends the demise of metaphysics. Vattimo's line of reasoning in a chapter entitled "Crisis of Humanism" derives much from Nietzsche and Heidegger and hangs on the premise that humanism falsely assumes the centrality of the human subject. See Gianni Vattimo, *The End of Modernity* (Baltimore: The Johns Hopkins University Press, 1985), 32. Engelhardt refers only briefly to this tradition of the crisis in humanism while devoting almost one-third of his entire discussion to traditional expressions of humanism. I mention this, even though Engelhardt does not, because the change he suggests in the tradition, specifically the de-privileging of human distinctiveness, resembles the "crash diet" for the human subject which Vattimo offers.

27. John Stephens, *The Italian Renaissance: The Origins of Intellectual and Artistic Change before the Renaissance* (New York: Longman Inc., 1990), 14.

28. Paul O. Kristeller, *Renaissance Thought* (New York: Harper, 1961), 8, cited by Engelhardt, *Bioethics and Secular Humanism*, 48.

29. Early in the chapter, Engelhardt quotes the statement found on the writing chamber walls of Montaigne's chateau and attributed to Publius Terentius Afer (185-159 B.C.): "I am a human, anything that happens to a human touches me." Engelhardt expands upon Terence's statement: "Humanism involves not only an interest in the exemplary intellectual and aesthetic accomplishments and well-being, but also a concern for others" (p. 43). It is just this concern, however, that finally disappears, as Engelhardt draws down value, content, and finally all positive respect for humans as humans from his ethic, leaving only a negative and empty notion of "the non-use of others without their consent."

30. Engelhardt, *Bioethics and Secular Humanism*, 43. I follow Engelhardt's wording very closely throughout these definitions which appear on pages 45-48.

31. Engelhardt, *Bioethics and Secular Humanism*, 48.

32. Stephens, *The Italian Renaissance*, 15.

33. Engelhardt, *Bioethics and Secular Humanism*, 45.

34. Engelhardt, *Bioethics and Secular Humanism*, 45.

35. Engelhardt, *Bioethics and Secular Humanism*, 57.

36. Taylor, *Sources of the Self*, 15.

37. Robert E. Goodin, *Political Theory and Public Policy* (Chicago: University of Chicago Press, 1982), 81-94.

38. Engelhardt, *Bioethics and Secular Humanism*, 56.

39. Isocrates' role in establishing the practice and culture of rhetoric in Ancient Greece and the subsequent domination of rhetoric in education are discussed by Farrell and Oakley, respectively. Thomas B. Farrell, *Norms of Rhetorical Culture* (New Haven, CT: Yale University Press, 1993), 58. Francis Oakley, *Community of Learning: The American College and the Liberal Arts Tradition* (New York: Oxford University Press, 1992), 50.

40. This version of Augustine's accommodation of rhetoric to study of Scripture is from Bruce Kimball, *Orators and Philosophers: A History of the Idea of Liberal Education* (New York: College Entrance Examination Board, 1995), 40-42.

41. Richard McKeon, "Rhetoric in the Middle Ages," *Speculum* 17, no. 1 (January 1942): 6.

42. Engelhardt, *Bioethics and Secular Humanism*, 87.

43. Oakley, *Community of Learning*, 57.

44. Engelhardt, *Bioethics and Secular Humanism*, 23. The other meanings pertain to: the identification of clerics who are not members of religious orders; the process by which church lands and property becomes the property of the state or the belongings of church clerics become those of secular clerics; "attempts to limit or annul the powers...and influence of the church" (23); and capital S–Secularism as a movement which developed during the nineteenth century aimed at establishing secular societal structures. In this meaning secular takes on a sectarian connotation for the first time. This Secularism intersects with Humanism's meaning (g) is the form of Secular Humanism, a humanism that embraces a specific creed or set of values. Finally, there is the sense of secular as the "process by which a culture's or a society's sense of the religious or the transcendent is transformed into an immanent, worldly province of meaning"(23). This last sense is, Engelhardt says, "complex and controversial" (30). Secularization in this last sense has shaped our civic institutions, including health care. "A well-articulated language of secular moral and legal analysis has developed to serve as the basis for the secular discussions of health and medicine" (31). My point of argument is that Engelhardt's survey of secularization provides the non-religious moral justification his bioethic employs. Humanism does not contribute to this non-religious moral justification, and Engelhardt does not take from the humanist tradition any of what it would, by definition, add.

45. Renaissance scholar Paul Oskar Kristeller reasons that humanism is not a philosophy because it embodies no common philosophical doctrine, strictly speaking, except "a belief in the value of man and the humanities and in the revival of ancient learning." Paul Oskar Kristeller, *The Classics and Renaissance Thought* (Cambridge: Harvard University Press, 1955), 11.

46. Engelhardt, *Bioethics and Secular Humanism*, 136.

47. Engelhardt, *Bioethics and Secular Humanism,* 140. Engelhardt explains this comment in a footnote by saying that the human species is as it is only due to chance mutations, natural catastrophes and the like. Furthermore, given the potential of genetic engineering, species boundaries could become hazy. No characteristics ascribed to humanity by the humanist tradition are, therefore, in any sense *necessary*.

48. Beyond this argument for not including Engelhardt's bioethic in the humanist tradition, I suggest that the purely negative condition of non-use of others without their consent is an insufficient condition for grounding non-marketplace morality. Bioethical decisions concern life/death and personhood matters, and the parties involved are often not engaging freely and consensually in a marketplace.

49. Knox, *White European Males* 86-90.

50. William J. Bennett, *To Reclaim a Legacy* (Washington, D. C.: National Endowment for the Humanities, 1994), 2. Quoted by Engelhardt, *Bioethics and Secular Humanism*, 75-6. Using Bennett as a defender of this traditional humanism shows just how inclusive this "fruitful notion" is.

51. Engelhardt, *Bioethics and Secular Humanism*, 59.

52. Grassi, *Rhetoric as Philosophy*, 27.

53. For information about use of emotion and thinking about emotion in classical Greece, I depend upon Martha Nussbaum, *The Fragility of Goodness* (New York: Cambridge University Press, 1986).

54. Nussbaum, *The Fragility of Goodness*, 46.

55. Nussbaum, *The Fragility of Goodness*, 45.

56. Robert E. Proctor points out at length in a scholarly–and moving–way what we can learn about the history and psychology of humankind by comparing the emotional lives of Cicero and Petrarch. Robert E. Procter, *Education's Great Amnesia* (Bloomington, Indiana: Indiana University Press, 1988), 59-83.

57. Engelhardt, *Bioethics and Secular Humanism*, 140.

58. Engelhardt, *Bioethics and Secular Humanism*, 48.

15

The Foundations of Bioethics and Secular Humanism: Why is There no Canonical Moral Content?

H. Tristram Engelhardt, Jr.

Why Matters are so Fundamentally Different from What Many Essayists in this Volume had Hoped.

This volume's essays direct primary attention to *The Foundations of Bioethics* and *Bioethics and Secular Humanism: The Search for a Common Morality*.[1] As the reader will have noted, some speak principally to the first edition of *Foundations*. Others address the second edition and indeed compare the latter with the former. In what follows, my response builds on the second edition. I am honored by the attention these readers have given to my reflections. Even where they have misread me, I am grateful for the exploration of my arguments and the assessment of their weaknesses. They have shown how to be clearer. The contributors to this volume, I hope, will recognize in this essay my debt to them for this exchange, even when I respond to correct their misimpressions and to criticize their criticisms. I especially owe thanks to Brendan P. Minogue, Gabriel Palmer-Fernández, and James E. Reagan, for the conference out of which this volume developed, for this volume itself, for their friendship and collegiality, and for the great joy I have taken in exploring ideas with them over the years.[2]

Foundations, particularly the second edition, provides an assessment of secular morality that shows it to be so impoverished that many of the contributors appear unwilling to acknowledge the difficulties we face. *Foundations* explores the collapse of the modern moral philosophical project, the project of putting reason in the place of the Christian God. The modern moral philosophical project had been to secure by reason (1) the general substance of Christian morality as well as (2) a secular equivalent of a divine right of governance for the political realization of that morality without (3) having faith in Christ. The hope was to establish a very particular morality in very general terms. This appeal to reason presumes that within, from, or through reason we as humans can argue to a content-full, canonical moral vision, so that (1) all who disagree with that vision are irrational, (2) one has the authority of reason to impose that vision, and (3) all can in principle be disclosed as bound within one moral community defined by this rationally justifiable morality.

259

B. P. Minogue et al. (eds.), Reading Engelhardt, 259–285.

The claim was not necessarily that reason was the source of morality. Rather, reason provided its justification. The morality itself might draw its content from sentiments, dispositions, feelings, caring, and/or intuitions. As long as a rational account was available to show why the morality endorsed should be binding, it could claim generality. In this way, morality would advance more than *de facto* sentiments or the outcome of various reflective equilibria among various *de facto* sentiments. There would in principle be a rational morality to provide the *terminus ad quem* for the reasoned search for a common consensus regarding proper deportment and its enforcement.

The collapse of the Western Christian synthesis at the end of the Middle Ages made the modern philosophical project very attractive. Western Christianity had developed a faith not only in God, but in reason's ability to disclose the general lineaments of morality without an attempt to come into contact with Him.[3] Therefore, it seemed plausible that one could have a moral life without a proper religious life. Rather than regarding the study of natural law as situated within a dialogue with God through nature, secular human reason was regarded as able to discover deep moral structures in reality from a monologue with itself or from a dialogue with human intentions, sentiments, inclinations, moral senses, or the characteristics of human nature.[4] Morality was thought disclosable in general objective terms outside of either a proper relationship with God or a proper religious community. As a consequence, when the West fragmented in the bloody religious wars of the 16th and 17th centuries, reason seemed to offer a neutral ground for a common content-full morality and a universal community. Reason was to secure the general character of the morality which the fragmentation of Western Christianity imperiled. It would provide a general morality, even if one acted as if God were dead. For our contemporary reflections on bioethics, this meant that one should be able to (1) reach across the babble of diverse religious bioethics and (2) provide rationally authoritative guidance for secular health care policy.

The modern philosophical project was a response to moral estrangement: the encounter between moral communities that did not share sufficient moral premises, moral rules of evidence and inference, or moral authorities, so as to bring moral controversies to a closure. Of course, there had always been moral strangers in Western Europe. They had been marginalized, persecuted, suppressed, and ignored. The Reformation introduced moral strangeness as a central element of political, social, intellectual, and religious life. *Pace* Kevin Wildes, moral strangers need not be separated in world-views incommensurable in the sense of being beyond the mutual understanding of those engaged in a controversy. It is enough that they cannot in principle resolve their moral controversies by sound rational argument or by appeal to authority, as can the Franciscans and Dominicans, Kevin Wildes' remarks to the contrary notwithstanding.[5] On the other hand, the circumstance that there are some overlapping areas where similar words are used does not indicate concord. The Roman Catholics, the Orthodox, and the various Protestant religions, for example, can all speak of the Eucharist, but each means something quite different.[6] These differences are often difficult to perceive from within Roman Catholicism, given its robust commitment to reason and thus to construing itself and its rationality as the rationality.[7]

The development of a canonical secular philosophical moral vision has encountered significant difficulties. As long as God was recognized as the source of (1) being, (2) the good, (3) rationality, and (4) the right, morality was superbly integrated. Since all was grounded in God, Who created all and knew all, and in Whose justice and mercy no good deed would be forgotten, there was no ultimate tension between the right and the good, nor between the good of the individual and the good of all. Moreover, the genesis, justification, and motivation of morality were united in God. A secular morality grounded in reason could not do as well. Reason could not provide a standpoint with the ontological, epistemological, and moral power of the divine standpoint. Without such a unity of the genesis, justification, and motivation of morality, both morality and bioethics are at jeopardy, a point made in an exchange once between Alasdair MacIntyre and Paul Ramsey.[8] Once God is lost as the focal point of rationality, morality, and being, one also loses the coherence of the right, the long-term good of persons, the good of particular communities, and the good of particular moral agents. Not only can the right conflict with the good, but in many circumstances the best interests of individuals can conflict with the greatest good for the greatest number.

The modern philosophical project is not able to restore to morality the coherent rationale it possessed when philosophical morality acknowledged the centrality of God. Yet there is a hunger for such a divine point of universality and coherence. It is this perspective to which Rawls aspires at the end of *A Theory of Justice* when he advances a mundane view *sub specie aeternitatis*.[9] It is also the perspective to which some of the essayists in this volume aspire when they advance particular content-full accounts of justice, fairness, and equality as if they were generally canonical. The difficulties of securing a secular moral justification for this perspective are multiple, as indeed Rawls has recognized.[10]

The difficulties go deeper than Rawls, as indeed many of the essayists in this volume acknowledge, though the problems are well known. As Kant completed the First Critique, he recognized, following Leibniz, that he needed to achieve a connection between the kingdom of grace and the kingdom of nature. Kant appreciated a major challenge confronting secular morality: to have general rational plausibility, secular morality must establish a substantial accord between the good of the individual and the good of all, as well as between the right and the good. To achieve this, for the moral life to have a fully integrated rationality and to be in accord with rationality generally, the happiness of each individual must in the end be proportionate to the worthiness of being happy:[11]

> Since, therefore, the moral precept is at the same time my maxim (reason prescribing that it should be so), I inevitably believe in the existence of God and in a future life, and I am certain that nothing can shake this belief, since my moral principles would thereby be themselves overthrown, and I cannot disclaim them without becoming abhorrent in my own eyes.[12]

To avoid a deep tension in the moral life among diverse moral rationalities (e.g., the good and the right) and between the good of individuals and the good of all, one needed to assume a deep "...harmony of nature and freedom [that would] never fail."[13] This harmony could only be secured if one invoked the standpoint of the omnipotent being who guarantees the realization of this harmony, at least in a future life.

Therefore, Kant had to act as if God existed and as if we were immortal, even if Kant could not prove God's existence or our immortality. Morality required these commitments as integral to coherent moral praxis (i.e., so as not to be fractured by the various moral and prudential rationalities). At the threshold of the French Revolution, Kant confronted the incompleteness without God of a fully secular morality:

> [W]ithout a God and without a world invisible to us now but hoped for, the glorious ideas of morality are indeed objects of approval and admiration, but not springs of purpose and action. For they do not fulfil in its completeness that end which is natural to every rational being and which is determined a priori, and rendered necessary, by that same pure reason.[14]

The point is that the modern philosophical project of rationality, of discursively disclosing a canonical morality recognizable by all as binding all outside of a particular faith, culture, or history, could not unite the right, the general good, the good of communities, the good of the individual, the short-term good, and the long-range good, without presupposing an omnipotent point of coordination and unity: God. *Pace* Weiner and other essayists in this volume, the coincidence of motivation and justification they presuppose could not otherwise be secured.

"TELL ME IT ISN'T SO," OR "YOU DON'T JUSTIFY ALL THE MORAL CONTENT I WANT, SO YOU MUST BE WRONG"

The difficulty in providing reason with the unifying power possessed by the divine standpoint is acknowledged only briefly at the beginning of the second edition of *Foundations*.[15] It is a theme that deserved greater attention. It is joined with another element of the failure of the modern philosophical project: the failure to provide a canonical, content-full account of the moral life. The modern philosophical project failed not only because it could neither (1) fully integrate the genesis, justification, and motivation of morality, nor (2) guarantee a harmony between the good and the right, nor (3) secure a harmony among the good of the individual, particular communities, and the good of all (not to mention the short-term good of contemporary persons and the very, very long-term good of all persons, whatever that could unambiguously mean), but also because (4) content-full moral reason revealed itself as manifold. The modern philosophical project went aground on a polytheism of competing views of the good life, proper human nature, fairness, equality, justice, etc. It therefore begs the question. We are left with a range of content-full secular moral visions among which one cannot choose in a secularly canonical fashion.

Which guidance should one select? The question cannot be answered without an infinite regress or a *petitio principii*. If one invokes one set of prudential concerns in selecting a moral sense, those concerns in order to give value guidance must already implicitly incorporate a particular ranking or ordering of values. Again, in selecting such guidance, one must either beg the question or engage in an infinite regress. Nor will appeals to coherence models or reflective equilibria offer anything more in this regard than a much more complicated scheme for begging the question. Any such account must implicitly give differential weight to some intuitions, considerations, convictions, and/or judgments over others. If the weighting is without principle, it can be rejected with a contrary weighting. If it is by principle, the principle must be justified. Insofar as this requires endorsing one moral vision over another, one will have presupposed a background moral vision. Concrete choices require concrete guidance. The question is always: which or whose guidance?

One cannot break out of this impasse by an appeal to feelings, carings, or rhetoric. Faith Lagay, for example, appears to endorse the general exposition I provide of humanism, as well as my exploration of its ambiguities in secular humanism. But she objects to a philosophical exploration of the possibility of justifying humanism's claim on all, primarily because the exploration shows that such a justification cannot be secured. She objects because all cannot be secured that she would want to establish: "Too much is sacrificed when humanism is left behind."[16] She appears even to acknowledge that there is no general rational justification that can provide a philosophical justification for a humanist ethic. She therefore appeals to emotions and rhetoric to secure the humanism she wants. Yet, whose emotions and which rhetoric? In the presence of a transcendent God Who reveals Himself, style, rhetoric, and emotions can have an anchor in the unique source of being, purpose, motivation, and justification. Apart from that point of reference, all moral content dissolves into a diversity of perspectives, each with its own tradition of grace, style, rhetoric, and emotions. One may confess that "my sense is that such a bioethic will be in the rhetorical tradition, admitting of values and emotions and focusing on particulars."[17] Such a confession of content-full, secular faith is fated to yearn after a general justification it cannot secure. Or, it must settle for being one among many competing, secular, moral visions, none of which can ever claim canonicity outside of its particular embrace of emotion and rhetoric. If one has carings or feelings without reasons to know which carings or feelings should guide, one has in the absence of a principle available to all abandoned morality as intersubjectively disclosable. The same is the case, as just observed, with appeals to reflective moral equilibria. Yet if one appeals to reason, one receives no content-full guidance.

James Nelson appreciates the challenge we face in providing a non-arbitrary, immanent justification for a canonical secular morality.[18] Yet, he shies away from the consequences of our failure convincingly to justify such a morality. Moreover, he confuses the justification of a morality with the motivation to conform to it. So, too, does Rory Weiner in conflating acceptance and justification.[19] They conflate the categorical possibility of being able to think a moral structure with the motivation to conform to it. Once we find ourselves in a world without transcendent anchor, we can at best identify the grammar of a practice into which we can think ourselves (e.g., a content-less procedural secular morality or a content-less empirical scientific procedure). Such a moral practice can be categorically compelling under the circumstances of meeting as moral strangers, because this practice offers us a realm of intersubjectivity without requiring the adoption of any particular content-full moral vision. A content-less secular morality that draws its moral authority from permission discloses the only possibility for general secular moral inter-subjectivity. Such a practice cannot provide a canonical motivation for entering, though there are costs if one does not enter: one loses the possibility of intersubjective collaboration in the face of being moral strangers. But persons must tally those costs within the particular moral visions they bring to this practice. This point is a categorical and dialectical one.[20] One cannot require permission to carry with it any particular content or will to beneficence without undermining the project itself by begging the question.[21]

Like many of the authors in this volume, Nelson recoils from the implications of the modern philosophical project's failure: the failure of the project of discovering within or through our moral rationality, sentiments, intuitions, and/or experiences a basis for establishing a canonical morality without begging the question or engaging in an infinite regress. But, is it possible without begging the question to determine with any normative force who should count as "mainstream moral theorists"?[22] One must first know where the right mainstream is and then how to find its middle. Again, such determinations will always beg the question or invoke an infinite regress if they do not frankly acknowledge their particularity. In the end, Nelson cannot repair this failure save with a secularly pious promissory note that "the rest of us...may take some heart from a trenchant observation with which Derek Parfit concludes his *Reasons and Persons*: nonreligious moral philosophy is a very young study."[23] However unpleasant, we must recognize the depth of the problems we face.

Yet there are limited solutions. Comparisons with secular empirical science are helpful, *pace* Nelson.[24] In *Foundations* I compare the practice of empirical science that has as its foundations the agreement of those who fashion intersub-jective terms for gauging and comparing the character of their observations and the practice of a morality that has as its foundation the agreement of those who participate in achieving an intersubjective domain of moral collaboration through permission.[25] Without agreeing why there is anything or concurring regarding the deep roots of its *de facto* coherence, metaphysical strangers can agree that insofar as they are interested in establishing intersubjectively assessable claims regarding the character of the world, the principle of induction will function as a guide insofar as the world remains coherent (for whatever deep reasons about which these metaphysical strangers need share no agreement). Such an approach does not commit the participants in this practice to any particular observations. They need only agree, insofar as they wish to collaborate, regarding how they will make observations and how in particular they will come to agreements about them. They will need to stipulate common *ceteris paribus* conditions. They will also need to make agreements about how to characterize and apply the principle of induction. The authority of empirical science is derived from the intersubjective agreement of those who participate in making and assessing observations, all without presupposing any particular deep metaphysics.

Similarly, insofar as persons meet as moral strangers, not recognizing the common and deep roots of the genesis, justification, and motivation of the moral life, and insofar as these strangers for whatever reasons wish to enter into a practice of intersubjective morality without presupposing any particular content-full morality as canonical, secular morality can have general authority insofar as the participants draw this authority from their common agreement to enter into this practice. It is enough for the project of justification that the framework is itself a categorical possibility. Such a secular morality has a generality as close to the Enlightenment hope as is possible, given secular reason's inability to identify the canonical content-full ranking or account of goods, values, or right and wrong-making conditions. Like those who must enter the market drawn by their own motivations, so, too, participants in general secular morality must enter with their own motivations as content-full views of the moral and prudential significance of the market. None of these motivations or views will be secularly canonical. Each view will in its own terms motivate participation and provide interpretations of what is undertaken. The diversity of motivations and understandings will be united in a single categorical possibility of common moral authority. One will surely want more. But in principle there is no secular philosophical way to secure secular canonical moral content. Nor do the essayists in this volume show how secular moralists can pull a canonical, content-full, moral rabbit out of the immanent hat of secular philosophical reflection without rigging the trick by begging the question.

LIVING WITH POLYTHEISM

In reason's stead, *Foundations* offers a general secular moral authority drawn from an appeal to the permission of those who would resolve controversies intersubjectively in the absence of a common moral vision. The claim is not that those who are bound in content-full moral communities need regard themselves as resolving their controversies in this fashion. Given this account of permission, the claim is not that, *pace* Weiner,[26] all will see good grounds to participate in the moral practice of providing moral authority for the intersubjective resolution of controversies among moral strangers. Members of religious communities, who regard themselves as living in the clear presence of God and who in addition hold that they need not act peaceably with moral strangers, will not enter into this secular practice. Neither will members of philosophical communities directed by particular intuitions of justice, fairness, and equality, who also hold themselves authorized to use coercive force to impose their philosophical moral visions on unconsenting others. None of these will ask the question that leads to the possibility of an intersubjective morality binding moral strangers in the absence of a particular vision of values: can a morality be articulated that can bind all despite diverse moral visions in terms that do not depend on a particular content-full moral understanding? Those who do not invoke such an intersubjective morality and coercively impose their particular morality will use force and justify it in a way that cannot in principle bind moral strangers generally.

Nor can one disclose a content-full, canonical, hypothetical contracting position, as Robison endeavors, and even strives to attribute to me, so as then to criticize me for not coming to the conclusions that might then be obvious, were one to have conceded such a view regarding *prima facie* propriety.[27] He has confused hypothetical moral agents with actual moral agents. In general secular morality one is left with actual persons defined as those actual agents who can give actual permission, however I might join with Margaret Hogan in lamenting this circumstance. Since the solution to the problem of acquiring moral authority in the absence of a canonical moral vision depends on avoiding the importation of content and the consequent conversion of a general perspective into a particular moral perspective, one must maintain the focus on persons as sources of permission. They must be construed as sparsely as possible. Yet, they have full authority to withdraw their authority from any practices imposed on them–they cannot be crippled by accident, as Robison suggests.[28] As the second edition of *Foundations* acknowledges with deep regret, this offers us at best a shadow morality in which much we recognize as wrong and unfair cannot be so characterized in general secular moral terms.

Foundations is best understood as attempting to save something from the failure of the modern philosophical project. *Foundations* is to be regarded as indicating the enduring remnant of the Enlightenment hope to disclose across moral communities the possibility for authoritative collaboration. The authority at stake is not that of God, reason, or human nature, but the sparse authority of permission. For those religious and philosophical communities who would impose their visions with conviction on others without a justification which moral strangers can in principle accept, the project of *Foundations* will be of little or no interest. Since no source of secular, moral authority is available but sparse permission, there is no way to take account of the inequalities and differences in power and position characterizing the status of the various persons who will find themselves about to collaborate as moral strangers. Some of the essayists, Robison for one, wish nevertheless to import their own particular sentiments about what appears to them right and good in such circumstances of inequality. Robison asserts: "Manipulating others, even peaceably, *seems prima facie* at odds with the sort of respect for others that one might think would underpin any theory of morality which relies upon getting permissions of the parties involved for any joint project" [emphasis added].[29] By regarding inequalities within a particular content-full moral vision, one again at best begs.[30] One cannot bootstrap oneself up into a canonical content-full understanding of morality, justice, or fairness.

Foundations and *Secular Humanism* do not pretend to draw out all of the implications of the views I advance in these volumes for problems of personal identity, etc. Rather, the goal has been to show why the project of secular morality cannot succeed as it has been understood. The foundations of secular morality must be reconceived. A more modest account of secular morality can be disclosed, while still recognizing that much more work will need to be undertaken. One will have to address many moral philosophical problems anew from a new point of departure and follow matters as far as they go. When all is examined and assessed, some problems will always remain opaque to secular solutions. They will remain TEYKU.[31] It is for this reason that I clearly acknowledge that there remains a role for democratic decision-making in clarifying boundaries and property holdings.[32] In this case, what is important is the nature of the claim which is to be clarified, namely, property as having its source in the character of persons as the origin of secular moral authority. Concern with clarifying boundaries will be more acute with regard to real property rather than the talents, energies, and services with regard to the owner-ship people have of their own. In our contemporary world it is these that are ever the more important element of possession. Also, there will be no way to rectify harms to past persons who died without explicit heirs unless one embraces a racism that would require racial rectifications, etc., a position not allowed by *Foundations*.

What can I say of Richard Owsley's engaging account of *The Magic Mountain*?[33] It is intriguing, fruitful, yet when he makes the remark that my phenomenology of illness is grounded in an account of gonorrhea,[34] I can but point to the essay he cites, which not only ties that disease into the history of its clinical experience as recorded by Thomas Sydenham and William Cullen, but then moves to explore the experience of myocardial infarction and the placement of both acute and chronic diseases (e.g., hypertension and diabetes) within explanatory accounts.[35] I will not join the contest as to whether any disease can equal tuberculosis, nor do I understand gonorrhea as paradigmatic of the disease experience. Instead, I address the central challenge of under-standing how different, taken-for-granted meanings, explanations, and ex-planatory systems constitute for us different ways of experiencing illness and disease. Within different socio-cultural and scientific expectations, diseases will be constituted for us and experienced differently. The polytheism that besets morality expresses itself as well in the phenomenology of illness and disease. So also, with regard to feminism, there will be many feminisms. The space that Mary Ann Cutter recognizes that *Foundations* offers for feminism is so unavoidably expansive that there can never be only one. The feminisms will even include traditional Christian feminism, which recognizes the Theotokos as the true arch-feminist of all time. So, too, there will be innumer-able secular accounts of gender. Once a point of transcendent orientation is lost, there is no unambiguous account of sex, gender, child-rearing, marriage, human welfare, or health care policy.

A similar point can be made with regard to John Moskop's reflections on the status of young children. It is difficult outside of a particular intact moral community to understand why one should have children, how one should raise children, and what the purpose and moral standing of families are. Furthermore, it will not be possible to find the background consensus for which Moskop yearns and for which he thinks he discerns some grounding in John Rawls' recent reflections.[36] In *Political Liberalism*, Rawls is very careful to have just the right persons and groups with just the right "ideological, philosophical, or religious commitments." Rawls, for example, specifies that "Such a consensus consists of all the reasonable opposing religious, philosophical, and moral doctrines likely to persist over generations and to gain a sizable body of adherents in a more or less just constitutional regime, a regime in which the criterion of justice is that political conception itself."[37] For Rawls, a great deal is packed into what counts as "reasonable" and "just," as well as his guess regarding what doctrines will persist over time (not to mention what should count as a "constitutional regime"). Crucial questions are begged and borders drawn in order to create a manageable consensus. Finally, let me observe with regard to Moskop's very helpful paper that my first forays into writing regarding abortion were undertaken not to defend the morality of abortion, but quite the opposite. Unexpectedly and to my displeasure, I found that such a general secular argument could not be secured. In general secular morality, I discovered that one could not even provide a non-consequentialist argument against infanticide.[38]

The multiplicity of moral and value visions, which express themselves in a multiplicity of experiences of illness and constructions of feminism, will manifest itself as well in a multiplicity of understandings of proper health care. Brendan Minogue diagnoses what is a tension within most two-tier accounts of health care. He also correctly sees where even the second edition of *Foundations* could have been more forthright in underscoring the stark nature of secular morality and of that health care policy that could be justified in terms of that morality.[39] The point that I advanced in *Foundations* is that, if societies have justly acquired common resources (and societies, by the way, will face the same difficulty as individuals in justifying their ownership of property), they may according to their established rules and procedures create various welfare systems, including mechanisms for supporting a basic level of health care for all. However, large-scale, geographically located governments will never have the moral authority to impose any one particular form of access to health care on all. Particular groups or associations will always be able to offer rival approaches. This understanding is rooted in a fundamental insight to which Hegel's account of society and state points, but which Hegel himself does not acknowledge.

> The pluralism of moral narratives cannot be overcome in a higher level content-full moral narrative. It can only be overcome in a mode of social organization that does not require further moral content. Hegel's account of the political unity of a pluralistic society offers a categorical justification of a political unity in the face of moral diversity, rather than an attempt to justify yet another particular content-full moral vision.... Hegel accomplishes more than he realizes, but such is the cunning of reason.[40]

The dialectical tension that Brendan Minogue adroitly diagnoses is precisely that which must move us to the acceptance of the state as a limited democracy and no more. It is this categorical claim that is fundamental to the accounts given of the state and of health care policy in *Foundations*. It is also the account that Ruiping Fan recognizes as morally unavoidable in our contemporary world.[41] It is unavoidable in principle.

The dialectical difference between society and state, which constrains one to affirm a limited democracy, allows this Hegelian approach to avoid the problems that Hegel diagnosed in Kant's account of ethics. Moral reason does not have a canonical content so that one can discover how persons ought universally to choose for themselves and for others. *Pace* Cynthia Brincat, my criticism of Kant is therefore harsher and more fundamental than she acknowledges. Rather than being able to appeal to reason as the core of autonomy, as Kant does throughout his treatment of freedom and morality, there is only permission. If Kant could have squared the circle, if he could have found a moral reason without content that could still give moral guidance, he would not have begged the question as to which moral rationality should guide. In appealing to permission as actual permission, one is not constrained to choose among permissions. All are equal. Any permission, however sparse, is a source of authority. The question is not begged.

To have more, one must beg the question or encounter God's grace. I have much sympathy for the agony Margaret Hogan feels with respect to what little secular morality can offer for fetuses and infants.[42] She quite correctly knows that there should be more, though she is not able to show how secular morality can provide more. To have enough to lead to the conclusions that she wants, she would need to find a moral community within which there are not only real relationships to others, but the right relationships with others. It is for this reason that the second edition of *Foundations* underscores repeatedly the disappointment one should feel with that little that secular morality can justify as the bond that can compass moral strangers.

LET US NOT FORGET THIS CENTURY'S BITTER LESSONS

If secular ethics could deliver canonical moral content, how can one adequately explain this century's horrors? If secular rationality could discover how humans ought to act, how can one account for how these horrors were philosophically defended? Even more, how could one account for this century's history if secular rationality is able not only to discover what one ought to do, but also to show why one ought to do it, in the sense of disclosing a motivation for proper deportment? In this regard, the essay by Ruiping Fan provides an important judgment regarding misplaced and unjustified faith in collectivist accounts of justice.

There is, of course, real evil. There are truly evil choices, which are not just intellectual mistakes. There is obdurate hatred and pride. There are undertakings so wrong that they carry the satanic imprint. Anyone who reads Adolph Hitler's *Mein Kampf* encounters the arrogant, demonic hatred that fueled much of the evil wrought by the National Socialists. Just because one knows the good, *pace* Plato, it does not follow that one will pursue the good. One need not hold that Hitler neither knew nor was able to know how he ought to act in order to account for the evil choices he made. However, there are moral mistakes that have their roots in intellectual difficulties. Even if there is a way in principle for knowing what one ought to do, one may not know how to accomplish this knowing. As there have been sustained controversies in science, so, too, one might expect analogous controversies in moral theory and regarding the nature of morality and moral knowledge.

One can concede all of this regarding this century's evil as well as the misguided choices that have brought us much harm and still point to the failure of secular morality. There are not just real and substantial disagreements about the good moral life or about how one can identify its character and justify its substance. In principle, one cannot resolve those controversies without begging the question or engaging in an infinite regress. As *Foundations* argues, we are left without content-full canonical secular moral guidance in matters that matter most because such cannot be secured. Many of the essayists in the volume find this circumstance so shocking, nightmarish, and uncomfortable that they suggest we pretend we have a secular, canonical morality. They suggest that we make do with accepting and explicating the moral sentiments and views we share with our moral friends. Nelson offers as a criticism of *Foundations* that by facing the failure of the modern philosophical project it is "shockingly out of step." The history of this century indicates that much is to be gained from being out of step with those who would with force achieve fairness and equality. Human history in general, and the history of this century in particular, show that more is needed other than such pious secular faith. As Ruiping Fan notes, "The history of this century has witnessed how enthusiastically pursuing so-called collective interests at the price of individual liberty under a centrally-planned economic system has caused human disasters, one after another, in all Marxist-Socialist countries."[43]

The Foundations of Bioethics and *Bioethics and Secular Humanism: The Search for a Common Morality* were written against the background of the failure of the various secular chiliastic promises that had marked this century from a "War to End all Wars" to the revolution that was to secure a workers' utopia. The manuscripts took shape in a city destroyed through the evils of National Socialism. They took on their unity when Berlin was still divided by an international socialism which had in its own right killed tens of millions. Given the moral catastrophes of this century and the tens of millions slaughtered by both national and international socialism, it will not do simply to acquiesce in a contingency of sentiments with which we may agree, or in a *de facto* consensus that appears to be prevailing.[44] No account of moral philosophy or bioethics can be complete without taking cognizance of the service philosophy provided for these tyrannies,[45] or of the ways philosophy supported the proclamation of "truths" that were empirically false about matters of global significance.[46]

Some lament that if all we have as a generally justifiable secular morality is content-less, as *Foundations* argues, this will not allow one with secular moral authority to forbid consensual gladiatorial games, infanticide, or the sale of private health care insurance. But if such had been all that secular morality had tolerated in this century, we would have been much better off, according to the avowed moral sentiments of many if not all of the essayists in this volume. All of this is the case without mentioning the slaughter of millions of innocent unborn children, which slaughter traditional Christians will put on a par with the killing of infants. We must recognize the evils to which particular philosophical arguments led, as well as the evils undertaken by persons well educated in the humanist traditions of Europe. We must also acknowledge how radically in our very century human consciences and moral sentiments have differed. Our century does not reveal a clear moral consensus regarding the nature of the good life.[47] Nor does it disclose a consensus about how one might establish such a consensus. This century's history discloses how difficult it has been for secular thinkers in a principled fashion to identify whose "widely shared moral convictions"[48] should be normative. Moreover, any contingent particularity if forced upon all will have only become the source of a new aspirant myth for the twentieth if not for the twenty-first century, to recall the title of a volume of justly ill fame.[49]

One finds repeated in many of the essays an optimism that has been shown to be unwarranted, and that in principle is unjustified. This century opened with the promise of bringing the triumph of Enlightenment secularity to the whole world. The bonds of superstition were finally to be broken so that social justice could be realized. Freed of the expectation of a world to come, one would bring the expectations of heaven to earth. As Christians looked to the Second Coming, so now non-believers could look to an ever better world.

> The world is growing better. And in the Future–in the long, long ages to come–IT WILL BE REDEEMED! The same spirit of sympathy and fraternity that broke the black man's manacles and is today melting the white woman's chains will tomorrow emancipate the working man and the ox; and, as the ages bloom and the great wheels of the centuries grind on, the same spirit shall banish Selfishness from the earth, and convert the planet finally into one unbroken and unparalleled spectacle of PEACE, JUSTICE, and SOLIDARITY.[50]

This confidence in the future foundered on the battlefields of the First World War, it arose anew and with full vigor in the October Revolution. Secular philosophical rationality combined with twentieth century sciences and technologies was to transform the world, finally achieving justice and equality in concrete and immanent terms.[51]

To accomplish this transformation, one needed ice-cold virtues, including a kind of steely courage. Such chthonic courage was supported as a philosophical task through which the truly human was to be realized. Philosophers provided rationales for the bloody achievement of a new humanism, which was to transform the world, finally setting aside alienation, exploitation, and unjust inequalities. Because "everything includes itself in power," this humanism was with force to bring power to the powerless. In so doing, the meaning of humanism was recast.

> Marxism rejected the abstract supraclass approach to the problems of humanism and placed them instead on a realistic historical foundation, formulating a new conception of humanism, that of proletarian, or social, humanism, which included in itself all the best achievements of humanist thought of the past. Marx first showed the realistic way

toward realizing the ideals of humanism by linking it with the scientific theory of social development, with the revolutionary movement of the proletariat, and with the struggle for communism.[52]

Revolutionary terror was to accomplish the redeeming sacrifice, the transubstantiation of the world from its religious and exploitative past to the humanism of its secular future.

The bloody sacrifice of the innocent could be accepted, so the argument went, because terror was not pursued for its own sake. It was accepted because of the future it would secure.

> It is certain that neither Bukharin nor Trotsky nor Stalin regarded Terror as intrinsically valuable. Each one imagined he was using it to realize a genuinely human history which had not yet started but which provides the justification for revolutionary violence. In other words, as Marxists, all three confess that there is a meaning to such violence–that it is possible to understand it, to read into it a rational development and to draw from it a humane future.[53]

Such philosophical considerations on behalf of the achievement by force of a humane future have had as their conclusion the death of tens of millions in the high-minded pursuit of justice, fairness, and equality.

As Friedrich Hayek appreciated, drawing on the reflections of Andrei Sakharov, the Soviet Union provided the case example of a regime based on a well-developed canonical morality, where coercion was dressed in "the slogan of social justice."[54] It is not bad enough that secular rational argument led to such bloody and abhorrent conclusions. It was not just that politicians used philosophy for slogans: philosophers took the justification of such slogans seriously. In addition, secular reflection did not motivate to benignity but supported structures that gave us the horrors of the Holocaust and the killing fields of Pol Pot's Cambodia. As the last shows, we have not learned the lessons of this century regarding state authority and moral diversity. As the history of this century demonstrates, *pace* Cynthia Brincat, we have little ground to think that we have only the "violent fanatical fringe to fear...[while the] majority of us...engage in moral discourse[.]"[55] Destructive Marxist mobs have often not constituted the fanatical fringe but the dominant consensus of a society, as Ruiping Fan indicates.[56]

The history of this century shows that philosophical reflection does not necessarily conclude to the social democratic and liberal consensus which Rorty and Rawls in concert with Fukuyama would have us believe stands central to the moral sentiments of reasonable moderns.[57]   The canonical, secular, moral consensus appears illusive. But were it to arrive and be less than unanimous, what would have been established? On the one hand, there has been and remains deep disagreement about what matters most. On the other hand, firm convictions regarding the content-full character of justice and the rational authority coercively to achieve it have been singularly destructive, especially of minority moral visions. Any consideration of securing and imposing a content-full secular bioethics on the basis of either a taken-for-granted common morality or of a philosophically justifying argument must face the history of how dangerous such attempts have been. Yet, despite the bloody carnage of this century, the theoretical failures of the modern philosophical project, and the broken promises of utopia realized, there remains for many the hope of rationally discovering a canonical, content-full secular moral vision of fairness, justice, and proper deportment and then of imposing it coercively on all with the authority of reason.

CONTENT FROM A CONTENT-LESS VIEW

Beyond an appeal to the principle of permission, we have no way to discover which among the content-full views of fairness should translate unfortunate circumstances into unfair circumstances. The little that we do secure does not give the content that many want. In this regard, many of the contributors to this volume often fail fully to appreciate the radical character of *Foundations'* vision. Hauerwas, for example, does not attend to the essential distinction between a liberal and a limited democracy when he connects *Foundations* to the political structures of democracy. Liberal democracies impose on their citizens one among the many views of freedom. In contrast, a limited democracy is limited in its authority even to achieve a particular view of freedom. The freedom it achieves is by default. Though limited democracy is not justified in any particular ranking or ordering of goods or values, the grounding of moral authority in permission has content-full implications because of the limits it places on secular moral authority. The position is libertarian by default, not by design. The position is not committed to some good of freedom or to a libertarian moral sense, however thin. For those in this volume who yearn for examples of what such policy would be like in practice, *Foundations* can at best suggest societies that approached some of the characteristics of an ideal polity (e.g., Iceland and the Republic of Texas).[58] *Foundations* looks as much to the future as the past.

Foundations has radical implications. It provides the secular rationale for the passing of the nation-state. Though in most passages *Foundations* directs itself to a critique of health care policy as we find it, *Foundations* also indicates how things ought to be, were that realizable. Haavi Morreim is correct in characterizing my position as opposing legal and medical monopolies achieved by licensure.[59] And Robison is incorrect in suggesting that physicians are members of one moral community.[60] Ideally, welfare, including health welfare, would rarely, if ever, be provided by geographically located states, but rather through various non-geographically located communities. One might imagine an international Vaticare system providing social benefits for Roman Catholics from child care and welfare to retirement and health care. Aside from the Vatican City itself, there would be no polity where only Vaticare benefits would be provided. The same would be the case with regard to much of health care civil and criminal law. Much of civil and criminal law would be attached to particular communities. Such community law would be realized in the relationships among the members of a community. It would also be enforced on all of the various premises a community might own across the world. Thus, there would likely be severe criminal, not to mention civil, penalties for someone performing an abortion in a Roman Catholic health care facility. This ideal, however unrealizable, serves to indicate the boundaries of generally justifiable secular moral and political obligations.[61] It is an ideal for which Roman Catholics who have traditionally conflated society and community have little sympathy.

For those who judge that such a state of affairs would cause more harm than benefit, there is in principle no answer from the perspective of *Foundations*. The arguments in *Foundations* are not consequentialist. Yet, one can be brought to consider the arguments in *Foundations* by attending to the consequences of attempting to discover and impose a content-full secular moral vision. If one examines the bloody carnage born of excessive expectations engendered by the modern moral philosophical project, and if one has the values expressed in many of the essays in this volume, one may be disposed to acquiesce in the limits of secular morality.

CHRISTIANITY RECONSIDERED, OR, DID BLESSED AUGUSTINE OF HIPPO COMMIT THE INVOLUNTARY SIN OF BEING A PROTO-METHODIST?

All of Western Christianity's evils cannot possibly be traced to Blessed Augustine of Hippo, however plausible that might seem at first inspection.

After all, we have houses of worship dedicated to his intercession.[62] Still, some of what he said about predestination and original sin has reached out to torment the West ever since. Some of Augustine's misguiding influence may even lie behind Hauerwas's concern that my portrayal of becoming a Christian is far too voluntaristic. After all, Methodists at least in Wales were for a while termed Methodist-Calvinists. Therefore, I find Hauerwas' criticism on this point reassuring. I have enough sins without taking on my head the condemnations of the Holy Fathers who sat at the Synod of Jerusalem (A.D. 1672) and condemned such ilk.[63] The point is that one is not born a Texan by one's free choice. The accepting of the grace to be Christian is something one does not achieve by physical birth or by inheritance. It involves not just someone's free choice at baptism, but one's own continued choices to repent and reclaim God's grace despite the broken and sinful biography of our lives.

This is stressed in the ritual for baptism. For example, the priest asks the catechumen (or the sponsor of the infant), "Dost thou renounce Satan, and all his Angels, and all his works, and all his service, and all his pride?" The catechumen or the sponsor then replies, "I do." The catechumen is then asked, "Hast thou united thyself unto Christ?" and the catechumen answers, "I have." The last question is asked four different times.[64] Though God's grace is un-merited, one must still choose it. Moreover, one must continually choose God's grace and act with it. One must again and again allow God to make one a Christian despite all one's sins. One must do this all one's life long. St. Symeon the New Theologian (949-1022) stresses this point against the Proto-Methodists of his time.

> It is not God's foreknowledge of those who, by their free choice and zeal, will prevail which is the cause of their victory, just as, again, it is not His knowing beforehand who will fall and be vanquished which is responsible for their defeat. Instead, it is the zeal, deliberate choice, and courage of each of us which effects the victory. Our faithlessness and sloth, our irresolution and indolence, on the other hand, comprise our defeat and perdition.[65]

This is not to say that works save. But choice can damn and choice can allow salvation. True enough, we find ourselves part of a new people, a new race born out of the common womb of baptism and united to a grace and redemption undeserved. Yet our place in the Body of Christ must be constantly chosen in an endless striving to our death and beyond. Prayer earns no interest. Once saved, not always saved. The struggle, as St. Paul understood, is that of a lifetime.

Christians can quite properly accept Christianity being a private opinion from the perspective of the secular state, while knowing that true holiness will transform all. The secular privatization of Christianity in a limited democracy is not the threat Hauerwas envisages. After all, one should not think of Christians as useful for inculcating the habits that can sustain stable and peaceable states, a legitimate point that Hauerwas raises regarding the stability of liberal (albeit not libertarian) polities in a post-Christian world.[66] Christians are the alternative to the world. We are also a disappointment for the secular world. What makes the Church good is God, not its members. The Church is good for nothing but holiness.

The Church is good not because of the love, morality, or decent behavior of Christians, but because repentance leads to God, Who makes love holy, as the parable of the publican and the pharisee discloses (Luke 18:9-14). Surely, our repentance should transfigure our sins into a loving desire for God expressed in a selfless love for all. In all of this Christianity is out of step with secular concerns and needs. Christians and Christianity do not exist to make the world better, democracy possible, or liberal governments feasible. Christos Yannaras speaks directly to this serious error, with which Hauerwas flirts, however briefly.[67]

> A host of people today, perhaps the majority in western societies, evaluate the Church's work by the yardstick of its social usefulness as compared with the social work of education, penitentiary systems or even the police. The natural result is that the Church is preserved as an institution essential for morals and organized like a worldly establishment in an increasingly bureaucratic fashion.[68]

A society will have great secular strength if it is full of pharisees. It will be at some considerable risk if it is filled with Christian publicans and prostitutes struggling with their repentance. No wonder the pagan Romans were well disposed to put us to death.

This view of Christianity is not one congenial to those who would want to employ finite reason to connect moral norms with the infinite God. It undercuts the hope that one can fashion an account of natural law outside of a proper religious life and then tie that law together with one's acknowledgment of God. Here one finds the roots of Kevin Wildes' misunderstanding of Christianity, a misunderstanding that would construe theology as faith seeking understanding rather than as faith seeking holiness.[69] The choice is not, as he and many in the Western tradition have thought, between reason and fideism. The Christian *tertium quid* is the very energies of God Himself. Theology seeks union with God through experiencing Him, not through reasoning to Him or about Him. This is not to say reasoning is useless or bad, but rather that it is peripheral to holiness. If one applied the biblical marital metaphor of knowing to this point at issue, it is as if Western Christianity confused writing good marital sex manuals with having good marital sex. Western Christianity, especially Roman Catholicism, confuses writing manuals about how one might know God with theology's task of experiencing God.[70] For Roman Catholics it is as if one had decided that one's marital love was underdeveloped if one had not written a marriage manual.

THE FOUNDATIONS OF BIOETHICS: A MORALITY FOR MODEST MORALISTS AFTER A BLOODY CENTURY

When persons meet as moral strangers, they are not bound in an experience of God. Instead, they meet in a sparse morality, which insofar as it remains secular, can neither unite the genesis, motivation, and justification of morality, nor identify as canonical a content-full account of the good or the right. The failure of reason to substitute for God is not only the undoing of the aspiration for a content-full secular morality. It calls into question all theologies that have hoped by means of sound argument to avoid faith. The failure of the project of grounding a content-full morality in reason thus reaches beyond the bounds of secular philosophy and undermines Western Christianity's thousand-year-old faith in reason and the whole edifice built upon it. One finds post-modernity not only in secular morality, but in Roman Catholic moral theological discussions. Still, the collapse is not so complete as to despoil us of any remnant of a general secular morality. In this sense, *Foundations* is optimistic. It does not lead us to the conclusion that, if God is not recognized, all is allowed. There is still a sparse fabric that we can invoke when we meet in the midst of unbelief.

Most, if not all, of the contributors to this volume know that there is more. Most even attempt to secure more by finding a way around the failures of the rational philosophical project to ground a content-full, canonical moral vision. When in the second edition of *Foundations* I return to lay out more starkly and forcefully why this cannot be accomplished, the reader should not conclude that I do not recognize that morality is more than my arguments can sustain. Nor should the reader think that I hold that we should live without community as atomic individuals in the sparse relationships that bind moral strangers. However, when we meet as moral strangers, our authority over each other is as sparse and as limited as the procedural morality with which we are left. If one wants more and seeks it in the wrong places, one runs the risk of recapitulating the bloody history of this century. Here is a special virtue of the sparse vision offered by *Foundations*: it reminds us, if we are not to repeat this history, that we must learn to live within the modest bonds of the secular morality with which we are left.

NOTES

1. H. T. Engelhardt, Jr., *The Foundations of Bioethics*, 2nd ed. (New York: Oxford University Press, 1996), 1st ed. (New York: Oxford University Press, 1986), and *Bioethics and Secular Humanism: The Search for a Common Morality* (Philadelphia: Trinity Press International, 1991).

2. Mark Cherry provided very helpful suggestions regarding the ancestral version of this paper, not all of which I followed.

3. John S. Romanides, *Franks, Romans, Feudalism, and Doctrine* (Brookline, Mass.: Holy Cross Orthodox Press, 1981).

4. Dumitru Staniloae, *The Experience of God* (Brookline, Mass.: Holy Cross, 1994).

5. Kevin Wm. Wildes, S.J., "Engelhardt's Communitarian Ethics: The Hidden Assumptions," in *Reading Engelhardt*, 88. Wildes appears to take the view that any differences within a community separates the members as moral strangers. "Moral stranger" is properly used to indicate a moral distance unresolvable in principle. Yet, the Dominicans and Franciscans both hold that the Pope in Rome has the authority to resolve all controversies bearing on faith and morals. Therefore, they are one religious and moral community. The acknowledgment of the Pope of Rome's authority guaranteed the unity of that community and that they are not moral strangers, even if they are not affective friends.

6. Kevin Wildes' reflections regarding the different significance of terms like "autonomy" within different moral communities show one word can be used with different meanings. His general position on this matter would appear straightforwardly to undercut his misunderstanding of me on pages 87-89 of his essay. *Foundations* recognizes that individuals may belong to various moral communities and employ words in common, though the words may have different meanings for each community.

7. Engelhardt, "Christian Bioethics as Non-Ecumenical," *Christian Bioethics* 1 (September 1995): 182-199.

8. Alasdair MacIntyre, "Can Medicine Dispense with a Theological Perspective on Human Natures," 119-138, and Paul Ramsey, "Kant's Moral Theology or a Religious Ethic?" 139-170, and MacIntyre, "A Rejoinder to a Rejoinder," 171-174, in *The Roots of Ethics*, ed. Daniel Callahan (New York: Plenum Press, 1981).

9. Rawls, *A Theory of Justice* (Cambridge, Mass.: Harvard University Press, 1971), 587.

10. Rawls, *Political Liberalism* (New York: Columbia University Press, 1993).

11. Immanuel Kant, *Immanuel Kant's Critique of Pure Reason*, trans. Norman Kemp Smith, (London: Macmillan, 1964), A812=B840

12. *The Critique of Pure Reason*, A828=B856, 650.

13. *Critique of Pure Reason*, A815=B894, 642.

14. *Critique of Pure Reason*, A813=B841, 640.

15. Engelhardt, *Foundations*, 2nd ed., 4.

16. Faith L. Lagay, "Secular? Yes; Humanism? No," in *Reading Engelhardt*, 238.

17. Lagay, "Secular? Yes," 252.

18. James Lindemann Nelson, "Everything Includes Itself in Power," in *Reading Engelhardt*, 15-29.

19. Rory B. Weiner, "Beyond Forbearance as the Moral Foundation for a Health Care System," in *Reading Engelhardt*, 113-138.

20. H. T. Engelhardt, Jr., "*Sittlichkeit* and Post-Modernity: An Hegelian Reconstruction of the State," in *Hegel Reconsidered*, eds. H. T. Engelhardt, Jr., and Terry Pinkard (Dordrecht: Kluwer, 1994), 211-224. For my account of the dialectic, see *Mind-Body: A Categorial Relation* (The Hague: Martinus Nijhoff, 1973), 89-126.

21. Weiner, "Beyond Forbearance," 128-129.

22. Nelson, "Everything Includes Itself in Power," 18.

23. Nelson, "Everything Includes Itself in Power," 18, 28. Moreover, Parfit's claim seems suspect, since the ancient Graeco-Roman world compassed many non-religious moral theorists.

24. Nelson, "Everything Includes Itself in Power," 23.

25. Engelhardt, *Foundations*, 2nd ed., 104.

26. Weiner, "Beyond Forbearance," 113-138.

27. Wade L. Robison, "*Monopoly* with Sick Moral Strangers," in *Reading Engelhardt*, 107. Without a sufficient background argument, an assertion about what is *prima facie* right, wrong, or just is only a covert way of demanding that others agree. Robison also takes me to be defending a position that *Foundations* shows to be indefensible. "What may come to mind when we think of an instance of what Engelhardt considers the basis of morality are individuals, fully rational and fully informed, negotiating with each other, in respectful ways, to find some solution to a common problem." Robison, 100. The position of *Foundations* is thus recharacterized in quasi-hypothetical contractor terms so that it can be criticized for not coming to the conclusions that would follow from such a quasi-Rawlsian position, were it defensible

28. Robison, in developing an account of *Monopoly* as a heuristic for understanding social actions, would need to note that, like Rawls's arguments, *Monopoly* presupposes a background set of rules (i.e., the thin theory of game-playing that underlies *Monopoly*), which dictates how the players who enter must play. In real life, real persons are free to develop new ways of collaborating with others who join with them in fashioning their own "monopoly games." Which is to say, Robison does not note that there are multiple senses of society and community. Robison has in the background the rationalist assumption that society and moral community are univocal. Robison also fails to draw a distinction among tacit consent, implicit consent, and acquiescing in having a wrong done to one. If one acquiesces in a mugger taking one's assets, one does not by that acquiescence convey permission or authorize the transfer. It is for this reason that non-limited democracies do not have the secular moral authority they claim over their citizens, no matter how long they have been at the project of coercing the citizens within their

boundaries, but beyond the limits of secular moral authority. *Monopoly* imposes one canonical, content-full account of what it means to win. Such a canonical, content-full account is not available from general secular morality.

29. Robison, "*Monopoly*," 100. Robison also affirms claims concerning what *seems prima facie* fair to him in a crucial passage on page 107 of his essay. Unfortunately, when moral strangers meet, manipulation that is peaceable cannot be counted out as being improper. See *Foundations*, 2nd ed., 308-309.

30. Rory B. Weiner, "Beyond Forbearance," 116.

31. Engelhardt, *Foundations*, 2nd ed., 129-134.

32. Engelhardt, *Foundations*, 2nd ed., 179f.

33. Richard M. Owsley, "The Magic Mountain: A Prelude to Engelhardt's Phenomenology of Illness," in *Reading Engelhardt*, 149-161.

34. "The disease the accompanying experience of which Engelhardt utilizes for a phenomenology of illness is gonorrhea." Owsley, "The Magic Mountain," 160.

35. A phenomenology of disease would require a phenomenology of embodiment. I have elsewhere suggested the general lineaments of the phenomenology of embodiment. Engelhardt, *Mind-Body: A Categorial Relation.*

36. John C. Moskop, "Persons, Property or Both? Engelhardt on the Moral Status of Young Children," in *Reading Engelhardt*, 169.

37. John Rawls, *Political Liberalism*, 15.

38. Perhaps John Moskop misreads me if he takes the argument in *Foundations* as being sufficient to give a non-consequentialist argument against infanticide, rather than a non-consequentialist argument against harming but not killing infants in ways that will harm the persons whom they will be. Moskop, "Persons, Property or Both?" 166.

39. I speak forthrightly to these points in the passages about utopia. See *Foundations*, 2nd ed., 175-180, and 400-401.

40. Engelhardt, "Hegelian Reconsiderations of the State," in *Hegel Reconsidered*, 222.

41. Ruiping Fan, "The Unjustifiability of Substantive Liberalisms and the Inevitability of Engelhardtian Procedural Liberalism," in *Reading Engelhardt*, 221-233.

42. Margaret Monahan Hogan, "Tris Engelhardt and the Queen of Hearts: Sentence First, Verdict Afterwards," in *Reading Engelhardt*, 175-187.

43. Fan, "The Unjustifiability of Substantive Liberalisms," 221.

44. Richard Rorty, *Contingency, Irony, and Solidarity* (Cambridge: Cambridge University Press, 1989).

45. The communist tyrannies were philosophical. They were undertaken and maintained with reflective, philosophically buttressed, moral conviction. Though National Socialism produced philosophical reflections rarely seriously considered beyond German borders, Marxism-Leninism engendered a continued, worldwide philosophical interest and following. It likely secured the largest influence secular philosophy has ever enjoyed. It also justified terror on a scale never before realized. Consider the following statement concerning the philosophy's contribution to communist revolutions and therefore to the carnage they unleashed. "The victorious socialist revolutions performed in a number of countries, the construction of socialism and the building of a communist society have become realities due to the fact that this titanic effort on the part of the masses has for its theoretical foundation the philosophy of Marxism-Leninism, which is the

world outlook of the communist parties.... It was no accident that Marx, Engels and Lenin, who were great revolutionaries, politicians and economists and active members of the revolutionary movement, were also great philosophers who paid constant attention to the study and development of philosophy. That enabled them in times of social upheavals to find correct solutions and correctly determine the trend of social developments." B. M. Boguslavsky, V. A. Karpushin, A. I. Rakitov, V. Y. Chertikhim, and G. I. Ezrin, *ABC of Dialectical and Historical Materialism* (Moscow: Progress Publishers, 1978), 509-510.

46. The facts of the matter to the contrary notwithstanding, in his volume on Marxist-Leninist philosophy, distributed abroad during the 1970's and 80's, Sheptulin asserts that "The communist socio-economic system is marked by an unprecedentedly high level of development of the productive forces, capable of ensuring the production of the abundant material wealth required to meet all society's demands." A. P. Sheptulin, *Marxist-Leninist Philosophy* (Moscow: Progress Publishers, 1978), 488. Within a guiding moral and metaphysical framework, the facts had been recast. Consider the following quote from Leonid Brezhnev in a volume concerning material dialectics. "Whatever discipline the Soviet scientists work in, they are always characterized by a typical feature: their high communist consciousness and their Soviet patriotism. The Soviet scientist (if, certainly, it is a truly Soviet scientist) bases his whole scientific activity on the scientific ideology of Marxism-Leninism, is an active champion of communism, fights any reactionary and obscurantist forces. Our scientists subject all their practical activity to the task of realization of the noble communist ideals." L. I. Brezhnev, "Leninskim kursom" [Following Lenin's Course] (vol. 5, Politizdat, Moscow, 1976), 364, in M. E. Omelyanovsky, *Dialectics in Modern Physics* (Moscow: Progress Publishers, 1979), 383.

47. There remain diverse moral communities. There are dedicated communists, socialists, social democrats, Christian democrats, libertarians, and religious fundamentalists. They are separated by substantially different views of the good and the right, even if one excludes from consideration the separations among communities rooted in religious understandings which divide moralities through their differing understandings of the deep metaphysics of the world. Secular political debates recurrently disclose fundamental moral disagreements and real moral diversity.

48. Nelson, "Everything Includes Itself in Power," 18.

49. Alfred Rosenberg, *Der Mythus des 20. Jahrhunderts* (Munich: Hoheneichen Verlag, 1934).

50. Howard Moore, *The Universal Kinship* (London: George Bell, 1906), 328f.

51. The society created by the October Revolution was considered the preeminent realization of equality and justice despite the immense injustices it produced. Those who sought justice through its structures held that everything includes itself in power. They brought to history a content-full moral program for the empowerment of the disempowered. They sought by force to redress inequalities of circumstance. Barely a decade before the collapse of the Soviet Union, its leaders could proclaim "The establishment of the principles of social equality and justice is one of the greatest achievements of the October Revolution. We have every right to say that no other society in the world has done or could have done as much for the masses, for the working people, as has been done by socialism!" L. I. Brezhnev, "The Great October Revolution and Mankind's Progress," *New Times* 45 (November 1977), 6.

52. *Great Soviet Encyclopedia*, 3rd ed., vol. 7, 551.

53. Maurice Merleau-Ponty, *Humanism and Terror*, trans. John O'Neill (Boston: Beacon Press, 1969), 97.

54. Friedrich Hayek, *The Mirage of Social Justice* (Chicago: University of Chicago Press, 1976), 66.

55. Cynthia A. Brincat, "The Foundations of *The Foundations of Bioethics*: Engelhardt's Kantian Underpinnings," in *Reading Engelhardt*, 189.

56. Fan, "The Unjustifiability of Substantive Liberalisms," 221.

57. Rorty, *Contingency*; Rawls, *Political Liberalism*; Francis Fukuyama, *The End of History and the Last Man* (New York: Free Press, 1992).

58. *Foundations*, 2nd ed., 97-99, 175, 188.

59. Haavi Morreim, "Medicine's Monopoly: From Trust-Busting to Trust," in *Reading Engelhardt*, 45-75.

60. Robison, "*Monopoly*," 105.

61. For my sketch of "secular utopia," see *Foundations*, 2nd ed., 174-180. The issue of non-geographically based moral communities is addressed in passing in 357-358 and 400-401.

62. Seraphim Rose, *The Place of Blessed Augustine in the Orthodox Church* (Platina, Calif.: Saint Herman of Alaska Brotherhood, 1983).

63. *The Acts and Decrees of the Synod of Jerusalem Sometimes Called the Council of Bethlehem*, trans. J. N. W. B. Robertson (London: Thomas, 1899).

64. *Service Book of the Holy Orthodox-Catholic Apostolic Church*, trans. Isabel Florence Hapgood, 6th rev. ed. (Englewood. N.J.: Antiochian Orthodox Christian Archdiocese, 1983), 274f.

65. *St. Symeon the New Theologian, On the Mystical Life: The Ethical Discourses*, trans. Alexander Golitzin (Crestwood, N.Y.: St. Vladimir's Seminary Press, 1995), 87.

66. Stanley Hauerwas, "Not All Peace Is Peace: Why Christians Cannot Make Peace With Engelhardt's Peace," in *Reading Engelhardt*, 41.

67. Hauerwas suggests that liberal accounts of social cooperation presuppose continuing Christian habits and institutions for their material possibility. Hauerwas, "Not All Peace is Peace," 41. There are good grounds to think that he is wrong, given the case of liberal democracy in Japan. One might also consider the democratic institutions of ancient pagan Germanic Europe. But such issues are matters beyond the scope of this essay. It is enough to stress that Christianity should resist being understood in instrumental terms towards a better world.

68. Christos Yannaras, *The Freedom of Morality* (Crestwood, N.Y.: St. Vladimir's Seminary Press, 1984), 123.

69. Wildes," Engelhardt's Communitarian Ethics," 89.

70. Hierotheos Vlachos, *Orthodox Spirituality*, trans. Effie Mavromichali (Levadia, Greece: Birth of the Theotokos Monastery, 1994).

CYNTHIA A. BRINCAT is Co-Director of the Dr. James Dale Ethics Center and Assistant Professor in the Department of Philosophy and Religious Studies at Youngstown State University.

MARY ANN GARDELL CUTTER is Associate Professor of Philosophy at The University of Colorado at Colorado Springs. From 1980 to 1988 she worked with Professor Engelhardt. She publishes on topics in the philosophy of medicine, biomedical ethics, and applied ethics (when her three young children are preoccupied).

RUIPING FAN is currently a Ph.D. candidate in the Department of Philosophy at Rice University and Co-Managing Editor of the *Journal of Medicine and Philosophy*. He translated *The Foundations of Bioethics* by H. Tristram Engelhardt, Jr. into Chinese (Changsha, China: Hunan Science and Technology Press, 1996).

STANLEY HAUERWAS is Gilbert T. Rowe Professor of Theological Ethics at the Divinity School, Duke University. He is the author of numerous articles and books. Among his books are *Character and the Christian Life, A Community of Character, Against the Nations, The Peaceable Kingdom, After Christendom, Naming the Silences: God, Medicine, and the Problem of Suffering*, and *Dispatches from the Front: Theological Engagements with the Secular*. He is co-editor with Alasdair MacIntyre of the series *Revisions*, published by the University of Notre Dame Press and associate editor of the *Encyclopedia of Bioethics*.

MARGARET MONAHAN HOGAN is Director of the Center for Ethics and Public Life, and Assistant Professor in the Department of Philosophy, King's College. She is the author of *Finality and Marriage*.

FAITH L. LAGAY is a doctoral candidate at the Institute for the Medical Humanities at the University of Texas Medical Branch in Galveston. Her research interests lie in bringing the humanist tradition and specifically the medical humanities to bear on ethical questions arising from the Human Genome Project and the technological potential for genetic engineering. She is the author of "Deliberative Rhetoric and Public Discourse: The Human Gene Therapy Example," *Cambridge Quarterly of Healthcare Ethics*.

LAURENCE B. McCULLOUGH is Professor of Medicine, Community Medicine, and Medical Ethics, in the Center for Medical Ethics and Health Policy at the Baylor College of Medicine, in Houston, Texas. He is also Adjunct Professor of Ethics in Obstetrics and Gynecology at Cornell University Medical College in New York. He is co-author, with Frank A. Chervenak, M.D., of *Ethics in Obstetrics and Gynecology* (Oxford University Press, 1994) and co-editor with Nancy L. Wilson of *Long-Term Care Decisions: Ethical and Conceptual Dimensions* (Johns Hopkins University Press, 1995). His *John Gregory and the Invention of Professional Medical Ethics and the Profession of Medicine* will be published by Kluwer Academic Publishers in 1997. He served as Tris Engelhardt's research assistant at the Institute for the Medical Humanities at the University of Texas Medical Branch from 1974 to 1975.

E. HAAVI MOREEIM is Professor in the College of Medicine, University of Tennessee, in the Department of Human Values and Ethics. For twelve years there, and for the four previous years at the University of Virginia School of Medicine, she has done clinical teaching and consulting in medical ethics. Although her research spans a variety of topics, it particularly focuses on the ethical and legal implications of medicine's changing economics. She has over seventy publications in journals of law, medicine, and ethics, including the *Journal of the American Medical Association*, *Archives of Internal Medicine*, *California Law Review*, *Hastings Center Report*, and the *Wall Street Journal*. Her book, *Balancing Act: The New Medical Ethics of Medicine's New Economics*, first appeared in 1991 and has been republished in paperback by Georgetown University Press in 1995.

JOHN C. MOSKOP is Professor of Medical Humanities at the East Carolina University School of Medicine in Greenville, North Carolina, where he has taught since 1979, and Director of the Bioethics Center, University Medical Center of Eastern Carolina. He has been a visiting professor at the University of Calgary (1979), the University of Montana (1988), and the Medical College of Wisconsin (1994). He served as Chair of the Faculty at East Carolina University from 1991 to 1993. His publications include the co-edited volumes *Ethics and Mental Retardation*, *Ethics and Critical Care Medicine*, and *Children and Health Care: Moral and Social Issues*.

JAMES LINDEMANN NELSON is Professor of Philosophy at the University of Tennessee at Knoxville, a Fellow of the University's Center for Applied and Professional Ethics and Clinical Associate at the University of Tennessee Medical Center at Knoxville. He has also taught at Vassar, New York University, Michigan State University, and St. John's University, and from 1990-1995 was Associate for Ethical Studies at The Hastings Center. Co-author with Hilde Lindemann Nelson of *The Patient in the Family* (Routledge, 1995) and *Alzheimer's: Hard Questions for Families* (Doubleday, 1996), Nelson is also general co-editor of *Reflective Bioethics*, a new series of monographs forthcoming from Routledge.

RICHARD M. OWSLEY has taught philosophy for the last thirty years at the University of North Texas. Previous to this, he taught at Auburn University and Indiana University. His recent publications include papers on Karl Jaspers, Martin Heidegger, and William Whewell. Owsley just completed a term as President of the New Mexico/West Texas Philosophical Association, and is currently writing a book on the philosophy of Erwin W. Straus.

WADE L. ROBISON is the Ezra A. Hale Professor in Applied Ethics at Rochester Institute of Technology. He has co-edited two books in applied ethics, *Medical Responsibility* and *Profits and Professions*, and a book on David Hume. He has published numerous articles in the history of philosophy, on David Hume especially, in the philosophy of law, and in practical and professional ethics. His book on making moral and rational decisions about the environment, *Decisions in Doubt: The Environment and Public Policy*, won the Nelson A. Rockefeller Prize in Social Science and Public Policy.

RORY B. WEINER is Lecturer in Philosophy at Northeastern University and the University of Connecticut where he teaches courses in medical ethics and moral and political philosophy. He was a Visiting Assistant Professor at the University of Florida's Center for Studies in Criminology and Law where he taught philosophy of law, and a Teaching Fellow in courses on moral and political philosophy at Harvard University's Committee on the Core Program. He has published and presented papers on moral theory, health policy, health law, and professional ethics. He is currently completing a book tentatively titled *A Moral Foundation for the United State's Health Care System.*

KEVIN WM. WILDES, S.J, is Associate Director of the Kennedy Institute of Ethics and Assistant Professor in the Department of Philosophy, Georgetown University. He holds a secondary appointment as Assistant Professor in the Department of Medicine at the Georgetown University School of Medicine. He is also a Senior Scholar of the Kennedy Institute of Ethics and the Center for Clinical Bioethics at Georgetown. He serves as Associate Editor of *The Journal of Medicine and Philosophy* and of the book series, *The Philosophy of Medicine*, as well as Co-Editor of *The Journal of Christian Bioethics* and of the book series, *Clinical Medical Ethics* and *Philosophical Studies in Contemporary Culture*. Father Wildes is the editor of *Birth, Suffering and Death: Catholic Perspectives at the Edges of Life* and *Critical Choices and Critical Care: Catholic Perspectives on Allocating Resources in Intensive Care Medicine*. He is finishing his own book on methodology in secular bioethics.

BRENDAN P. MINOGUE is Professor in the Department of Philosophy and Religious Studies and former Director of the Dr. James Dale Ethics Center at Youngstown State University. He serves as clinical ethicist at Western Reserve Care System and is a founding member and past President of the Bioethics Network of Ohio. He is the author of various articles on the philosophy of science and medical ethics, and recently published *Bioethics: A Committee Approach.*

GABRIEL PALMER-FERNÁNDEZ is Co-Director of the Dr. James Dale Ethics Center, Director of the Peace and Conflict Studies Program, and Associate Professor in the Department of Philosophy and Religious Studies at Youngstown State University. Among his publications are journal articles on the history of modern Christian ethics, the moral doctrine of war and medical ethics, and two books, *Deterrence and the Crisis in Moral Theory* and *Moral Issues: Philosophical and Religious Perspectives.* He is also General Editor of the monograph series *Religion, Politics, and Public Life.*

JAMES E. REAGAN is medical ethicist at the National Center for Clinical Ethics of the Department of Veterans Affairs. He provides ethics consultation and educational program support to VA facilities nationwide. He has published and lectured on ethical issues regarding consent, confidentiality, care for the dying, advance directives, ethics committees and case consultation, health care reform and artificial human reproduction. He is a co-founder and past Executive Director of the Bioethics Network of Ohio, and from 1987-1995 was medical ethicist at St. Elizabeth Hospital Medical Center in Youngstown, OH.

PUBLICATIONS BY H. TRISTRAM ENGELHARDT, JR.

BOOKS

Mind-Body: A Categorial Relation (The Hague, Holland: Martinus Nijhoff, 1973).

The Foundations of Bioethics (New York: Oxford University Press, 1986).
This volume appeared in Japanese, translated by Hisatake Kato and Nobuyuki Iida (Tokyo: Asahi Publishers Inc., 1989). An Italian translation appeared as *Manuale di bioetica*, introduction by Umberto Veronesi, trans. Massimo Meroni (Milan: Il Saggiatore, 1991).

The Foundations of Bioethics, 2nd. ed. (New York: Oxford University Press, 1996).
A Spanish translation appeared as *Los fundamentos de la bioética* (Barcelona: Ediciones Paidos, 1995).

Bioethics: Readings and Cases, Baruch A. Brody and H. Tristram Engelhardt, Jr. (Englewood Cliffs, N.J.: Prentice-Hall, Inc., 1987).

Bioethics and Secular Humanism: The Search for a Common Morality (Philadelphia: Trinity Press International; London: SCM Press, 1991).

BOOK-LENGTH WORK

"Philosophy of Medicine," H. Tristram Engelhardt, Jr., with Edmund L. Erde, in *A Guide to the Culture of Science, Technology, and Medicine*, ed. Paul T. Durbin (New York: Macmillan Free Press, 1980), 364-461. Second edition with updating, 1984, 675-677.

BOOK TRANSLATED

The Structures of the Life-World, by Alfred Schutz and Thomas Luckmann, translated and introduced by Richard M. Zaner and H. Tristram Engelhardt, Jr. (Evanston: Northwestern University Press, 1973).

BOOKS IN PREPARATION

Diseases and Health: The Role of Values in Medical Explanations; in preparation.

VOLUMES EDITED

The Humanities and Medicine, edited and introduced by Chester R. Burns and H. Tristram Engelhardt, Jr., a special issue of *Texas Reports on Biology and Medicine*, Spring, 1974.

Evaluation and Explanation in the Biomedical Sciences, edited and introduced by H. Tristram Engelhardt, Jr. and Stuart F. Spicker (Dordrecht, Holland: D. Reidel Publishing Company, 1975).

Philosophical Dimensions of the Neuro-Medical Sciences, edited and introduced by Stuart F. Spicker and H. Tristram Engelhardt, Jr. (Dordrecht, Holland: D. Reidel Publishing Company, 1976).

Science, Ethics, and Medicine, edited by H. Tristram Engelhardt, Jr. and Daniel Callahan, with an introduction by H. Tristram Engelhardt, Jr. (Hastings-on-Hudson, New York: Hastings Center, 1976).

Philosophical Medical Ethics: Its Nature and Significance, edited and introduced by Stuart F. Spicker and H. Tristram Engelhardt, Jr. (Dordrecht, Holland: D. Reidel Publishing Company, 1977).

Knowledge, Value, and Belief, edited by H. Tristram Engelhardt, Jr., and Daniel Callahan, with an introduction by H. Tristram Engelhardt, Jr. (Hastings-on-Hudson, New York: Hastings Center, 1977).

Mental Health: Philosophical Perspectives, edited by H. Tristram Engelhardt, Jr., and Stuart F. Spicker, with an introduction by H. Tristram Engelhardt, Jr. (Dordrecht, Holland: D. Reidel Publishing Company, 1978).

Morals, Science, and Sociality, edited by H. Tristram Engelhardt, Jr. and Daniel Callahan, with an introduction by H. Tristram Engelhardt, Jr. (Hastings-on-Hudson, New York: Hastings Center, 1978).

Clinical Judgment, edited by H. Tristram Engelhardt, Jr., Stuart F.Spicker, and Bernard Towers, with an introduction by H. Tristram Engelhardt, Jr. (Dordrecht, Holland: D. Reidel Publishing Company, 1979.

Mental Illness: Law and Public Policy, edited by Baruch A. Brody and H. Tristram Engelhardt, Jr., with an introduction by H. Tristram Engelhardt, Jr. (Dordrecht, Holland D. Reidel Publishing Company, 1980).

Knowing and Valuing: The Search for Common Roots, edited by H. Tristram Engelhardt, Jr., and Daniel Callahan, with an introduction by H. Tristram Engelhardt, Jr. (Hastings-on-Hudson, New York: Hastings Center, 1980).

The Law-Medicine Relation: A Philosophical Exploration, edited and introduced by H. Tristram Engelhardt, Jr., Joseph M. Healey, and Stuart F. Spicker (Dordrecht, Holland: D. Reidel Publishing Company, 1981).

Concepts of Health and Disease, edited and introduced by Arthur Caplan, H. Tristram Engelhardt, Jr., and James McCartney (Massachusetts: Addison-Wesley Publishing Company, 1981).

The Roots of Ethics: Science, Religion, and Values, edited by Daniel Callahan and H. Tristram Engelhardt, Jr. (New York: Plenum Press, 1981). (A selection of essays from "Volumes Edited" 4, 6, 8 and 11)

New Knowledge in the Biomedical Sciences, edited by William B. Bondeson, H. Tristram Engelhardt, Jr., Stuart F. Spicker, and Joseph M. White, Jr., with an introduction by H. Tristram Engelhardt, Jr. (Dordrecht, Holland: D. Reidel Publishing Company, 1982).

Abortion and the Status of the Fetus, edited by William B. Bondeson, H. Tristram Engelhardt, Jr., Stuart F. Spicker, and Daniel Winship with an introduction by H. Tristram Engelhardt, Jr. (Dordrecht, Holland: D. Reidel Publishing Company, 1983). Second printing with updating, 1984.

Scientific Controversies: A Study in the Resolution and Closure of Disputes Concerning Science and Technology, edited and introduced by H. Tristram Engelhardt, Jr., and Arthur Caplan (New York: Cambridge University Press, 1987).

Euthanasia and the Newborn, edited by Richard C. McMillan, H. Tristram Engelhardt, Jr., and Stuart F. Spicker (Dordrecht, Holland: D. Reidel Publishing Company, 1987).

The Contraceptive Ethos, edited by Stuart F. Spicker, William B. Bondeson, and H. T. Engelhardt, Jr. (Dordrecht, Holland: D. Reidel, 1987).

The Use of Human Beings in Research, edited by Stuart Spicker, Ilai Alon, Andre de Vries, and H. Tristram Engelhardt, Jr. (Dordrecht: Kluwer, 1988).

Sicherheit und Freiheit: Zur Ethik des Wohlfahrtsstaates, eds. Christoph Sachße and H. Tristram Engelhardt Jr. (Frankfurt/M: Suhrkamp, 1990).

Theological Developments in Bioethics: 1988-1990, B. A. Brody, B. A. Lustig, H. T. Engelhardt, Jr., and L.B. McCullough (Dordrecht: Kluwer, 1991).

Philosophy and Medicine, eds. with a preface by S. F. Spicker and H. Tristram Engelhardt Jr. (Tokyo, Japan: Jiku, 1992); appeared in Japanese, ed. Ryūji Ishiwata.

Regional Developments in Bioethics: 1989-1991, eds. B. A. Brody, B. A. Lustig, H. T. Engelhardt, Jr. and L. B. McCullough (Dordrecht: Kluwer, 1992).

Theological Developments in Bioethics: 1990-1992, eds. B. A. Lustig, B. A. Brody, H. T. Engelhardt, Jr., and L. B. McCullough (Dordrecht: Kluwer, 1993).

Hegel Reconsidered: Beyond Metaphysics and the Authoritarian State, eds. H. T. Engelhardt, Jr. and Terry Pinkard, with an introduction by H. Tristram Engelhardt Jr., (Dordrecht: Kluwer, 1994).

ARTICLES AND CHAPTERS OF BOOKS

"Viability, Abortion, and the Difference Between a Fetus and an Infant," *American Journal of Obstetrics and Gynecology* 116 (June, 1973): 429-34.

"The Philosophy of Medicine: A New Endeavor," *Texas Reports on Biology and Medicine* 31 (Fall, 1973): 443-52.

"The Beginnings of Personhood: Philosophical Considerations," *Perkins Journal* 27 (Fall, 1973): 20-27.

"Psychotherapy as Meta-ethics," *Psychiatry* 36 (November, 1973): 440-45.

"Kantian Knowledge of Other Persons–An Exploration," *Akten des 4.Internationalen Kant-Kongresses* (Proceedings ofthe Fourth International Kant-Congress), ed. G. Funke and J. Kopper (Berlin: Walter DeGruyter, 1974), Vol.VII, 2, 576-81.

"The Ontology of Abortion," *Ethics* 84 (April, 1974): 217-34.

"Explanatory Models in Medicine: Facts, Theories, and Values," *Texas Reports on Biology and Medicine* 32 (Spring, 1974): 225-39.

"Solitude and Sociality," *Humanities* 10 (November, 1974): 227-87.

"The Disease of Masturbation: Values and the Concept of Disease," *Bulletin of the History of Medicine* 48 (Summer, 1974): 234-48.

"The Concept of Bereavement," *Death and Ministry*, ed. J. D. Bane, A. H. Kutscher, *et al.* (New York: Seabury Press, 1974), 217-220.

"Elective Abortion: Issues in a Moral Dilemma," H. Tristram Engelhardt, Jr., *et al.*, in *Continuing Education* 3 (March, 1975): 20-25.

"The Counsels of Finitude," *The Hastings Center Report* 5 (April, 1975): 29-36.

"The Concepts of Health and Disease," in *Evaluation and Explanation in the Biomedical Sciences*, ed. H. Tristram Engelhardt, Jr. and Stuart F. Spicker (Dordrecht, Holland: D. Reidel Publishing Company, 1975), 125-41.

"A Demand to Die" (a commentary on a case history), *The Hastings Center Report* 5 (June, 1975): 10, 47.

"Ethical Issues in Aiding the Death of Small Children," in *Beneficent Euthanasia*, ed. Marvin Kohl (Buffalo: Prometheus Books, 1975), 180-192.

"John Hughlings Jackson and the Mind-Body Relation," *Bulletin of the History of Medicine* 49 (Summer, 1975): 137-51.

"Bioethics and the Process of Embodiment," *Perspectives in Biology and Medicine* 18 (Summer, 1975): 486-500.

"The History and Philosophy of Medicine: A Report on a Postgraduate Seminar on the Humanities in Medicine," *Clio Medica* 19 (September, 1975): 57-63.

"The Patient as Person–An Empty Phrase?" *Texas Medicine* 71 (September, 1975): 57-63.

"Defining Death: A Philosophical Problem for Medicine and Law," *American Review of Respiratory Disease* 112 (November, 1975): 587-590.

"On the Bounds of Freedom: From the Treatment of Fetuses to Euthanasia," *Connecticut Medicine* 40 (January, 1976): 51-54, 57.

"Individuals and Communities, Present and Future: Towards a Morality in a Time of Famine," *Soundings* 59 (Spring, 1976): 70-83.

"Fear of Flying," (a commentary on a case history) *Hastings Center Report* 6 (February, 1976): 20.

"Philosophy and Medicine," *Journal of Medicine and Philosophy* 1 (March, 1976): 93-100.

"Reflections on our Condition: The Geography of Embodiment," in *Philosophical Dimensions of the Neuro-Medical Sciences*, eds. Stuart F. Spicker and H. Tristram Engelhardt, Jr. (Dordrecht, Holland: D. Reidel Publishing Company, 1976), 59-68.

"Human Well-Being and Medicine: Some Basic Value-Judgments in the Biomedical Sciences," in *Science, Ethics, and Medicine*, eds. H. Tristram Engelhardt, Jr. and Daniel Callahan (Hastings-on-Hudson, New York: Hastings Center, 1976), 120-139.

"The Roots of Science and Ethics," *Hastings Center Report* 6 (June, 1976): 35-38.

"The Meaning of Extraordinary in Extraordinary Care," in *Proceedings Conference on Emerging Medical, Moral, and Legal Concerns*, eds. A. W. Seimsen and Ira Greifer (Honolulu, Hawaii: Institute of Renal Disease, 1976), 47-62.

"Ideology and Etiology," *Journal of Medicine and Philosophy* 1 (September, 1976): 256-68.

"Concept of Health," *Encyclopedia Britannica*; 1977 *Medical and Health Annual* (Chicago: Encyclopedia Britannica), 1976, 100-08.

"The Dialectic as a Meta-Ontological Method," *Hegel-Jahrbuch*, 1975 (Koln: Pahl-Rugenstein Verlag, 1976), 424-29.

"Husserl and the Mind-Brain Relation," in *Selected Studies in Phenomenology and Existential Philosophy* 6 Phenomenology and the Sciences, eds. D. Ihde and R. Zaner (The Hague: Martinus Nijhoff, 1977), 51-70.

"Some Persons are Humans, Some Humans are Persons, and the World Is What We Humans Make of It," in *Philosophical Medical Ethics: Its Nature and Significance*, eds. Stuart F. Spicker and H. Tristram Engelhardt, Jr. (Dordrecht, Holland: D. Reidel Publishing Company, 1977), 183-94.

"Ontology and Ontogeny," *The Monist* 60 (January, 1977): 16-28.

"Is There a Philosophy of Medicine?" *Proceedings of the Philosophy of Science Association 1976*, Vol. 2, eds. Frederick Suppe and Peter D. Asquith (Ann Arbor, Michigan: Edwards Brothers, 1977), 94-108.

"Splitting the Brain, Dividing the Soul: Being of Two Minds," *Journal of Medicine and Philosophy* 2 (June, 1977): 89-100.

"Issues and Attitudes in Research and Treatment of Variant Forms of Human Sexual Behavior," in *Ethical Issues in Sex Therapy and Research*, eds. William H. Masters, Virginia E. Johnson, and Robert C. Kolodny (Boston: Little, Brown, 1977), 132-137.

"Errors in Medicine: Let Me Count the Ways," in *Knowledge, Value and Belief*, eds. H. Tristram Engelhardt, Jr., and Daniel Callahan (Hastings-on-Hudson, New York: Hastings Center, 1977), 310-320.

"Suicide," Karen Lebacqz and H. Tristram Engelhardt, Jr., in *Death, Dying, and Euthanasia*, eds. Dennis J. Horan and David Mall (Washington, D.C.: University Publications of America, 1977), 669-705.

"A Study of the Federal Government's Ethical Obligations to Provide Compensation for Persons Injured in the Course of their Participation in Research Supported by Funds Administered by the Secretary of Health, Education, and Welfare," *HEW Secretary's Task Force on the Compensation of Injured Research Subjects*, Appendix A (Bethesda, Maryland: National Institutes of Health, 1977), 666-672.

"Observations of a Physician-Patient," Michael Berger and H. Tristram Engelhardt, Jr., *Southern Medical Journal* 70 (August, 1977): 98.

"Defining Occupational Therapy: The Meaning of Therapy and the Virtues of Occupation," *The American Journal of Occupational Therapy* (November/December, 1977): 122-125.

"Medicine and the Concept of Person," in *Ethical Issues in Death and Dying*, eds. Tom L. Beauchamp and Seymour Perlin (Englewood Cliffs, New Jersey: Prentice Hall, Inc., 1978), 271-284.

"Rights and Responsibilities of Patients and Physicians," in *Medical Treatment of the Dying: Moral Issues*, eds. Michael D. Bayles and M. H. Dallas (Cambridge, Massachusetts: Schenkman Publishing Company, 1978), 9-28.

"The Doctor's Role in the Evolution of Human Society," in *Limits of Medicine*, eds. Stewart G. Wolf and Beatrice Bishop Berle (New York: Plenum Press, 1978), 1-10, 17-21.

"Definitions of Death: Where to Draw the Line and Why," in *Death and Decision*, ed. Ernan McMullin (Boulder, Colorado: Westview Press for the American Association for the Advancement of Science, Selected Symposia Series, No. 18, 1978), 15-34.

"To Treat or Not to Treat–The Dilemma," H. Tristram Engelhardt, Jr., *et al.*, *Heart and Lung* 7 (May/June, 1978): 499-504.

"La Experiencia de la Enfermedad y el Problema del Cuerpo," *Quiron* 9 (Marzo/Junio, 1978): 57-66.

"Health and Disease: Philosophical Perspectives," in *Encyclopedia of Bioethics*, ed. Warren Reich (New York: Macmillan Free Press, 1978), 599-606.

"Philosophy of Medicine," H. Tristram Engelhardt, Jr. and Edmund L. Erde in *Encyclopedia of Bioethics*, ed. Warren Reich (New York: Macmillan Free Press, 1978), 1049-1054.

"Moral Autonomy and the Polis: Response to Gerald Dworkin and Gregory Vlastos," in *Morals, Science, and Sociality*, eds. H. Tristram Engelhardt, Jr. and Daniel Callahan (Hastings-on-Hudson, New York: Hastings Center, 1978), 202-214.

"Taking Risks: Some Background Issues in the Debate Concerning Recombinant DNA Research," *Southern California Law Review* 51 (September, 1978): 1141-1151.

"Basic Ethical Principles in the Conduct of Biomedical and Behavioral Research Involving Human Subjects," *The Belmont Report*, Appendix Vol. l, Department of Health, Education, and Welfare, Publication Number (12) 78-0013, section 8, 1-45.

"Bioethics," *Colliers Encyclopedia*, Vol. 4 (New York: Macmillan Educational Corporation, 1979), 163-164.

"The Ethics of Suicide: A Secular View," John C. Moskop and H. Tristram Engelhardt, Jr., in *Suicide: Theory and Clinical Aspects*, ed. L. D. Hancoff (Littleton, Massachusetts: Publishing Sciences Group, 1979), 49-57.

"Is Aging a Disease?" in *Life Span: Values and Life-Expanding Technologies*, ed. Robert M. Veatch (San Francisco: Harper and Row, 1979), 184-194.

"Confidentiality in the Consultation-Liaison Process: Ethical Dimensions and Conflicts," H. Tristram Engelhardt, Jr. and Laurence B. McCullough, *Psychiatric Clinics of North America* 2 (August, 1979): 403-413.

"Rights to Health Care: A Critical Appraisal," *The Journal of Medicine and Philosophy* 4 (June, 1979): 113-117.

"Mentally Retarded Hepatitis B Carriers in Public Schools," *Hastings Center Report* 9 (December, 1979): 16-17.

"Philosophical Problems in Biomedicine: Towards a Philosophy of Medicine," *Current Research in Philosophy of Science*, eds. P.D. Asquith and H. E. Kyburg, Jr. (East Lansing: Philosophy of Science Association, 1979), 436-449.

"Causal Accounts in Medicine: A Commentary on Stephen Toulmin," reprinted in *Changing Values in Medicine*, eds. Mark Siegler and Eric Cassell (Frederick, Maryland: University Publications of America, Inc., 1979), 73-81.

"Ethical Issues in Diagnosis," *Metamedicine* 1 (February, 1980): 39-50.

"Doctoring the Disease, Treating the Complaint, Helping the Patient: Some of the Works of Hygeia and Panacea," *Knowing and Valuing*, eds. H. Tristram Engelhardt, Jr. and Daniel Callahan (Hastings-on-Hudson: Hastings Center, 1980), 225-249.

"Tractatus Artis Bene Moriendi Vivendique: Choosing Styles of Dying and Living," in *Frontiers in Medical Ethics: Applications in a Medical Setting*, ed. Virginia Abernethy (Cambridge, Massachusetts: Ballinger Publishing Company, 1980), 9-26.

"Bioethics in the People's Republic of China," *Hastings Center Report* 10 (April, 1980): 7-10.

"Ethical Issues in Pain Management," in *Pain and Society*, eds. H. W. Kosterlitz and L. Y. Terenius (Weinheim, West Germany: Chemie, 1980), 483-500.

"The Principles of Pain Management Group Report," H. Mersky and H. Tristram Engelhardt, Jr., *et al.*, in *Pain and Society*, eds. H. W. Kosterlitz and L. Y. Terenius (Weinheim, West Germany: Chemie, 1980), 483-500.

"Value Imperialism and Exploitation in Sex Therapy," in *Ethical Issues in Sex Therapy and Research*, Vol. II, eds. William H. Masters, Virginia E. Johnson, and Robert C. Kolodny (Boston: Little, Brown, and Company, 1980), 109-137.

"Personal Health Care or Preventive Care: Distributing Scarce Medical Resources," *Soundings* 63, 3 (Fall, 1980): 234-256.

"Philosophy and Medicine: Some Reflections on a Critical Assessment by Caroline Whitbeck," in *Research in Philosophy and Technology*, ed. P. Durbin (Greenwich, Connecticut: JAI Press, Inc., 1980), 127-130.

"Health Care Allocations: Responses to the Unjust, the Unfortunate, and the Undesirable," in *Justice and Health Care*, ed. Earl Shelp (Dordrecht, Holland: D F. Reidel Publishing Company, 1981), 121-137.

"Ethics in Psychiatry," H. Tristram Engelhardt, Jr. and Laurence B. McCullough, in *American Handbook of Psychiatry* (Second Edition, Vol. 7), Editor in Chief - Silvan Arieti, with H. Keith and H. Brodie (New York: Basic Books, Inc., 1981), 795-818.

"Relevant Causes: Their Designation in Medicine and Law," in *The Law-Medicine Relation: A Philosophical Exploration* (Vol. 9, *Philosophy and Medicine Series*), eds. Stuart F.Spicker, Joseph M. Healy, Jr., and H. Tristram Engelhardt, Jr. (Dordrecht, Holland: D. Reidel Publishing Company, 1981), 123-127.

"Physicians and the Community of Physicians: An Account of Collective Responsibilities," *The University of Dayton Review* 15 (Winter, 1981-1982): 41-52.

"Clinical Judgment," *Metamedicine* 2 (October, 1981): 301-317.

"Why New Technology is More Problematic Than Old Technology" in *New Knowledge in the Biomedical Sciences*, eds. William B. Bondeson, H. Tristram Engelhardt, Jr., Stuart F. Spicker, and Joseph M. White, Jr. (Dordrecht, Holland: D. Reidel Publishing Company, 1982), 179-183.

"The Role of Values in the Discovery of Illness," in *Contemporary Issues in Bioethics*, 2nd edition, eds. Tom Beauchamp and LeRoy Walters (Belmont, California: Wadsworth, 1982), 73-75.

"Bioethics," in *Health and Medical Horizons*, 1982, eds. D. F. Klein, *et. al.* (NewYork: Macmillan Educational Company, 1982), 186-188.

"Philosophy, Health Care, and Public Policy," *Mobius* 2 (July, 1982): 17-22.

"Suicide and Assisting Suicide: A Critique of Legal Sanctions" H. Tristram Engelhardt, Jr. and Michele Malloy, *Southwestern Law Review* 36 (November, 1982): 1003-1037.

"Goals of Medical Care, A Reappraisal," in *Who Decides: Conflicts of Rights in Health Care*, ed. Nora K. Bell (Clifton, NJ: Humana Press, 1982), 49-66.

"Understanding Faith Traditions in the Context of Health Care: Philosophy as a Guide for the Perplexed," in *Health/Medicine and the Faith Traditions*, eds. Martin E. Marty and Kenneth L. Vaux (Philadelphia: Fortress Press, 1982), 163-184.

"Old Problems, New Technologies, and the Changing Values: The Challenge of Biomedicine," in *The Philosophical Society of Texas Proceedings*, ed. D. H. Winfrey (Austin, Texas: The Philosophical Society of Texas, 1982), 9-18

"Ethical Issues and Genetic Renal Disease," in *Controversies in Nephrology*, eds. George E. Schreiner, James F. Winchester, and Betty F. Mendelson (Washington, D.C.: Georgetown University Press, 1982), 185-200.

"Bioethics in Pluralist Societies," *Perspectives in Biology and Medicine* 26 (Autumn, 1982): 64-78.

"Illnesses, Diseases, and Sicknesses," in *The Humanity of the Ill*, ed. Victor Kestenbaum, (Knoxville, Tenn: The University of Tennessee Press, 1982), 142-156.

"The Subordination of the Clinic," *Value Conflicts in Health Care Delivery*, eds. Bart Gruzalski and Carl Nelson (Cambridge, Mass: Ballinger Publishing Company, 1982), 41-57.

"Occupational Therapists As Technologists and Custodians of Meaning," in *Health Through Occupation: Theory and Practice in Occupational Therapy*, ed. Gary Keilhofner (Philadelphia: F. A. Davis Co., 1983), 139-145.

"Viability and the Use of the Fetus," in *Abortion and the Status of the Fetus*, eds. William B. Bondeson, H. Tristram Engelhardt, Jr., Stuart F. Spicker, and Daniel Winship (Dordrecht, Holland: D. Reidel Publishing Company, 1983), 183-208.

"The Physician-Patient Relationship in a Secular, Pluralist Society," in *The Clinical Encounter*, ed. Earl Shelp (Dordrecht, Holland: D. Reidel Publishing Company, 1983), 253-266.

"Joseph Margolis, John Rawls, and the Mentally Retarded," in *Ethics and Mental Retardation*, eds. Loretta Kopelman and John C. Moskop (Dordrecht, Holland: D. Reidel Publishing Company, 1984), 37-42.

"Medizinische Technik und ethische Probleme," in *Wandlung von Verantwortungen und Werten in unserer Zeit* (Bonn: Deutsche UNESCO Kommission, 1983), 93-105.

"Clinical Problems and the Concept of Disease," in *Health, Disease, and Causal Explanations in Medicine*, eds. Lennart Nordenfelt and B. Ingemar Lindahl (Dordrecht: D. Reidel Publishing Company, 1984), 27-41.

"Comments on Wulff's 'The Causal Basis of the Current Disease Classification'," in *Health, Disease, and Causal Explanations in Medicine*, eds. Lennart Nordenfelt and B. Ingemar Lindahl (Dordrecht: D. Reidel Publishing Company, 1984), 179-182.

"Causes, Effects, and Side Effects: Choosing Between the Better and the Best," H. Tristram Engelhardt, Jr. and Stuart F. Spicker, in *Health, Disease, and Causal Explanations in Medicine*, eds. Lennart Nordenfelt and B. Ingemar Lindahl (Dordrecht, Holland: D. Reidel Publishing Company, 1984), 225-233.

"Allocating Scarce Medical Resources," *New England Journal of Medicine* 311 (July 5, 1984): 66-71.

"Genetic Engineering: Prospects and Recommendations," Bernard Davis and H. Tristram Engelhardt, Jr., *Zygon: Journal of Religion and Science*, (September, 1984): 277-280.

"Persons and Humans: Refashioning Ourselves in a Better Image and Likeness," *Zygon: Journal of Religion and Science* 19 (September, 1984): 281-295.

"Current Controversies in Obstetrics: Wrongful Life and Forced Fetal Surgical Procedures," *American Journal of Obstetrics and Gynecology* 151 (February 1, 1985): 313-318.

"Humanism and the Profession(al)," *Journal of Dental Education* 49 (April 1985): 202-206.

"Physicians, Patients, Health Care Institutions–and the People in Between: Nurses," in *Caring, Curing, Coping*, eds. Anne H. Bishop and John R. Scudder, Jr. (Tuscaloosa, Alabama: The University of Alabama Press, 1985), 62-79.

"Medical Decisions in a Context of Conflicts," *Chest* 88 (September, 1985, Supplement): 172S-174S.

"Moral Tensions in Critical Care Medicine: Absurdities as Indications of Finitude," in *Ethics and Critical Care Medicine*, eds. John C. Moskop and Loretta Kopelman (Dordrecht, Holland: D. Reidel Publishing Company, 1985), 23-33.

"Hartshorne, Theology, and the Nameless God," in *Theology and Bioethics*, ed. Earl E. Shelp (Dordrecht, Holland: D. Reidel Publishing Company, 1985), 45-48.

"Looking for God and Finding the Abyss: Bioethics and Natural Theology," in *Theology and Bioethics*, ed. Earl E. Shelp (Dordrecht, Holland: D. Reidel Publishing Company, 1985), 79-91.

"Typologies of Disease: Nosologies Revisited," in *Logic of Discovery and Diagnosis in Medicine*, ed. Kenneth F. Schaffner (Berkeley, California: University of California Press, 1985), 56-71.

"Etica Biomedia: Viejo y Nuevo Panorama," in *Retardo Mental* (Caracas: AVEPANE, 1985), 399-405.

"Reason," in *Powers That Make Us Human*, ed. Kenneth Vaux (Chicago, Illinois: University of Illinois Press, 1985), 75-91.

"From Philosophy and Medicine to Philosophy of Medicine," *The Journal of Medicine and Philosophy* 11 (February, 1986): 3-8.

"Suicide and the Cancer Patient," in *Ca-A Cancer Journal for Clinicians* 36 (March/April, 1986): 105-109.

"Intensive Care Units, Scarce Resources, and Conflicting Principles of Justice," H. Tristram Engelhardt, Jr. and Michael A. Rie, *Journal of the American Medical Association* 255 (March 1986): 1159-1164.

"Ensuring Against Tragedy: The Decision to Treat the Severely Head Injured," in *Neurotrauma Treatment, Rehabilitation and Related Issues*, eds. Michael E. Miner and Karen A. Wagner (Boston: Butterworths, 1986), 19-26.

"The Social Meanings of Illness," *Second Opinion* 1 (July, 1986): 27-39.

"The Lessons of Finitude," The *Western Journal of Medicine* 145 (August, 1986): 187-188.

"Clinical Complaints and the Ens Morbi," *The Journal of Medicine and Philosophy* 11 (August, 1986): 207-214.

"Humanidades en la Educacion Medica Americana," *JANO: Medicina Y Humanidades* 31 (5-10 November, 1986): 49-50, 53-54, 57-58, 61.

"Editorial Comment," *Obstetrics and Gynecology* 68 (November, 1986): 724-725.

"Bioethik in der pluralistischen Gesellschaft," *Medizin Mensch Gesellschaft* 11 (December, 1986): 236-241.

"Problems in the Availability of Health Care: Bioethics Reexamined," *Unitas* 60 (June, 1987): 139-150.

"Licensing, Certification, and the Restraint of Trade: The Creation of Differences Among the Health Care Professions," Susan Costello, H. Tristram Engelhardt, Jr., and Mary Ann Gardell in *Bioethics: Readings and Cases* (Englewood Cliffs, New Jersey: Prentice-Hall, Inc., 1987), 89-95.

"Infanticide in a Post-Christian Age," in *Euthanasia and the Newborn*, eds. Richard C. McMillan, H. Tristram Engelhardt, Jr. and S. F. Spicker (Dordrecht, Holland: D. Reidel Publishing Company, 1987), 81-86.

"The Baby Doe Controversy: An Outline of Some points in Its Development," Mary Ann Gardell and H. Tristram Engelhardt, Jr., in *Euthanasia and the Newborn*, eds. Richard C. McMillan, H. Tristram Engelhardt, Jr., and S. F. Spicker (Dordrecht, Holland: D. Reidel Publishing Company, 1987), 293-299.

"Health Care Institutions," in *Health Care Ethics*, eds. Donald Van DeVeer and Tom Regan (Philadelphia: Temple University Press, 1987), 428-453.

"Having Sex and Making Love: The Search for Morality in Eros," in *Sexuality in Medicine*, Vol. 2, ed. Earl E. Shelp (Dordrecht, Holland: D. Reidel Publishing Company, 1987), 51-66.

"Entscheidungsprobleme konkurrierender Interessen von Mutter und Foetus," in *Ethische und rechtliche Fragen der Gentechnologie und der Reproduktionsmedizin*, ed. V. Braun, D. Mieth, and K. Steigleder (Munich, Germany: J. Schweitzer Verlag, 1987), 150-159.

"Gentherapie an menschlichen Keimbahnzellen: Kann und soll die 'schöne neue Welt' verhindert werden?" in *Ethische und rechtliche Fragen der Gentechnologie und der Reproduk-*

tionsmedizin, ed. V. Braun, D. Mieth, and K. Steigleder (Munich, Germany: J. Schweitzer Verlag, 1987), 255-262.

"The Bad, the Ugly, and the Unfortunate," in *Ethical Dimensions of Geriatric Care*, eds. S. F. Spicker, S. R. Ingman, and I. R. Lawson (Dordrecht: D. Reidel, 1987), 263-270.

"Persons, Sex, and Contraceptives," in *The Contraceptive Ethos*, eds. S. F. Spicker, *et al.* (Dordrecht: D. Reidel, 1987), 39-45.

"Human Reproductive Technologies," in *Der Stand der bioethischen Discussion in den USA mit besonderer Beruecksichtigung der Problemstellungen in der Bundesrepublik*, ed. Hans-Martin Sass (Bonn, Western Germany: Studie im Auftrage des Bundesministeriums fuer Forschung und Technologie, 1987), 363-403.

"The Foundations of Bioethics," *Revue de Metaphysique et de Morale* 92 (1987): 387-399.

"Information and Authenticity," *Journal of General Internal Medicine* 3 (January 1988): 91-93.

"Biological Nihilism and Modern Moral and Political Theory," *Politics and the Life Sciences* 6 (February 1988): 202-205.

"The Authority of the Captain," in *The Physician as Captain of the Ship*, eds. Nancy M. P. King, Larry R. Churchill, and Alan W. Cross (Dordrecht, Holland: D. Reidel, 1988), 67-73.

"Reexamining the Definition of Death and Becoming Clearer about What it is to be Alive," in *Death: Beyond Whole-Brain Criteria*, ed. Richard M. Zaner (Dordrecht: Kluwer, 1988), 91-98.

"Diagnosing Well and Treating Prudently," in *The Use of Human Beings in Research*, ed. S. F. Spicker, *et al.* (Dordrecht: Kluwer, 1988), 123-141.

"National Health Care Systems: Conflicting Visions," in *Health Care Systems*, ed. Hans-Martin Sass and Robert Massey (Dordrecht: Kluwer, 1988), 3-13.

"Withholding Medical Treatment from the Severely Demented Patient," in *Archives of Internal Medicine*, N. Wray *et al.* and H. Tristram Engelhardt, Jr. *et al.* 148 (September 1988): 1980-1984.

"Morality for the Medical-Industrial Complex," H. T. Engelhardt, Jr. and Michael A. Rie, *New England Journal of Medicine* 319 (October 20, 1988): 1086-1089.

"Foundations, Persons, and the Battle for the Millennium," *Journal of Medicine and Philosophy* 13 (Nov. 1988): 387-391.

"Fashioning an Ethic for Life and Death in a Post-Modern Society," *Hastings Center Report* 19 (January/February 1989): 7-9.

"The Use of Anencephalic Tissue for Transplantation," Robert Cefalo and H. T. Engelhardt, Jr., *Journal of Medicine and Philosophy* 14 (Feb. 1989): 25-43.

"Pain, Suffering, Addiction,and Cancer," in *Drug Treatment of Cancer Pain in a Drug-Oriented Society*, ed. C. S. Hill, Jr., and W. S. Fields (New York: Raven, 1989), 27-36.

"Taking the Family Seriously: Beyond Best Interest," in *Children and Health Care*, ed. Loretta Kopelman and John Moskop (Dordrecht: Kluwer, 1989), 231-237.

"Advocacy: Some Reflections on an Ambiguous Term," in *Children and Health Care*, ed. Loretta Kopelman and John Moskop (Dordrecht: Kluwer, 1989), 317-321.

"Foundations: Why They Provide so Little," *Journal of the British Society for Phenomenology* 20 (May 1989): 67-69.

"Freedom vs. Best Interest: A Conflict at the Roots of Health Care," in *Dax's Case: Essays in Medical Ethics and Human Meanings*, ed. Lonnie D. Kliever (Dallas, Texas: Southern Methodist University Press, 1989), 79-96.

"The Financial Enforcement of Living Wills: Putting Teeth into Natural Death Statutes," Michael Rie and H. T. Engelhardt, Jr., *Advance Directives in Medicine*, eds. Chris Hackler, Ray Moseley, and Dorothy E. Vawter (New York: Praeger Publishers, 1989), 85-92.

"Advance Directives and The Right to Be Left Alone," *Advance Directive in Medicine*, eds. Chris Hackler, Ray Moseley, and Dorothy E. Vawter (New York: Praeger Publishers, 1989), 141-154.

"Applied Philosophy in the Post-Modern Age: An Augury," *Journal of Social Philosophy* 20 (June 2 1989): 42-48.

"Can Ethics Take Pluralism Seriously?" *Hastings Center Report* 19 (September/October, 1989): 33-34.

"Comments of the Recommendation Regarding Section 504 of the Rehabilitation Act of 1973 and the Child Abuse Amendments of 1984," in *A Report of the U.S. Commission of Civil Rights*, Medical Discrimination Against Children with Disabilities (September 1989): 158-165.

"Entwicklungen der medizinischen Ethik in den USA: Die Verführung durch die Technik und der Irrtum einer Lebenserhaltung um jeden Preis," H. Tristram Engelhardt Jr. and Thomas J. Bole, *Arzt und Christ*, 36:2 (1990): 113-121.

"The Birth of the Medical Humanities and the Rebirth of the Philosophy of Medicine," *Journal of Medicine and Philosophy* 15 (June, 1990): 237-241.

"Some Reflections on the Definition of Death," translated into Japanese as "Shi no Teigi o Megutte," *Igaku-Tetsugaku Igaku-Rinri* (*Annals of the Japanese Association for Philosophical and Ethical Research in Medicine*) 8 (1990): 117-128.

"Taking Pluralism Seriously, or Is the Ethics Manual of the American College of Physicians Unsympathetic to Physicians with Religious Objections to Abortion?" *Linacre Quarterly* 57 (August, 1990): 11-14.

"Medical Knowledge and Medical Vision," in *The Growth of Medical Knowledge*, ed. H. A. ten Have, G. K. Kimsma, and S. F. Spicker (Dordrecht: Kluwer, 1990), 63-71.

"Ethics in Cardiovascular Medicine: Background and General Principles," William W. Parmley, Robert C. Schlant, Gordon L. Crelinsten, H. Tristram Engelhardt Jr., *et al.*, in *Journal of American College of Cardiology* 16 (July 1990): 7-10.

"Human Nature Technologically Revisited," *Social Philosophy & Policy* 8 (1990): 180-191.

"Developing Health Care Policy in Secular Pluralist Societies," in *Bio-Ethiek*, ed. Ch. Suzanne and J. Stuy (Brussels: VUB Press, 1990), 19-30.

"From Prenatal Screening to Foregoing Life-Prolonging Treatment: Justifying Health Care Policy in the 21st Century," in *Bioethics and Medical Economics in the 21st Century*, eds. Kazumasa Hoshino and Takao Saito (Tokyo: Sokyusha, Co. Ltd., 1990), 1-23.

"Die Einfuerung von Zugangsbeschränkungen für kosten-intensive lebensrettende medizinische Behandlung," in *Sicherheit und Freiheit*, eds. Christoph Sachße, H. T. Engelhardt Jr. (Frankfurt/Main: Suhrkamp, 1990), 289-312.

"Texas: Messages, Morals, and Myths," *Journal of the American Studies Association of Texas* 21 (October 1990): 33-49.

"Integrity, Humaneness and Institutions in Secular Pluralist Societies," in *Integrity in Health Care Institutions*, eds. Ruth E. Bulger and Stanley J. Reiser (Iowa City, Iowa: University of Iowa Press, 1991), 33-43.

"Ethics in Critical Care Medicine: Morality in the Face of Finitude," in *Critical Care*, eds. R. W. Taylor and W. C. Shoemaker (Fullerton, California: Society of Critical Care Medicine, 1991), 103-119.

"Autonomie und Selbstbestimmung: Grundlegende Konzepte der Bioethik in der Psychiatrie," in *Ethik in der Psychiatrie*, eds. W. Poelinger and W. Wagner (Berlin, Germany: Springer-Verlag, 1991), 61-71.

"Medical Ethics for the 21st Century," *Journal of American College of Cardiology* 18 (July 1991): 303-307.

"Natural Theology and Bioethics," in *The Philosophy of Charles Hartshorne* [the Library of Living Philosophers, Vol. 20], ed. Lewis E. Hahn (La Salle, Ill.: Open Court, 1991), 159-168.

"Rights to Health Care: Created, Not Discovered," in *Rights to Health Care*, eds. T. J. Bole and W. B. Bondeson (Dordrecht, Holland: Kluwer, 1991), 103-111.

"Virtue for Hire: Some Reflections on Free Choice and the Profit Motive in the Delivery of Health Care," in *Rights to Health Care*, eds. T. J. Bole and W. B. Bondeson. (Dordrecht, Holland: Kluwer, 1991), 327-353.

"Is There a Universal System of Ethics or are Ethics Culture-Specific?" in *Organ Replacement Therapy: Ethics, Justice and Commerce*, eds. W. Land, J. B. Dossetor (Berlin Heidelberg: Springer-Verlag, 1991), 147-153.

"The Artificial Donation of Human Gametes," H. T. Engelhardt Jr. and K. Wm. Wildes, S.J. in *Bailliere's Clinical Obstetrics and Gynaecology* 5 (September 1991): 637-658.

"Bioethics" (in Japanese), in *Human Being, Science, Religion*, ed. Committee for Academic Planning (Kyoto: Ryukoku University, 1991), 353-372.

"Why a Two-Tier System of Health Care Delivery is Morally Unavoidable," in *Rationing America's Medical Care*, eds. M. A. Strosberg, J. M. Wiener, and R. Baker (Washington, D.C.: Brookings Institution, 1992), 196-207.

"The Foundations of Bioethics: Themes of Autonomy and Control," *Towards a New Replenishment of Medical Education and Hospital Service*, ed. Institute of Medical Humanities (Tokyo: Shin-zau-sha, 1992), 357-374.

"Bioethique: Jusqu'ou faut-il legiferer?" in *Bioethique: Jusqu'ou Faut-il Legiferer?* (Paris:Institut EURO 92, 1992), 3-27.

"Observer Bias: The Emergence of the Ethics of Diagnosis," in *The Ethics of Diagnosis*, eds. J.L. Peset and D. Gracia (Dordrecht, Kluwer, 1992), 63-71.

"The Search for a Universal System of Ethics," in *Ethical Problems in Dialysis and Transplantation*, eds. C. M. Kjellstrand and J. B. Dossetor (Dordrecht:Kluwer, 1992), 3-19.

"Selling Virtue: Ethics as a Profit Maximizing Strategy in Health Care Delivery," H. Tristram Engelhardt, Jr. and M. A. Rie, *Journal of Health & Social Policy* 4 (1992): 27-35.

"Bioethics in the Post Modern World: Belief and Secularity," *Politeia* 51 (1992): 1-24.

"Advance Directives on Hospital Admission," A. W. Broadwell, E. V. Boisaubin, J. K. Dunn, and H. T. Engelhardt, Jr., *Southern Medical Journal* 86 (Feb. 1993): 165-168.

"Il concetto di persona e il fondamento di un'autoritá morale laica," H. T. Engelhardt, Jr. and K. Wm. Wildes *Bioetica E Persona*, ed. Evandro Agazzi (Milano: Franco Angeli, 1993), 13-26.

"National Health Care Policy: The Moral Issues," *Bulletin of the American College of Surgeons* 78 (April 1993): 10-14.

"Ethical Decision Making in Critical Care," in *Principles and Practice of Medical Intensive Care*, ed. R. W. Carson and M. S. Geheb (Philadelphia: W.B. Saunders 1993), 1724-1730.

"Western Bioethics and the Post-Modern World," *Journal of Seizon and Life Sciences* 4 (June 1993): 1-12.

"Personhood, Moral Strangers and The Evil of Abortion," *Journal of Medicine and Philosophy* 18 (August 1993): 419-421.

"Bioetica: laica e religosa," *Bioetica* (1993): 346-350.

"AIDS and HIV Infection: Some Ethical Reflections on a New Disease," in *A Study of Applied Ethics*, ed. Nobuyuki Iida (Chiba University Press, 1993), Vol. 2, 397-401.

"The Psychiatric Admission Index: Deciding When to Admit A Patient," H. Tristram Engelhardt, Jr., and John H. Coverdale, *Journal of Clinical Ethics* 4 (Winter 1993): 315-318.

"Cases and Social Reality: Making the Decision to Admit," H. T. Engelhardt, Jr., and John H. Coverdale, *Journal of Clinical Ethics* 4 (Winter 1993): 354-356.

"Il corpo in vendita: dilemmi morali della secolarizzazione," in *Questioni di bioetica*, ed.S. Rodotà (Rome: Laterza and Figli, 1993), 123-138.

"The Four Principles of Health Care Ethics and Post-Modernity: Why a Libertarian Interpretation is Unavoidable," H. Tristram Engelhardt, Jr. and Kevin Wm. Wildes, S.J., *Principles of Health Care Ethics*, ed. Raanan Gillon (New York: John Wiley, 1994), 135-147.

"Human Reproductive Technology: Why All the Moral Fuss?" in *The Beginning of Human Life*, eds. Fritz Beller and Rober Weir (Dordrecht; Kluwer, 1994), 89-100.

"*Sittlichkeit* and Post-Modernity: An Hegelian Reconstruction of the State," *Hegel Reconsidered*, eds. H. T. Engelhardt, Jr. and Terry Pinkard (Dordrecht: Kluwer, 1994), 211-224.

"Klaus Hartmann and G.W. F. Hegel: A Personal Postscript," *Hegel Reconsidered*, eds. H. T. Engelhardt, Jr. and Terry Pinkard (Dordrecht: Kluwer, 1994), 225-229.

"Postmodernity and Limits on the Human Body: Libertarianism by Default," H T. Engelhardt Jr. and Kevin Wm. Wildes, S.J. in *Medicine Unbound*, eds. R. H. Blank and A.L. Bonnicksen (New York: Columbia University Press, 1994), 61-71.

"Consensus: How Much Can We Hope For?" in *The Concept of Moral Consensus*, ed. Kurt Bayertz (Dordrecht: Kluwer, 1994), 19-40.

"A Skeptical Postscript," in *The Concept of Moral Consensus*, ed. Kurt Bayertz (Dordrecht: Kluwer, 1994), 235-240.

"Attitudes of Critical Care Professionals Concerning Distribution of Intensive Care Resources," Society of Critical Care Medicine Ethics Committee, H. T. Engelhardt Jr., member, *Critical Care Medicine* 22 (Feb. 1994): 358-362.

"Health Care Reform: A Study in Moral Malfeasance," *Journal of Medicine and Philosophy* 19 (October 1994): 501-516.

"The Emergence of Secular Bioethics," H. Tristram Engelhardt, Jr. and Kevin Wm. Wildes, S.J. in *Principles of Medical Biology*, eds. E. E. Bittar and N. Bittar (Greenwich, Conn.: Jai Press, 1994), 1-15.

"The Search for Untainted Money," *American Journal of Respiratory Cell and Molecular Biology* 12 (February 1995): 123-124.

"Towards a Christian Bioethics," *Christian Bioethics* 1 (March 1995): 1-10.

"Moral Content, Tradition, and Grace: Rethinking the Possibility of a Christian Bioethics," *Christian Bioethics* 1 (March 1995): 29-47.

"Bioethics in Japan and the West: An Investigation in Moral Diversity," in *The Dignity of Death*, ed. Kazumasa Hoshino (Kyoto: Shibunkaku, 1995), 347-358 (in Japanese).

"Health and Disease: Philosophical Perspectives," H. T. Engelhardt Jr. and Kevin Wm. Wildes, S.J. in *Encyclopedia of Bioethics*, rev. ed., ed. Warren Reich (New York: Macmillan, 1995), vol. 3, 1101-1106.

"Philosophy of Medicine," H. T. Engelhardt, Jr. and Kevin Wm. Wildes, S.J. in *Encyclopedia of Bioethics*, rev. ed., ed. Warren Reich (New York, Macmillan 1995), vol. 4, 1680-1684.

"Solidarity: Post-Modern Perspectives," *Rechtsphilosophische Hefte* 4 (1995): 49-63.

"Futile Care for the Critically Ill Patient," H. T. Engelhardt, Jr. and George Khushf, *Current Opinion in Critical Care* 1 (1995): 329-333.

"Models of Medical Explanation, or the Passing of Traditional European Medicine," International Prospects of Medical Ethics, eds. Ren-zong Qui, H.M. Sass, Dapu Shi (Xian: People's Education Press of Shangxi, 1995), 9-23 (in Chinese).

"Reproductive Ethics: Conflicts of Vision and Authority," in *International Prospects of Medical Ethics*, eds. Ren-zong Qiu, H. M. Sass, Dapu Shi (Xian: People's Education Press of Shangxi, 1995), 145-167 (in Chinese).

"Human Reproduction: Conflicts at the Roots of Bioethics and Health Care Policy," in *Ethical Aspects of Human Reproduction*, eds. Claude Sureau and Françoise Shenfield (Montrouge, France: John Libbey, 1995), 49-60.

"Vecchiaia, eutanasia, e diversità morale: la creazione di opzioni morali nell' assistenza sanitaria," *Bioetica* (1995), No. 1: 74-84.

"Christian Bioethics as Non-Ecumenical," *Christian Bioethics* 1 (September 1995): 182-199.

"La Bioética: Hito de las humanidades Médicas," H. T. Engelhardt, Jr. and Mark S. Cherry, *Cuadernos de Bioética* 1 (Sept. 1995): 55-64.

"Bioethics After the Failure of Reason," *European Philosophy of Medicine and Health Care* 3 (1995), special issue on CD-ROM.

"Sanctity of Life and Menschenwürde: Can these Concepts Help Direct the Use of Resources in Critical Care?" in *Sanctity of Life and Human Dignity*, ed. Kurt Bayertz (Dordrecht: Kluwer, 1996), 201-219.

"From Pagan Greece to Post-Modern Europe," H. Tristram Engelhardt, Jr. and Mark J.Cherry, *European Philosophy of Medicine and Health Care* 4 (1996): 5-12.

"Manners in the Ruins of Community," in *Gentility Recalled*, ed. Digby Anderson (London: The Social Affairs Unit, 1996), 181-194.

DATE DUE